Praise for Ann Douglas

"Douglas writes about pregnancy in an easy ~~~~~~~~~~~~~~~~ >ook's strength is its woman-centredness, all the way from the ~~~~~~~~~~~ rtum."

—*Today's Parent*

"Thank you, Ann Douglas, for *The Mother of All Pregnancy Books*. Canada can now hold its own in the glutted pregnancy book field.... Comprehensive, informative, up-to-date, and brazenly neutral."

—*Toronto Star*

"A book that lives up to its name.... Incredibly comprehensive yet easy to follow."

—*Chicago Tribune*

"The must-read pregnancy book! Ann Douglas has created the most comprehensive guide to pregnancy we've ever seen."

—Denise and Alan Fields, authors, *Baby Bargains*

"At long last, a new pregnancy bible for women of my generation and younger has emerged in the form of *The Mother of All Pregnancy Books*. With humor, sensitivity, an easy, no-jargon style, and a million 'extras' that the leading pregnancy books don't cover, Ann Douglas holds nothing back. Not only do I love this book, but I will use it as a valuable tool in my own work as a women's health author."

—M. Sara Rosenthal, author of *The Pregnancy Sourcebook* and *The Breastfeeding Sourcebook*, and founder of www.sarahealth.com

"Start reading this treasure trove even before you get pregnant so you can make it through every jam-packed page before your baby arrives."

—Paula Spencer, "The Mom Next Door" columnist, *Woman's Day Magazine*; author of *Everything ELSE You Need to Know When You're Expecting*

"This is truly 'the mother of all pregnancy books'—an intelligent resource that covers every pregnancy-related topic imaginable in a fun, reassuring way. Ann Douglas has done an exceptional job of arming parents-to-be with the facts they need to make the healthiest possible choices from preconception through postpartum. A must-have!"

—Susan Newman, Ph.D., author of *Parenting an Only Child: The Joys and Challenges of Raising Your One and Only*

"Not preachy and bossy.... It's upfront and fun."

—*Toronto Sun*

"Finally, a pregnancy book that includes essential pre-pregnancy concerns, such as planning and physical and emotional preparation! Ann Douglas has written her masterwork *The Mother of All Pregnancy Books* in the same unpretentious, concise style as her Unofficial Guide. She also stays true to her goal of informing parents and prospective parents as completely as possible, so they will be well-equipped to sort through the pros and cons of their own life choices as they see them. Not one to forgo difficult issues, her chapter entitled "When Pregnancy Isn't Perfect" is one of the best I've read, both for its sensitivity and for its emphasis on coping and prevention. This is a book that will serve women and their families well."

—A. Christine Harris, Ph.D., author of *The Pregnancy Journal*

"*The Mother of All Pregnancy Books* is a comprehensive and incredibly informative resource about pregnancy (and what comes before and after!). Ann Douglas tells all in her witty style, entertaining readers along the way. Unlike other pregnancy books, Douglas combines thorough research and reporting with the human touch, offering her own experiences and insight while educating her readers at one of the most important times in their lives. This book is not to be missed!"

—Elisa Ast All, Editor-in-Chief, *Pregnancy* magazine,
Baby Years magazine, and iParenting.com

"If you're looking for an all-in-one 'Tell me everything, and tell it like it is' book for your pregnancy, *The Mother of All Pregnancy Books* is it. Not only is this hefty volume filled with facts about fertility, pregnancy and birth, it also contains hundreds of anecdotes from moms who lived—and maybe even loved—pregnancy. Author Ann Douglas knows her stuff, and is wise but not preachy friendly but not overbearing. Keep this book close at hand for instant guidance through the highs and the lows of this extraordinary time!"

—Nancy Price, ePregnancy.com

"Here's a book that's packed with up-to-date information and practical advice on almost every aspect of pregnancy—from prenatal testing to proper nutrition, from infertility procedures to financial planning, from bedrest to breastfeeding. Yet despite its breadth and depth, the text is not dry or dull. Instead, Ann Douglas's reassuring style and insightful anecdotes make readers feel like they're chatting with a savvy, smart, sympathetic friend."

—Tamara Eberlein, coauthor of *When You're Expecting Twins,
Triplets, or Quads* and *Program Your Baby's Health*

"If you're looking for the inside scoop on what it's really like to have a baby, you've come to the right place. *The Mother of All Pregnancy Books* takes on tough topics most pregnancy books shy away from. It's a totally comprehensive guide that features a non-bossy, fresh, and fun approach to the greatest adventure life has to offer. Based on the best advice from over 100 Canadian parents, this information is served up with a uniquely Canadian spin."

—*The Hamilton Spectator*

THE MOTHER OF ALL
PREGNANCY
BOOKS

An All-Canadian Guide to Conception,
Birth, and Everything in Between

THIRD EDITION

ANN DOUGLAS

Collins

Medical Disclaimer:

This book is designed to provide you with general information about pregnancy so that you can be a better informed health consumer. It does not contain medical advice. This book is not intended to provide a complete or exhaustive treatment of this subject; nor is it a substitute for advice from your physician or midwife, who know you best. Seek medical attention promptly for any specific medical condition or problem that you may be experiencing. Do not take any medication without obtaining medical advice. All efforts were made to ensure the accuracy of the information contained in this publication as of the date of writing. The author and the publisher expressly disclaim any responsibility for any adverse effects arising from the use or application of the information contained herein. While the parties believe that the contents of this publication are accurate, a licensed medical practitioner should be consulted in the event that medical advice is desired. The information contained in this book does not constitute a recommendation or endorsement with respect to any company or product.

Contents

Chapter 6: Your Incredible Growing Baby / 172

The First Trimester: The Beginnings of Life, and the Start of a Whole New Way of Life / 173

Before Ovulation / 173;
Pre-embryonic stage: The first three weeks of development / 173; Embryonic stage: Your baby begins to develop human characteristics / 176; Fetal stage: Your baby's body systems mature / 179

The Second Trimester: Goodbye Nausea, Hello Maternity Jeans / 180
On the grow / 180

The Third Trimester: Your Incredible Growing Belly / 182
The final sprint / 182

Chapter 7: The Pregnancy Road Map / 186

The Complaints Department / 186
What's normal and what's not / 187

Pregnancy Complaints from A to Z / 187
Abdominal muscle separation / 187; Acne / 192; Backache / 192; Belly button soreness / 194; Bleeding gums / 194; Bleeding and spotting, vaginal / 195; Braxton Hicks contractions / 195; Breast tenderness and enlargement / 196; Breathlessness / 198; Carpal tunnel syndrome / 198; Constipation / 199; Cramping / 199; Cravings / 200; Ear changes / 200; Eye changes / 200; Faintness and dizziness / 201; Fatigue / 202; Food aversions / 202; Gassiness and bloating / 203; Headaches / 203; Heartburn (a.k.a. reflux) / 204; Hernia, hiatal / 205; Hemorrhoids / 205; Hip soreness / 206; Insomnia / 206; Itchiness (abdominal) / 207; Laryngitis and voice changes / 208; Leg cramps / 208; Morning sickness (a.k.a. nausea and vomiting of pregnancy) / 209; Nasal changes / 214; Perineal aching / 215; Pubic-bone pain (osteitis pubis) / 215; Rashes / 216; Restless leg syndrome (RLS) / 217; Round ligament pain / 217; Saliva, excessive (ptyalism) / 218; Sciatica / 219; Skin changes / 219; Smell, heightened sense of / 221; Stretch marks / 222; Sweating / 222; Swelling and fluid retention / 223; Thirstiness / 224; Urinary incontinence / 224; Urination, increased frequency of / 224; Vagina, changes to the / 225; Vaginal secretions, increased / 225; Varicose veins / 226; Weepiness / 227; Yeast infections / 227

Chapter 8: This Is Your (Soon-to-Be) Life / 229

Decisions, Decisions . . . / 230
Pregnant and chic / 230; Prenatal classes: Who needs them? / 233; Umbilical cord blood banking / 235; The circumcision decision / 237;

Decision Time / 349

The Top Labour-Related Worries / 372

Going Overdue / 384

What Labour Is Really Like / 387

Parting Words / 403

Introduction

The bookstore shelves are overflowing with books on conception, pregnancy, and birth. In fact, the last time I was in one of the big chain superstores, there was almost an entire aisle devoted to the business of making babies. (Clearly, the pregnancy book world has been experiencing a population explosion of its own.)

While some folks might argue that the last thing the world needs is another pregnancy book, I beg to differ. You see, what's been missing from bookstore shelves is a fun yet informative guide to pregnancy written for and by Canadians.

That's why I decided to write this book.

Why a Canadian Pregnancy Book?

Flip through a typical American pregnancy book and you'll find pages and pages of material that simply doesn't apply to Canadian parents: chapters on such topics as coping with health insurance nightmares (a U.S. phenomenon, thank heaven) or your rights under the Family and Medical Leave Act (the American government's maternity leave legislation). And even those chapters that are relevant to Canadian parents suffer from a major failing: the expert sources that get cited time and time again in these books are American.

What Canadian parents need is a book that reflects what it's like to give birth here in Canada—a book that talks about the unique challenges that Canadian parents face (the chronic shortage of obstetricians in rural Canada, for example) and that contains up-to-date advice from Canadian health authorities such as the Society of Obstetricians and Gynaecologists of Canada and the Canadian Paediatric Society. (Believe it or not, health authorities on both sides of the border don't always see eye to eye on everything.)

Of course, it wouldn't be possible—or even advisable—to write a pregnancy book that completely ignores what's happening south of the border. After all, some of the most significant medical breakthroughs in the treatment of pregnancy loss and infertility in recent years have happened in medical labs in the United States. What Canadian parents need, however, is a pregnancy book that looks at that information through Canadian eyes and that interprets it for a Canadian audience. That's what *The Mother of All Pregnancy Books* is all about.

A One-of-a-Kind Pregnancy Book

As you've no doubt noticed by now, pregnancy books tend to fall into one of two distinct categories: bossy books that treat pregnancy as a nine-month exercise in deprivation and that leave you feeling like a bad person if you ingest so much as a single glass of diet pop during your entire pregnancy; and humorous books that treat pregnancy and birth as one big joke. (Hey, I enjoy a laugh as much as the next gal, but there are times when I'd prefer a hefty serving of hard medical facts.)

The Mother of All Pregnancy Books doesn't fall into either of these classic pregnancy book traps. It arms you with the facts so that you can make up your own mind about such important issues as nutrition during pregnancy, prenatal testing, pain relief during labour, and circumcision.

Why the Mother of All Pregnancy Books?

It isn't difficult to figure out why we chose to call this book *The Mother of All Pregnancy Books*. This is one comprehensive book, after all. If you take a quick flip through the pages of this updated third edition, you'll discover a lot of valuable information packed between the covers, including

- a frank discussion of what it's really like to have a baby—the emotional and physical challenges of pregnancy, the career and financial costs of starting a family, and other big-picture issues that many pregnancy books don't delve into;
- what you need to know to start preparing your body for pregnancy (including a discussion of the latest research about the father's role in maximizing the likelihood of a healthy conception);
- need-to-know information about the roles of alternative and complementary therapies, both prior to and during your pregnancy;
- practical advice on what you can do to boost your odds of conceiving quickly;
- useful tips on choosing a caregiver and a place to give birth (assuming, of course, that you have the luxury of choice);
- friendly and reassuring advice on establishing a pregnancy-friendly lifestyle and giving your baby the healthiest possible start in life;
- fascinating facts about how your baby and your body change during pregnancy;
- a summary of the latest research about the influence of the pre-birth environment on the health of the developing baby over a lifetime and, in some cases, across generations;

- timely reassurance, from mothers who have been there, about the pregnancy worries that may be keeping you up at night;
- advice on coping with a smorgasbord of pregnancy-related aches and pains (including some that you swear couldn't have anything to do with pregnancy);
- the inside scoop on what labour is *really* like and practical advice on planning for the birth you want;
- tips on coping with a high-risk pregnancy from moms who've been there and who want you to benefit from what they learned along the way;
- a roundup of the latest research on mood disorders during pregnancy;
- a sneak peek at life after baby, including practical advice on easing the transition to parenthood for both you and your partner.

What makes this book really special, however, is the fact that it's based on interviews with more than 100 Canadian parents and parents-to-be. These folks passed on their best advice on a variety of different pregnancy-related topics—everything from keeping the romance in your relationship while you're trying to conceive to keeping your breakfast down once you manage to get pregnant. (This completely revised third edition has also benefited from the feedback of readers like you: readers who cared enough about the book to write in and tell me what they loved about it and what I could do to improve it. Thank you so much for the amazing input, everyone.) It's this real-world perspective that makes *The Mother of All Pregnancy Books* unique and relevant. After all, who better to talk about the ins and outs of conception, pregnancy, and birth than people who've been there, done that, and lived to tell?

As you've no doubt gathered by now, *The Mother of All Pregnancy Books* is unlike any other pregnancy book you've read. It's comprehensive, it's fun to read, and, best of all, it's "made in Canada."

I hope you enjoy the book.

ANN DOUGLAS

P.S. My editors and I would like to make the next edition of *The Mother of All Pregnancy Books* as helpful as we can for Canadian parents. If you have any comments to pass along, we'd love to hear what you have to say. You can contact me via my websites (www.having-a-baby.com and www.anndouglas.ca.)

CHAPTER 1

Are You Really Ready to Have a Baby?

"There's never a 'perfect' time to have a baby. Realistically, some times are better than others, but if you keep waiting for the perfect time, you'll be waiting forever."

—LORI, 29, MOTHER OF FOUR

"There's never a truly 'right time' to have a baby. Something always comes up. Simply hold each other's hands, smile, and jump on the train!"

—ALEXANDRA, 33, MOTHER OF TWO

So you're thinking of having a baby—of trading your relatively sane and orderly life for the chance to hop on board what can best be described as an 18-year-long roller-coaster ride. (Actually, friends of mine who have kids in their twenties tell me that the ride lasts a heck of a lot longer than 18 years, but I have to confess, I'm still in denial.)

Well, before you do anything rash, like tossing the birth control out the window or reaching for the thermometer and the temperature graph, you might want to slam on the brakes for a moment. After all, don't you owe it to yourself to find out what it's *really* like to become a parent before you sign yourself up for the mother of all commitments?

If it's the scoop on parenthood that you're after, you've come to the right place. I mean, if there's one thing I've learned during my years in the motherhood trenches, it's that you've got to be prepared to tell the God's-honest truth when other parents come around looking for advice and answers. Anything else is a clear violation of the Mom Code—and, trust me, you don't want to mess with *that*. Glossing over what labour or new-mom sleep deprivation really feels like isn't nice and it isn't fair. It's also a sure-fire way to win you some very hormonal enemies.

I've always been one to spill the beans on things (good, bad, and ugly), and I'm not about to change my tell-all ways just because I'm writing a book. Besides, I wouldn't exactly be holding up my end of the deal—giving you the inside scoop on having a baby—if I only talked about how great newborn babies' heads smell and how much fun you'll have filling the hard drive in your computer with snap-shots of your baby doing one cute thing after another. In the interest of full disclosure, I owe it to you to spell out the other things you should be thinking about, such as how much this little cherub is going to set you back in first-year acqui-sition costs (diapers, a stroller, food, and the latest and greatest digital camera).

But wait—that's assuming you're going to go ahead with the deal in the first place; that you've weighed the career costs and the relationship fallout (babies do not bring couples closer together, at least in the short term—that's a bald-faced lie) and decided that having a baby is still a lovely idea.

And if you do decide you want to have a baby, you've still got to decide whether you want to be serious about those baby-making plans tonight, next week, or sometime in the next decade. Of course, before you make that decision, you'll want to make sure you're fully up to speed on the latest facts about biological clocks—both his and hers. (Yep. Even guys have a reproductive best-before date.)

I'll wrap up the chapter by discussing how you may feel about starting a family and what to do if you and your partner aren't exactly on the same page when it comes to the whole baby-making issue.

Just one small footnote before we move on to the real nitty-gritty. There are a number of important health-related issues to consider when you're planning a pregnancy. Rather than starting out with a heavy-duty biology lecture that might evoke frightening flashbacks to your grade-nine health class, I thought I'd ease you into the book gently. That's why I've chosen to postpone the dis-cussion of pre-conception health issues until Chapter 2. (Stay tuned.)

A Question of Timing

If you're waiting for some sort of magical signal that will tell you in no uncer-tain terms that this is really-and-truly-without-a-doubt the right time to have a baby, you could find yourself in for a pretty lengthy wait.

You see, there are always more reasons not to get pregnant than there are reasons to start a family. In fact, if you and your partner were to sit down with a pot of coffee and a pad of paper, you'd be bound to come up with a whole laundry list of reasons why you'd be insane to even think about getting pregnant right now. Here are a few of the reasons that might very well find their way on to your list:

- You've just bought a house and you're up to your eyeballs in debt. You figure that if you scrimp and save and do without unnecessary frills like groceries and clothes, you just might manage to pay for the damned thing before it's time to retire.
- You've just sprung for a hot new sports car—and the interior isn't exactly baby friendly. Even worse, there's no place to attach a car seat tether strap.
- You've just booked one of those truly decadent couples cruise-ship vacations and you know your partner would be less than thrilled if you were to spend most of the vacation holed up in the washroom, battling morning sickness.
- You've just changed jobs and you don't want to have to announce to your new employer that you're "in the family way" before you even get your first paycheque.
- You're approaching the busy season at work and you don't want to risk having to take any time off just because your stomach starts churning every time you come within 20 feet of the coffee pot.
- You and your partner are getting along so famously that you're reluctant to risk ruining a perfectly good relationship by adding a baby to the mix. (There's an alternative scenario to consider, just in case the phrase "marital bliss" isn't the first thing that comes to mind when you think of your partner. If you and your mate aren't getting along at all, you may wonder if having a baby would prove to be the final straw for your relationship.)
- You've agreed to serve in your best friend's wedding party eight months from now and she's already picked out the matching dresses for her seven bridal attendants. Judging by the cut of the dress, there isn't much room for expansion. What if she were to ask you to relinquish your dress to a surrogate matron of honour?
- If you were to conceive tonight, you could end up giving birth in the midst of a midwinter blizzard or a midsummer heat wave. (Hey, if there's one thing we Canadians can depend upon, it's weather extremes.)
- You need to lose weight and you'd like to drop those extra pounds before you start your family. (Or, conversely, you've just finished losing a ton of weight and you'd like to enjoy the sensation of having a flat stomach before you agree to sublet your belly to someone else.)
- You find the sound of children screaming in restaurants to be annoying

rather than endearing—which makes you question whether you've really got what it takes to become a parent. (Of course, this experience can sometimes elicit the opposite reaction: it can convince you that you're bound to do a better job at parenting than that imbecile in the next booth. Hope springs eternal.)

Yes, there are always a million and one reasons not to have a baby. And some of them actually make a lot of sense. I mean, if you and your partner are thinking about calling it quits, a positive pregnancy test may not be welcome at this stage of the game. Likewise, it's probably not a great idea to announce you're pregnant when you're just a week or two into a new job—unless, of course, you happen to be self-employed. But as for waiting until your financial affairs are in order, your calendar is clear for the next nine months, you've reached your ideal weight, and you feel psychologically fit to become a parent (whatever that means), you could find yourself waiting a very long time to plan that perfectly timed pregnancy. (Heck, I've got four kids and I'm still not 100 per cent sure that I'm up to the challenge.)

What it really costs to raise children

There's no denying it. The latest stats about the cost of raising children are enough to convince you to put your baby-making plans on hold for at least the foreseeable future—or to start auctioning off baby-naming rights in order to help underwrite the cost of Junior's upbringing. According to a recent report published in *MoneySense* magazine, you can expect to spend $243,660 to raise a child from birth through age 18. And that doesn't even account for the cost of post-secondary education.

So where does the money go? Childcare will take a big bite out of your budget, with daycare fees ranging from $9,000 per year for an infant to $5,100 per year for a school-aged child. You're also likely to spend more per year on housing (more space equals higher rent or mortgage payments), furnishings ($210 per child for furniture and related equipment), transportation (families with kids spend an extra $2,065 on transportation as compared to families without), recreation ($855 per child), lessons ($205), personal care items ($250), health care ($245), clothing ($785), and food (which ranges from $1,140 for a toddler to $2,400 for a teen).

Of course, "very few Canadians will find they are spending exactly the average, just as very few Canadians make exactly the average income," journalist Camilla Cornell notes in the introduction to her report. "A wealthy two-parent couple will no doubt spend more than our figure, and a money-conscious single

1.1　What It Costs to Raise a Baby from Birth to Age One	
Food	$1,507
Clothing	1,720
Health care	141
Child care (for employed single parent)	4,568
Shelter, furnishings, household operations	2,157
Total	**$10,093**

Source: Centre for International Statistics at the Canadian Council on Social Development (2004), the last year for which such figures are available.

Notes:
- You will spend considerably less on food than indicated in this table if you breastfeed. (These figures include the costs of infant formula for an entire year. What's more, health care costs for formula-fed babies tend to be higher than for breastfed babies.)
- A significant number of mothers are employed during their baby's first year of life. The Canadian *Maternity Experiences Survey* (2009) found that 11 per cent of new mothers had returned to work by the time their child was 6 months old, either for financial or career reasons.

parent will likely spend less. Studies also indicate that the more children you have, the less you spend on each one of them and the amount spent will vary from province to province and by the size of the city you live in."

Statistics like these are proof that a little knowledge can be a dangerous thing. Not only do they fail to remind you that you're not required to have the entire $243,660 on hand before you lose the birth control, they also neglect to point out that there are ways of paring down your child-rearing costs without practically guaranteeing that your child will end up on the talk show circuit singing the "I Had a Deprived Childhood" blues.

As you've no doubt noticed by now, prospective fathers tend to be particularly shell-shocked by these types of statistics. In fact, the vast majority of men I know would rather reach for the condoms than risk being shacked up in some unheated shanty with a wife and a brood of children they can't afford to feed. (Clearly this provider thing is hard-wired into men's brains.)

Myrna, a 32-year-old mother of one, remembers her partner experiencing these very types of money-related worries before they decided to take the plunge. "My husband is very practical," she explains. "He's very much into saving money and paying off our mortgage—so every time we thought about having kids, he'd get anxious about how much money it was going to cost to send them to university!"

While you don't want to embark on a pregnancy without giving any thought to how you're going to pay for a car seat, baby clothes, and other first-year essentials, you don't necessarily have to start freaking out right now about how you're going to finance Junior's postgraduate studies at McGill. Think short term: can you afford to take some time off work and do you have the cash on hand to cover the basics?

That's the pragmatic approach that Marinda, 30, and her partner chose when they started planning for their first pregnancy. "Although we didn't have much money, we both believed that if we waited to be completely financially stable before having children, we might never have them. Being self-employed, I knew I wouldn't receive any financial compensation from anyone (employer or government) for staying at home, other than the baby bonus, so during my pregnancy I saved enough money to cover half the rent for exactly one year. This [combined with my husband's income] allowed me to stay home for an entire year with my baby."

"Don't plan your family around finances. Personally, I think a woman's internal clock is a more reliable guide to family planning! If you have access to free used baby stuff—perhaps from friends or older siblings—babies are not that expensive. I spent less than $2,400 on my pregnancy and my baby's first year of life."

– MARIA, 31, MOTHER OF TWO

Career considerations

As if money-related worries weren't enough, you've also got your career to consider—and this advice applies regardless of whether you're planning to stay at home or go back to work immediately, a year after the birth, or five to ten years down the road.

While it would be nice to think that only a few Neanderthal employers still take the view that switching to the "Mommy Track" is proof that you're no longer as committed to your career as your childless counterparts, most women find there are still some career costs associated with having a baby. If you're not willing to put in 60 or more hours a week to prove to the powers that be that you're on the fast track to the executive suite, you could find yourself being overlooked come promotion time, particularly if you work in a profession such as law, where billable hours tend to determine who's hot and who's not.

And then there are all the intangible opportunities that may be lost if you choose to work less-than-full-time hours, or if you decide to drop out of the workforce altogether for a couple of years after your baby's arrival. Joanne Thomas Yaccato, author of *Balancing Act: A Canadian Woman's Financial Success Guide*, discusses this point in an article that ran in *Chatelaine* magazine shortly after the birth of her daughter: "Time off work means time out of circulation; if I lose too many contacts now, I can be a long time getting them back."

Does this mean the situation is hopeless? That switching to the Mommy Track will automatically derail your career?

Not necessarily, says Lori M. Bamber, author of *Financial Serenity: Successful Financial Planning and Investment for Women*. She argues that the career hit can be lessened if both parents help to cushion the blow: "Having a child does mean sacrificing a degree of career advancement and financial well-being, but the damage can be lessened dramatically by applying the power of two—two loving partners who work together to share the costs."

According to Bamber, that means ensuring that you and your partner are equally aware of the career sacrifices required after your baby arrives, and that the two of you are willing to plan accordingly. "Splitting the maternity leave so that Dad can have some bonding time with the baby is a wonderful idea and will signal to both employers that, yes, your priorities have changed—and, yes, you can still be counted on because your partner is also there to support you."

Career costs aside, one of the biggest challenges that working parents—and working moms in particular—face is in juggling their various work and family commitments. There's never enough time or energy to get everything done—to pull off the daily tightrope act that means balancing the needs of your job against the needs of your family, and vice versa. That's where the much-talked-about "mommy guilt" fits in: feeling like you're always shortchanging someone, somewhere. Eventually you learn to accept that fact—that mothers are mere mortals and that they can't be expected to be everything to everyone at one time—but until you reach that realization, you can do quite a number on yourself trying to prove otherwise. Frankly, it can be pretty exhausting.

Lori Bamber offers these words of wisdom to women who are trying to decide whether to return to work after their babies arrive: "I wish I had known that the period in which I was consumed by motherhood would be such a relatively short one relative to my career. At the time, it seemed like I was giving up so much and as if those sacrifices were forever. My children are already at an age where they are as much a help to me as a responsibility, and I am only now entering my prime career years. If I could have known then what I know now, I think I would have relaxed a bit and enjoyed things all the more."

shift careers

Instead of trying to make your old career fit your new life as a parent, why not consider switching to a career that meshes better with motherhood? Think about ways you can build upon the skills you acquired during your pre-baby life while anticipating the career you hope to have when your kids are a little older.

The age issue

Another issue that many prospective parents find themselves grappling with is whether or not there's a "perfect age" at which to have a baby.

Some parents choose to start their families when they're still in their twenties, believing that the physical demands of parenting will be easier to handle if they have their babies sooner rather than later. Sometimes they think ahead about the kind of life they want for themselves and their children in years to come. (Jennifer, a 31-year-old mother of two boys, ages 3 and 1, decided to start her family early: "I had visions of my child being 20 and me seeming really old," she recalls.)

Others prefer to wait until they're a little older and more established so that they'll have fewer financial worries and a lot more life experience to bring to the parenting table.

A growing number of women are opting to postpone motherhood until later in life. The latest figures from Statistics Canada indicate that the average age of a woman giving birth in Canada in 2010 was 29.6 years and that over half of all mothers (51.2%) who gave birth in 2010 were 30 years of age or older. So, is postponing motherhood until your late thirties or early forties in the best interests of both mother and baby? Not according to the Society of Obstetricians and Gynaecologists of Canada, which has been spreading the word that waiting too long to start a family may mean missing out on parenthood entirely.

The female biological clock

You see, unlike men, who have the ability to manufacture sperm throughout their reproductive lives, women are born with all the eggs they will ever have. The quality of those eggs deteriorates over time—something that can lead to fertility problems and an increased chance of pregnancy loss as a woman ages. By the time a woman reaches 40, for example, nearly half of her eggs will be chromosomally abnormal—a significant increase over age 35, when just one-third of a woman's eggs are abnormal. What's more, according to a study reported in the *British Medical Journal*, by age 45, her odds of having her pregnancy end in miscarriage are close to 75 per cent.

While you might not consciously choose to postpone a pregnancy until you're into your forties, you could find yourself on the far side of 40 by accident. You might find, for example, that after switching into baby-making mode at age 35 it takes you a couple of years to conceive, or that an undiagnosed medical condition (for example, a sexually transmitted infection, fibroids, polycystic ovaries, or endometriosis) has taken its toll on your fertility. There's also the other piece of the process to consider—your partner. Until the two of you start trying to conceive, you have no idea how the baby-making equation is going to work out: sometimes one plus one doesn't add up to a baby (at least not quickly or easily). While many of these problems can be resolved, fertility treatments take time—time that may no longer be on your side if you've waited too long to start trying.

Here are some other things you should know if you're planning to put your pregnancy plans on hold for now:

- Your odds of conceiving decrease as you age. While a woman in her early twenties has a 20 to 25 per cent chance of conceiving during a particular menstrual cycle, a woman in her late thirties has just an 8 to 10 per cent chance of becoming pregnant during any one cycle. (See Chapter 4 for a more detailed discussion of the effect of aging on a woman's fertility.) If she does conceive, the risk of spontaneous miscarriage is higher for a woman over the age of 35.
- Women who become pregnant later in life are more likely to conceive multiples. In addition, more women in their late thirties and their forties are now giving birth to twins and triplets—and even octuplets—as a result of fertility treatments. Given the higher rate of complications in pregnancies involving multiples, and the fact that multiples are more likely to be born prematurely and to weigh less than 5 pounds (2.3 kilograms) at birth, the news that there are two or more babies on the way can lead to worry as well as excitement.
- Older women are more likely than younger women to give birth to babies with chromosomal problems. While a 25-year-old woman faces 1 in 476 odds of giving birth to a baby with a chromosomal problem such as Down syndrome, a 45-year-old woman faces 1 in 21 odds.
- Women who become pregnant after age 40 are more likely to develop pregnancy-related complications such as pre-eclampsia (extremely high blood pressure), gestational diabetes (a form of diabetes that's triggered during pregnancy), premature birth (birth before the 37th completed week of pregnancy), and intrauterine growth restriction (when the

fetus is significantly smaller than what would be expected at a particular gestational age). Older mothers are also more likely to have pre-existing health problems (such as arthritis, heart problems, diabetes, or mental health issues) that may complicate their pregnancies.

•   Older mothers are more likely to require an operative vaginal delivery (for example, a delivery in which forceps or a vacuum extractor are used) or an induction (when labour is induced artificially). What's more, according to an article in the U.S. medical journal *Obstetrics and Gynecology*, women over the age of 44 are 7.5 times more likely than younger women to require a Caesarean delivery. (U.S. Caesarean rates are always higher than Canadian rates, but it's an interesting fact to note nonetheless.)

> "I've had six miscarriages and have always struggled with infertility problems. That's why it's taken me 20 years to have four children. If you're willing to wait until you're older to start a family, then you must also be willing to deal with the possibility of fertility problems. I'm so glad that I started my family at 20."
>
> —LIZ, 40, MOTHER OF FOUR

The male biological clock

The biological clock waits for no woman—and for no man either, it would seem. In recent years, fertility researchers have started to document the ways in which time takes its toll on the male reproductive system. Sure, the biological clock is a lot more forgiving of prospective fathers than it is of prospective mothers, but it doesn't hurt for a would-be dad to hedge his fertility bets, given these recent findings on the male reproductive front:

•   A man's fertility declines with age. While the drop-off isn't as dramatic for men as it is for women (men continue to manufacture sperm throughout their lives, while women have to make do with the supply of eggs they were born with), it's something that the fertility world is starting to take more seriously (after many years of operating under the notion that it was only women who had a best-before date). A study reported in the medical journal *Fertility and Sterility* involving 2,000 women found that women age 35 and older with partners age 45 and older took five times longer to conceive than those whose partners were age 25 or younger. The study also found that women age 25 and under take four times longer to conceive with older partners (over 45) than with younger partners (under 25).

- Sperm quality declines with age. A study published in *Fertility and Sterility* found that in men between the ages of 30 and 50, sperm volume declines by 30 per cent, sperm motility declines by 37 per cent (meaning that the sperm are slower swimmers), and sperm are five times more likely to be misshapen (something that can prevent conception from occurring in the first place or lead to a miscarriage or genetic problem in the developing baby).

- The risk of miscarriage is greater if a woman conceives with an older partner. Researchers at the Columbia University School of Public Health found that the miscarriage risk is 60 per cent greater for a woman conceiving with a partner age 40 or older as compared to a woman conceiving with a partner under the age of 25, regardless of her own age, because older men have more abnormal sperm than young men do.

While there's still more research to be done on the issue of the male biological clock, men who hope to become fathers would be wise to err on the side of caution and to heed the same advice that is often given to would-be mothers: if having a baby is important to you, start planning for your future family sooner rather than later.

what about dads?

Birth defects become more common as men age. Researchers at the University of California, Los Angeles, found that men age 50 and older were four times more likely than younger men to father a child with Down syndrome. Researchers at the University of California, Berkeley, found that older men were more likely to father children with dwarfism or multiple genetic and chromosomal problems. And researchers at the Mount Sinai School of Medicine in New York found that men in their forties are six times as likely as men between the ages of 15 and 29 to father autistic children. A study by a team of British and Swedish researchers has also found that children born to men over 50 are four or five times more likely to develop schizophrenia than children born to fathers age 21 to 24.

A Baby? Maybe . . . Protecting Your Fertility

So you'd like to have a baby someday—just not right now. First of all, congratulations for sneaking a peek in a pregnancy book to get the pregnancy-planning facts ahead of time. That's *way* forward thinking. Now carry that thought process into action mode so that you can safeguard your fertility—and encourage your partner to safeguard his—to ensure the necessary equipment will be in top working order when it's time to get with the baby-making program. In addition to flipping through the remainder of this chapter and the one that follows, you may want to talk to your doctor about your future plans for parenthood. Your doctor may want to flag some health or lifestyle issues for you before you lose the birth control for good.

---

how old are your eggs?

Fertility experts have recently started talking about female reproductive age in terms of a woman's "ovarian reserve" (the number of eggs a woman's ovaries have in reserve) or—as Sherman J. Silber, MD, author of *How to Get Pregnant*, likes to put it—the amount of time left on a woman's biological clock. The most accurate method of assessing a woman's ovarian reserve is to conduct an ultrasound examination and perform an antral follicle count. The test can be performed by a fertility doctor at any point in your menstrual cycle and won't be affected by any hormones you may be taking. The advantage in finding out just how old—or young—you are, reproductively speaking, is that you can make some informed decisions on that basis. As Silber notes in his book, if the test results reveal that you are approaching the end of your reproductive years, but you still don't feel ready for motherhood, you might decide to freeze some eggs for future retrieval. Likewise, if you discover that you have at least another two decades left on your biological clock, you might not feel quite so pressured to get pregnant this month.

Your plan

Choose a birth control method that is fertility enhancing rather than one that could cause you grief once you start trying to conceive. Most experts agree that the birth control pill is a good choice because it changes the consistency of your cervical mucus, thereby reducing the likelihood that bacteria will get into the uterus and tubes. Pill use has been proven to prevent ovarian cysts, to arrest the progression of endometriosis (a condition that can result in progressive scarring of the Fallopian tubes), to decrease the incidence of ovarian and uterine cancer, and to restore a normal hormonal balance in women who don't ovulate. The intrauterine device (IUD), on the other hand, isn't attracting such rave reviews. It's been linked to increased incidence of pelvic inflammatory disease (a major cause of infertility in women).

If you want a comprehensive—and Canadian—roundup of various types of birth control, including the lowdown on the latest generation of hormonal birth control options, pick up a copy of *Sex Sense* by the Society of Obstetricians and Gynaecologists of Canada and visit www.sexualityandu.ca.

Pay attention to your gynecological health. Don't neglect any strange symptoms or mildly annoying gyno issues just because you're not planning to have a baby in the immediate future. The time to resolve these problems is when they arise—not years after the fact. If, for example, you have a milky discharge from your breasts, you don't menstruate at all unless you're on the pill, or you experience increasing facial hair and acne into your twenties, you may not be ovulating regularly or you may have some sort of hormonal imbalance (for example, polycystic ovarian disease). Likewise, if you experience unusual pain and bleeding (heavy or breakthrough bleeding), you may be developing ovarian cysts (generally non-cancerous growths that can disrupt your menstrual cycles), endometriosis, or fibroids (non-cancerous growths in the uterus that can prevent pregnancy or increase your likelihood of miscarriage). The sooner you seek out treatment for these conditions, the greater your odds of being able to start your family when you finally decide it's time.

Find out about any reproductive red flags that may be hanging from your family tree or hiding in your family closet. If you have a close female relative who had trouble conceiving, or if there's a history of endometriosis, uterine fibroids, early menopause, or uterine anomalies in your family, it's possible that you could experience these problems too. Many of these conditions are treatable, so find out now which, if any, of them may be in the cards for you. In some families, obstetrical histories and gynecological conditions are the stuff of which the best-ever family reunions are made; in others, words like "period" and "pelvic exam" are still considered slightly shocking—shocking enough that everyone in the family learns to speak the language of euphemisms whenever the conversation turns to "women's complaints." (Yes, it still happens in the best of families.)

Know who you're hopping into bed with. If there's a baby in your future, you should plan to practise safe sex, starting right now. Be monogamous or limit your number of sexual partners. Use condoms and spermicide. And make a point of being tested regularly for sexually transmitted infections (STIs) such as chlamydia, gonorrhea, syphilis, human papilloma virus (HPV can cause genital warts and has been linked to both pre-cancerous and cancerous conditions of the cervix), herpes, HIV, and hepatitis B and C. These STIs can cause infertility by either contaminating the pelvic cavity or altering your body's immunological defences—something that can trigger pelvic inflammatory disease. And, of course, some of these STIs could also lead to some very serious health problems for both you and your baby-to-be. If you think you may have been exposed to an STI, seek the help of your health-care provider before you attempt conception, since effective treatment is available.

Quit smoking. Women who smoke are 30 per cent less fertile than women who don't smoke. What's more, they're at increased risk of developing pelvic inflammatory disease—one of the greatest threats to a woman's fertility (something you should be thinking about right now, even if you don't have visions of a car seat showing up in your vehicle anytime soon). You'll want to try to quit smoking before you start trying to conceive anyway: smoking during pregnancy has been linked to a laundry list of pregnancy complications and health problems in babies, including an increased risk of sudden infant death syndrome (SIDS). If the pill is your birth control option of choice, you should be talking to your doctor about other birth control options or methods to help you quit smoking: smoking while you take the pill is an especially dangerous combination, due to the increased risk of cardiovascular disease. If you want to research quit-smoking programs on your own, check out the websites of the Canadian Cancer Society (www.cancer.ca) and the Lung Association (www.lung.ca), as well as the Health Concerns section of the Health Canada website (www.hc-sc.gc.ca).

Create a healthy environment for the baby you hope to conceive. Minimize your exposure to toxins at work and at home, and work with your neighbours to safeguard the air, land, and water in your community.

Your partner's plan

Encourage your partner to safeguard his fertility, too. A man's reproductive system can be damaged as a result of sports injuries, cycling long distances (for example, more than 160 kilometres (99 miles) a week), exposure to toxic chemicals or radiation, and the use of anabolic steroids and certain types of medications that may hamper sperm production and/or reduce sperm counts. If he's serious about becoming a father some day, he should also plan to get rid of his spare tire: men who are significantly overweight tend to have an oversupply of the female sex hormone estrogen—something that can scramble the messages passing between the testes and the pituitary gland. He should also look at his use of alcohol, drugs, and cigarettes: these so-called lifestyle drugs may hamper his ability to ejaculate and/or affect his fertility. Finally, anything that causes persistent overheating of his testicles is bad news (whether that's having a laptop on his lap or driving a truck long distances or wearing underwear that's too tight).

Tell him to pay attention to uncomfortable sensations. If a man experiences itching, burning, or a feeling that something's just not right in his reproductive tract, he should get it checked out rather than hoping the symptoms will disappear on their own: even if he'd rather stand buck-naked in front of a group of his colleagues at work than have a heart-to-heart talk with the family doctor about his prostate or his urethra. A low-grade infection can kill off sperm—something that can hamper your baby-making plans. Fortunately, this condition is easily treated. A course of antibiotics will generally do the trick. Other common causes of male infertility—such as clogged ejaculatory ducts and enlarged veins in the scrotum (a.k.a. varicoceles)—can also be treated relatively easily, should that uncomfortable sensation in his nether regions prove to be one of the root causes of your future fertility problems.

butt out	So much for the myth that smoking makes a guy manly: smoking releases adrenaline and other compounds into the bloodstream that interfere with the flow of blood to the penis. The bottom line? It's harder for a smoker to achieve and maintain an erection than it is for a guy who chooses to butt out.

Make sure that your partner seeks treatment if he has persistent difficulty achieving and maintaining erections. Erections are, after all, a key barometer of male sexual health. A whole bunch of factors can come into play here: aging, general health (diabetes, high cholesterol, certain prescription medications), lifestyle (smoking, steroids, alcohol use, obesity, poor physical fitness). As Harry Fisch, author of *The Male Biological Clock*, likes to put it so succinctly, "What's bad for the heart is bad for the penis."

Now or never? The health wild card

Sometimes there are specific health considerations that need to be taken into account when you're deciding whether to start your family sooner rather than later.

Heather wasn't in any particular hurry to start trying to have a baby until her doctor gave her a bit of a push. "I have celiac disease and had struggled with poor immune function, extremely low weight, and poor nutritional status for many years," the 37-year-old mother of one explains. "So in early 1996, when my gynecologist told me, 'This is as healthy as I've ever seen you, and if you want to have a child, this is probably the time to do it,' we decided it was now or never. I was in the midst of completing doctoral studies and we hadn't bought a house yet—one of our goals before having a baby—but we knew it was the right time. Given my health, it might be the only time that would be right, so we both agreed that starting our family was the thing to do."

Jenny, a 31-year-old mother of one, had a similar experience: "I have a pre-existing medical condition called Alport syndrome, a form of hereditary kidney disease," she explains. "My nephrologist advised that if we wanted to have children, we should do so sooner rather than later. My husband and I agreed that we wanted children and acknowledged the seriousness of my doctor's recommendations."

I get so emotional, baby

Your age and your physical health aren't the only factors you'll want to consider when attempting to answer the mother (or father) of all queries: Is this the right time to have a baby? If they were, you could input this data into a computer and get a deliciously uncomplicated answer. As things stand, you will also need to take the pulse of your relationship with your partner (if you're embarking on pregnancy as a couple) before making the big decision.

You can get there from here, right?

Couples who stop to consider how having a baby will impact their relationship may find that it can be difficult to get other couples who have crossed "the great divide" into parenthood to speak frankly about what it's really like. Seasoned parents may joke about how much your life is going to change ("You'll never have sex again!"), or they may offer vague reassurances about how it's rough at first, but you'll get through it. *Get through it how?* you may wonder, looking for some sort of parenting road map (or at least a crumpled up napkin with notes pointing you toward a few key landmarks along the way). But they shrug their shoulders and laugh, saying, "Sometimes we wonder how we got through it. We fought about everything." And they're right: there is a lot more to fight about in your post-baby life as a couple—eight times as much, according to marriage researcher John Gottman, Ph.D., author of *Why Marriages Succeed or Fail.* Fortunately, there is plenty you can do to stay connected as a couple through pregnancy and beyond, and to make your transition to parenthood as smooth as possible for yourself, your partner, and your new baby. We'll be talking about that throughout the remainder of this book.

If you're entering into pregnancy with a partner, something you do need to consider from the get-go—even before you start trying to conceive—is whether you want to have a family with that person. In other words, is he or she Mr. or Ms. Right?

I know: it's a pretty blunt question (and one that you may not find spelled out in black and white in too many other places), but it's one that you owe it to yourself to mull over seriously before you start making decisions that will affect you and your baby for a lifetime. Think about the type of parent your partner is likely to make, given what you know about your partner as a person. Is your partner patient, loving, generous, democratic, or a bit of a control freak? If he or she doesn't have the necessary parenting skills in place right now (and, frankly, a lot of us benefit from some on-the-job training after baby arrives), go into best-guess scenario mode. Consider what you know about your partner's upbringing and how he or she treats other people. Think about the quality of your relationship today and how stable your relationship has been over the years. Can you see yourself with this person—or at least co-parenting with this person—forever? Can you see your partner being a loving and nurturing parent to your child? Which types of parenting issues could you see yourselves disagreeing over: potty training, allowances, or dating rules? (If you can't see yourselves disagreeing about anything, either you've hooked up with a saint or you've got an underactive imagination.) Have you and your partner ever talked about anything parenting-related?

And now on to the heavy stuff. *The really heavy stuff.* Has there been a history of abuse—whether physical or emotional—in the past, or is there likely to be abuse in the future? You don't have to answer this question for anyone but yourself—the answer that you know to be true is the only one that counts. But here's what you need to know. According to the Society of Obstetricians and Gynaecologists, between 6 and 8 per cent of Canadian women experience

"I always knew that I wanted children, but it wasn't a burning need. Once we'd been married for a few years, I started thinking about babies. Having them, holding them, and wanting one really badly. My husband was the same. That's when we knew that we were ready: we just thought about it all the time."

—JENNIFER, 31, MOTHER OF TWO

abuse in their relationships each year, and the incidence rate is believed to be higher for pregnant women. Violence during pregnancy can cause a woman to become depressed—even suicidal—and it can lead to pregnancy complications and even the death of the mother or the baby. For information and support, contact the National Clearinghouse on Family Violence: www.phac-aspc .gc.ca/ncfv-cnivf/. You can also find local agencies and phone numbers in the front of your local phone book. If you've admitted to yourself that you need to make this call, I want you to look at those statistics again: *at least 8 per cent of Canadian women are abused each year.* That number means you're not alone.

The Truth about Baby Fever: Not Everyone Catches It

Some couples report that, after years of not feeling any burning desire to have children, they're suddenly hit with "baby fever"—a powerful urge to go forth and multiply. That was certainly the case for 32-year-old Jennifer, who recently gave birth to her first baby: "Two years before, I couldn't see myself as anything but a career person and graduate student. A year before, I was comfortable with becoming a wife, but not a mother. Then, almost overnight, motherhood felt right."

Others worry that they don't have what it takes, particularly if they haven't been swept up by that much-talked-about tidal wave of pre-mommy and pre-daddy emotion. "We really had to make a conscious decision to have a baby," explains Mark, 32, whose wife, Debbie, 31, is expecting their first child. "Our lives are quite comfortable now and there was no real drive within us. We were kind of waiting to be hit by this uncontrollable urge, but it never came. Age was probably the biggest consideration for us, both for the baby's health and not wanting to be too old as the child was growing up."

Myrna, a 32-year-old mother of one, found herself experiencing similar feelings of ambivalence throughout her twenties. It took a family crisis to encourage her to give serious thought to having a baby: "What started me thinking about having a child was watching my father go through a very serious, acute illness," she recalls. "My parents have six children, and it really was a time that brought out the strengths in all our family members. I think it also reinforced in me the importance of family and the bond that I share with my parents and brothers and sisters. I finally became more aware of how much I would miss if I didn't have a child and experience that deep feeling of being a parent. I can't speak for Scott, but I think he was much more ready than I was: he had been secretly 'kid-watching' for quite a few months. So when we finally decided, it was actually a pretty quick decision."

When you and your partner don't agree

While Myrna and Scott arrived at their decision at roughly the same time, some couples find they're operating on entirely different timelines when it comes to embarking on that weird-yet-wonderful voyage to parenthood.

It's a phenomenon that author Marni Jackson describes in her book *The Mother Zone: Love, Sex, and Laundry in the Modern Family* when she recalls how she felt about her partner's reluctance to commit to starting a family: "I wanted him to want [a baby] in exactly the same way, and to the same degree, as I did," she writes. "It didn't occur to me that men might come at the idea of fatherhood from a different angle. Perhaps for men babies are just an idea, an abstraction until they hold them in their arms. But the initial urge, the detailed, irresistible, and irrational longing, was mine. It was physical, like hunger."

Jennifer, 26, remembers feeling impatient when it became obvious that her husband, Kirk, was less ready to start a family than she was. "Kirk took a little longer than me to feel that it was the 'right time,'" she explains. "He said that he wanted to learn to be a good husband before he also had to become a good father. Also, at the time, he was in a contract position that wasn't necessarily secure. His reasons were more logical than emotional, and they were very good reasons that needed to be considered.

"I have to be truthful and admit that it made me sad he wasn't ready. I probably pressured him more than I meant to. I worried about waiting too long, as I'd had a bout of cervical cancer in my early twenties and didn't want scarring to prove too formidable an obstacle to conception. If we did have trouble conceiving, I really wanted to leave myself enough time to follow other options like assisted conception and adoption."

In the end, it didn't take Kirk very long to come around. The couple is currently expecting their first child. Jennifer offers these words of wisdom to other couples who may find themselves at different points on the journey to parenthood: "Deciding you're ready to have a baby is a monumental decision in the relationship of a couple. Although it's hard to wait for your partner to be 'ready,' it's imperative that you give him the opportunity to get used to the idea, too. It's important to remember that your partner's reasons for waiting are just as valid as your own. You'll never be happier than when you first make love after agreeing that the time is right: that feeling alone is worth waiting for."

If you find that you and your partner are ready to do battle on the baby-making issue, it may be time to call a temporary truce. Here are a few quick tips:

Keep the lines of communication open. While it may be difficult—even painful—for you to hear your partner talk about his or her reluctance to start a family, it's important to encourage your partner to say what's holding him or her back. Is your partner worried about how having a child may affect your financial situation? Does he or she feel unprepared to take on the responsibility of caring for a tiny human being? The more you can find out about your partner's concerns, the easier it will be for you to help to address them.

> "Our only reason for waiting a bit was to give us time to adjust to being a couple. It was our belief that parenting is a challenge requiring a definite team effort, and we wanted to strengthen our team with some practise since we'd both been single for so long."
>
> —JENNIFER, 32, MOTHER OF ONE

Focus on other aspects of your relationship. Try to remember what it was about your partner that attracted you in the first place—something that's easier said than done, of course, if you're feeling angry and frustrated right now—and make a point of having fun together on a regular basis so that you can stay connected as a couple while you weather this difficult period in your relationship.

Accept the fact that you can't force someone to want a baby any more than you can force someone to fall in love with you. All you can do is give your partner the space and time he or she needs and hope for the best.

When Mother Nature has other plans

For some couples, the whole concept of planning a pregnancy is a moot point. Long before they get the chance to sit down to have "the big talk," the pregnancy test comes back positive.

That's what happened to Ken and Nicole, who welcomed their first baby two and a half years ago. Ken was thrilled at the prospect of becoming a father, but Nicole didn't initially share his enthusiasm. "I had a lot of adjusting to do," she recalls. "I wasn't sure if I was ready to be a mom yet, and I had to adjust to all the changes my life was about to undergo. Fortunately, time, love, and patience resolved the issues of readiness for me."

Bevin and Ben, parents of a 5-month-old baby girl, found themselves faced with a similar surprise. "Ben and I had actually decided that about four years from now would be the right time to have a baby," Bevin recalls. "Unfortunately, someone else had other plans! We were just starting the process of purchasing our first home, I was toiling away at university correspondence courses, Ben was very involved with his weekend passion of skydiving, and we were both working to get debts paid off before having kids. Still, if you pledge to love and care for the child and to do the best you can, then if the timing is off, it's not the end of the world."

LeeAnne, a 29-year-old mother of three, feels that it can actually be a blessing to not have to consciously plan a pregnancy. "I never did decide it was the 'right time' to have a baby: they just sort of arrived on their own schedule. That was probably for the best. I don't think we would have decided on our own to have children as early in our twenties as we did, but we're both very glad that it turned out that way. The kids are great ages in relation to one another (7, 5 and a half, and 3 and a half), and we both feel we have more energy and focus now than we might in our late thirties or early forties. (I could be wrong on that! Guess I'll find out when I get there, for sure!)"

"It was my husband who got the ball rolling. I always knew I wanted children, but was still a bit nervous about the whole thing. I wasn't sure I was ready. We were married when I was 25, and when I was 27 he gave me a card on Mother's Day that said, 'I'm ready when you are.' I think we talked about it for about six months after that."

–JANE, 33, MOTHER OF TWO

CHAPTER 2

Your Pre-game Plan

If you had called your doctor's office to schedule a pre-pregnancy checkup a generation ago, your doctor would have had you pegged as a hypochondriac. After all, back then it was highly unusual for a woman to show up in her doctor's waiting room before the start of the second trimester (at which point she could feel confident her pregnancy had "taken"), let alone before she'd even started trying to conceive.

Today, the thinking is entirely different. Prospective parents are encouraged to start acting pregnant from the moment they so much as whisper the word "baby" to one another. And a pre-conception checkup is considered *de rigueur.* After all, it's a lot easier to deal with any health-related problems if they are detected before the pregnancy test comes back positive rather than after the fact. Besides, one of the most critical periods of embryonic development occurs during the early days after conception—a time when most women aren't even aware that they're pregnant. The logic here is obvious: if you start playing the part of the health-conscious parent-to-be right from the get-go (as opposed to waiting for official word that there's a baby on board), you'll be getting your pregnancy off to the healthiest possible start. That's good news for you and baby.

Training for the Big Event

So you're ready to sign up for the mother of all marathons—that nine-month-long endurance event that culminates with the birth of a baby. Here are some things you can start doing right now to get your body ready:

Watch your weight—but not too carefully

While it's always a good idea to get to a healthy weight prior to attempting a pregnancy, the key word is "healthy," not "body of a supermodel." Believe it or not, the extra padding on your hips and thighs that drives you crazy on a day-to-day basis will serve you well as you embark on Project Baby. Women who have too little body fat tend to stop ovulating, which can wreak havoc on their plans to conceive, and those who do manage to conceive face an increased risk of becoming anemic (iron deficient) or having a low birth weight baby (one who weighs in at less than 5 pounds (2.3 kilograms) and who may be at increased risk of experiencing some potentially serious health problems).

That said, when it comes to body fat, you *can* have too much of a good thing. Women who start their pregnancy significantly overweight or who gain too much weight during pregnancy face a higher-than-average risk of experiencing a number of pregnancy- and birth-related complications, including pre-eclampsia (a serious medical condition characterized by extremely high blood pressure), gestational diabetes (a form of diabetes that occurs during pregnancy and that puts a woman at increased risk of developing diabetes later in life), or stillbirth. They may also require a labour induction and/or need a Caesarean section. What's more, overweight women are more likely to give birth to extremely large babies, babies with neural tube defects, and babies who are at increased risk of developing diabetes later in life.

And here's something else to think about: your heart has to work extra hard during pregnancy if you're carrying around a lot of extra weight. Research has shown that the cardiac output in obese women can jump by up to 50 per cent during pregnancy, as compared to the more typical 35 to 40 per cent experienced by non-obese women.

If you are significantly overweight, it's worth it to attempt to get within 15 pounds (6.8 kilograms) of your goal weight, and then to keep an eye on your portion sizes to maintain this weight before you start trying to conceive. (Yo-yo dieting—watching the scale swing up and down—isn't good for you, the baby you hope to conceive, or your self-esteem. So do yourself a favour: swear off those wacky fad diets that don't make anyone happy—except the wacky fad diet inventors.)

> *could you have diabetes?*
>
> Diabetes can sneak up on you. In fact, one-third of women with diabetes are so symptom-free that they aren't even aware that they have diabetes. That's why it's important to familiarize yourself with the risk factors for diabetes (being over-weight; not exercising regularly; having developed gestational diabetes during a previous pregnancy; being related to someone with diabetes; or being African American, Latina, Native American, Asian American, or Asian Indian) and to talk to your doctor about being tested for diabetes if you feel you could be at risk. If you do have diabetes, your odds of having a healthy pregnancy and a healthy baby are dramatically increased if you are able to get your blood sugar under control before you become pregnant. That means balancing eating with exercise, maintaining a healthy weight, and taking any medications that are prescribed by your doctor.

Don't let concerns about your weight prevent you from accessing pre-conception advice or prenatal care. If your doctor tends to focus on your weight and little else, consider changing health-care providers (perhaps midwifery care might be an option for you during your pregnancy) or come up with strategies for dealing with your caregiver's comments. Working with a counsellor who specializes in body image (and body image during pregnancy in particular) or attending a support group for women who are overweight during pregnancy may be very helpful in such a situation. Call your health unit for referrals to such services in your community.

With that said, here's an all-important point to consider before you start getting too obsessed about your weight: *maybe your weight is already in the healthy range.* Since most of us tend to be less than objective when sizing up our own bodies, rather than turning to the mirror for feedback, why not consider how your weight measures up on the Body Mass Index (BMI) (See Table 2.1: Are You at a Healthy Weight?) or in terms of waist-to-hip ratio? (For your waist-to-hip ratio, measure your waist at the navel and your hips at the widest part, then divide your waist measurement by your hip measurement. The ratio should be 0.80 or less for women; 0.81 to 0.85 indicates moderate risk of heart disease.) Or, ask your doctor for feedback on your weight-loss plans.

2.1 Are You at a Healthy Weight?

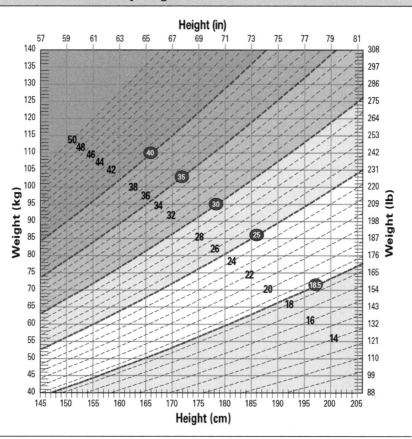

To calculate your BMI (kg/m²), use a straight edge to help locate the point on the chart where height (inches or centimetres) and weight (pounds or kilograms) intersect. Read the number on the dashed line closest to this point. For example, an individual who weighs 69 kilograms and is 173 centimetres tall has a BMI of approximately 23.

If your BMI is 18.5 or lower, you are considered underweight.

If your BMI is between 18.5 and 24.9, you are considered to be at a normal weight.

If your BMI is between 25.0 and 29.9, you are considered to be overweight.

If your BMI is 30.0 or higher, you are considered to be obese.

Source: *Canadian Guidelines for Body Weight Classification in Adults.* Health Canada, 2003.

If your BMI is higher than it should be and you'd like to lose a few pounds before you become pregnant, crash dieting is definitely out. Not only do you run the risk of depleting your body of the very types of nutrients it will need to build a healthy baby, your body may actually stop ovulating. (When your body is faced with famine-like conditions, it goes into self-preservation mode. After all, if there's barely enough food around to sustain you, your body isn't about to do something biologically reckless, like get pregnant.)

2.2 Health Risk Classification according to Body Mass Index (BMI)		
Health Risk Classification	**BMI Category (kg/m²)**	**Risk of Developing Health Problems**
Underweight	< 18.5	Increased
Normal weight	18.5–24.9	Least
Overweight	25.0–29.9	Increased
Obese class I	30.0–34.9	High
Obese class II	35.0–39.9	Very high
Obese class III	≧ 40.0	Extremely high

Source: Health Canada. *Canadian Guidelines for Body Weight Classification in Adults.* Ottawa: Minister of Public Works and Government Services Canada; 2003.

A far more sensible approach to dealing with any extra weight is to eat well, exercise regularly, and deal with any underlying issues that may have contributed to that weight gain in the first place. It may not be the quick fix or magic little weight-loss pill that gets pitched on late-night TV, but it's ultimately what works. To get started:

Ask for help. A family doctor, obstetrician, midwife, or public health nurse can refer you to a dietitian or nutritionist who can steer you in the right direction. It may be possible to meet with a dietitian or nutritionist at your local public health unit, or to have the services of such a professional covered by any extended health benefits you or your partner may carry.

Consult Canada's Food Guide for basic guidelines on eating well. For example, consuming five to six small, frequent meals each day; consuming plenty of whole grains; eating lean meats or alternatives (nuts, beans); eating lots of fruits and vegetables; and drinking lots of fluids.

Do a nutrient check

While you're engaged in this pre-baby nutritional navel-gazing, remember that it's just as important to focus on what you're eating as how much you're eating *get moving* Don't overlook the importance of being physically active if you're trying to lose weight. Exercise helps your body to burn calories, boosts your metabolic rate during and after a workout, encourages your body to build muscle tissue (which helps it to burn more fat), curbs your appetite, and can even help you to maintain your weight loss once you reach your goal weight. (One study from south of the border showed that 90 per cent of women who successfully maintained their weight loss for five years or more exercised three times each week for at least 30 minutes.) Health Canada has some related advice that makes a lot of sense: consider how active you have been until now and kick it up a notch, aiming for a minimum of 25 minutes per day of walking, swimming, dancing, or another type of physical activity.

(without getting totally obsessive, of course). Zero in on foods that pack the greatest possible nutritional punch. After all, you're trying to get your body ready for the biggest health challenge it will ever experience: sustaining another human being throughout the entire nine and a half months of pregnancy and during the time when you're breastfeeding.

Don't wait until your pregnancy is confirmed before you start eating for two (at least from a nutrient standpoint). While you don't have to consume more calories quite yet (unless, of course, you're seriously underweight and in weight-gain mode), you may want to give your diet a nutritional reno, starting today. Eat a variety of whole grains, fruits, and vegetables each day, and reduce your intake of trans fat. Boost your intake of foods that are rich in iron and calcium, and—if your health-care provider recommends it—consider taking a multivitamin supplement, too. (Just make sure you don't overdo it with vitamins A or D. Too much of either nutrient can be unhealthy for the baby you hope to conceive.) *Canada's Food Guide* is designed to meet the needs of Canadians from the preschool years on up. You can download a copy of the guide from www.myfoodguide.ca.

Find out which foods are—and aren't—considered safe during pregnancy. Fish that contain potentially risky levels of mercury should be eaten in moderation. Steer clear of foods that may be a risk for listeriosis and other food-borne illnesses, including raw fish; undercooked meat, poultry, seafood, hot dogs, and deli meats; refrigerated pâtés or meat spreads; refrigerated smoked seafood (unless it has been cooked); soft-scrambled eggs and all foods made with raw or lightly cooked eggs (such as homemade mayonnaise and some Caesar salads); unpasteurized soft cheeses (keeping in mind most Canadian soft cheeses are pasteurized); unpasteurized milk and foods made from unpasteurized milk; unpasteurized juices; and raw vegetable sprouts, including alfalfa, clover, and radish. (Chapter 5 has more information on food-borne illnesses.) Also avoid herbal supplements and teas, and foods that may trigger a food allergy in babies born to parents with a history of food allergies. (Consult a dietitian or public health nurse for details in planning your pregnancy diet if you or your partner has a history of food allergies.)

Folic acid

If the (Canadian) inventors of the hit board game *Trivial Pursuit* came out with a special Food and Nutrition edition, they'd have to work in dozens of trivia questions just to cover all the cool facts about folic acid.

Unless you're a total novice when it comes to the world of prenatal health (you've never flipped open a pregnancy magazine or picked up a prenatal health brochure anywhere, anytime), you've no doubt heard at least some of the good news about folic acid. Consuming an adequate amount of folic acid each day can significantly reduce your chances of giving birth to a baby with a neural tube defect (such as spina bifida or anencephaly). In fact, studies have shown that when folic acid is taken daily for at least three months prior to pregnancy, the risk of having a baby with a neural tube defect is reduced by 70 per cent. It's particularly important to take folic acid prior to pregnancy because the neural tube—the brain and spinal column in the developing embryo—develop very early in pregnancy, approximately 26 to 28 days after conception. But that's not all folic acid can do for a mom-to-be and her baby. It has also been proven to help reduce the incidence of other types of birth defects, the likelihood of a preterm birth, the risk of giving birth to a low birth weight baby, and the incidence of recurrent pregnancy loss.

This nutrient has scored such rave reviews with the nutritional powers that be that Health Canada and the Society of Obstetricians and Gynaecologists of Canada now advise *all women who could become pregnant* to take a supplement containing between 0.4 and 1.0 milligrams of folic acid daily, in addition to the amount of folic acid that is consumed through food sources.

It's smart advice. According to the Canadian Childbirth Trust, approximately 40 per cent of Canadian pregnancies are unplanned. And if you're counting on your diet—as healthy as it may be—to provide your daily quota of this nutrient, odds are it will fall short: a diet that follows *Canada's Food Guide* will only provide about 0.2 milligrams of folic acid per day.

The Society of Obstetricians and Gynaecologists of Canada recommends that all women who are planning a pregnancy consume a minimum of 0.4 milligrams of folic acid per day (the amount found in a standard prenatal vitamin) prior to conception and throughout the first 10 to 12 weeks of pregnancy—the point at which the baby's brain and spinal column are finished forming. Women who've previously had a baby with a neural tube defect may be advised to take 4 milligrams of folic acid daily. Women considered to be at moderate risk of giving birth to a baby with a neural tube defect—women who have a close relative with a neural tube defect, who have insulin-dependent diabetes, or who are epileptic and take the drugs valproic acid or carbamazepine, for example—should take 1 to 4 milligrams of folic acid daily. Your doctor or midwife will help you to determine what quantity of folic acid is recommended in your situation.

Iron

Folic acid isn't the only nutrient that a woman planning a pregnancy needs to be concerned about. Iron also plays an important role during pregnancy by helping to create the additional red blood cells needed to carry oxygen from your lungs to various parts of your body, as well as to your growing baby. If you have a severe case of anemia, your baby faces an increased risk of intrauterine growth restriction and fetal hypoxia during labour, and you'll be less able to handle the blood loss associated with a typical vaginal or Caesarean delivery.

Unfortunately, many women of childbearing age don't get enough iron in their diet. As a result, they may already be iron deficient (anemic) by the time they become pregnant. Because it's important to ensure that a pregnant woman has adequate iron reserves, your doctor will likely check your hemoglobin level at your pre-conception health checkup and throughout your pregnancy. If it's below normal, he or she may recommend an iron supplement and suggest that you make an effort to increase your intake of iron-rich foods (liver, kidney, and other organ meats; dried fruit; eggs—see Chapter 5 for other suggestions). You should plan to include these foods in your diet regularly, however, even if your hemoglobin result comes back normal, since your iron requirements double during pregnancy. That way, you'll have some iron reserves to draw upon if first-trimester morning sickness has you turning your nose up at anything more exotic than unsalted soda crackers.

Even if you do make a point of consuming iron-rich foods prior to pregnancy, you may still become iron deficient toward the end of pregnancy or after giving birth. If you find yourself feeling tired during pregnancy or after you've had your baby, it could be because your iron stores are low, in which case you'll want to talk to your doctor or midwife about taking an iron supplement.

Just a quick word to the wise: some iron supplements cause constipation and/or gastrointestinal upsets. While the side effects usually die down after a few days, some women find they have to switch to a slow-release or pediatric iron supplement. Your doctor, midwife, dietitian, or pharmacist will be able to help you to choose the iron supplement that's right for you.

You can also combat some of the constipating effects of iron supplements by drinking more fluids and increasing the amount of fibre in your diet.

Oh yeah, one final thing. Be careful about the type of beverage you use to wash down that iron supplement. While orange juice and other beverages that are high in vitamin C boost iron absorption, milk, tea, or coffee at meals can interfere with it.

Calcium

Even though Mother Nature does her best to ensure that you obtain adequate amounts of calcium from your food during pregnancy (a pregnant body is twice as efficient at absorbing calcium as a non-pregnant one), if you aren't obtaining enough calcium from food sources alone, your body will start to take calcium from your bones in order to meet the needs of your developing baby. (Yes, it's true: your baby is somewhat of a parasite. Your body will automatically do whatever it can to meet your baby's needs, and if that means depleting your calcium stores in order to ensure that the baby survives, then that's what it will do. It's romantic in a Robin Hood kind of way, isn't it? Other than the fact that the calcium depletion leaves you at an increased risk of osteoporosis and/or giving birth prematurely.)

While most women will get more than enough calcium by consuming four servings a day from the milk and milk products group of *Canada's Food Guide*, if you have a milk allergy, are lactose intolerant, or are a vegan who's chosen not to consume milk products, you may have difficulty getting enough calcium from your diet. In this case, you'll want to talk to your doctor, midwife, or registered dietitian about the advisability of taking a calcium supplement prior to and during pregnancy.

Be careful not to go overboard in the calcium department. Too much calcium during pregnancy (more than 2,500 milligrams daily from supplements and food sources combined, according to the folks at Health Canada) can put you at greater risk of developing a urinary tract infection (due to the increased amount of calcium that needs to be excreted in the urine) or kidney stones, and it can hamper your ability to absorb other nutrients such as iron, zinc, and magnesium.

If you're taking an iron supplement to combat anemia and a calcium supplement to boost your calcium stores, you might just end up with a Battle of the Nutrients going on in your very own body. Because iron tends to reduce your body's ability to absorb calcium, you'll have to give some thought to timing your iron and calcium supplements. One solution that some dietitians swear by is to take your iron supplement at night and your calcium supplement in the morning—assuming, of course, that morning sickness isn't preventing you from stomaching any supplement anytime.

what's in your drinking water? A glass of water can hide some pretty scary ingredients—like pesticides, industrial waste, arsenic, nitrates, and trihalomethanes (THMs), all of which are harmful or even deadly to the developing baby. If you're not sure about the quality of your drinking water, get it tested. Your provincial or territorial government can provide a list of approved labs.

Kick your smoking habit

If you're planning to get pregnant in the near future, you owe it to yourself and your baby-to-be to quit smoking now. Here's why. Smoking . . .

- **makes you less fertile.** A University of California, Berkeley, study found that smoking 10 cigarettes per day cuts a woman's chances of conceiving in half.
- **interferes with the absorption of vitamin C.** Since vitamin C has an important role to play in helping you to absorb iron, smoking can indirectly contribute to iron deficiency anemia.
- **disrupts the flow of oxygen to the baby.** Nicotine constricts the flow of blood through the blood vessels in the placenta, thereby reducing the amount of oxygen and nutrients that the baby receives.
- **can cause birth defects.** If you smoke 10 cigarettes per day, you're 50 per cent more likely to give birth to a baby with cleft palate and cleft lip. And if you smoke more than 21 cigarettes per day, you're 78 per cent more likely to give birth to a baby with these types of problems.
- **can harm your baby's lungs.** Mothers who smoke during pregnancy risk permanently altering the structure and function of their babies' lungs, which can make their babies more susceptible to respiratory disorders and infections during early childhood.
- **can cause certain pregnancy-related complications.** Women who smoke during pregnancy are more likely to experience placental abnormalities and bleeding.
- **increases your risk of giving birth prematurely.** Because babies who are born prematurely tend to experience more health problems than those

who are carried to term, this is yet another good reason to quit smoking before you start trying to conceive.

- **can be fatal to the developing baby.** Women who smoke during pregnancy face an increased risk of miscarriage, stillbirth, premature birth, and losing a baby to sudden infant death syndrome (SIDS).
- **can interfere with breastfeeding.** Smoking can decrease the quantity and quality of breast milk, which can lead to early weaning.
- **is bad for your baby's health.** Children who are exposed to second-hand smoke are more likely to develop asthma, bronchitis, and ear infections. What's more, exposure to second-hand smoke during childhood can cause lung cancer later in life.
- **is linked to childhood behavioural problems.** Toddlers whose mothers smoked during pregnancy are four times as likely to be impulsive and rebellious and to take risks.

Trying to kick your smoking habit before you start attempting to conceive? Make sure your menstrual cycle isn't working against you. A study reported in the February 1, 2000, issue of the *Journal of Consulting and Clinical Psychology* found that women who attempt to quit smoking during the first half of their menstrual cycles (prior to ovulation) experienced less severe symptoms of tobacco withdrawal and depression than women who tried to quit during the second half of their cycles (after ovulation).

While quitting is never easy, these tips can help you to join the non-smoking majority of moms-to-be:

Decide on a quitting strategy. Quitting cold turkey works well for some women, but not for others. If you can't make up your mind which way to go, here's a point to keep in mind: studies have shown that withdrawal symptoms disappear more quickly for smokers who quit completely rather than for those who gradually wean themselves off their habit.

Get your body in motion. A study conducted by researchers in Austria found that exercise can be a powerful aid in quitting smoking. The researchers found that 80 per cent of smokers who exercised managed to quit, as compared to 52 per cent of non-exercisers.

Expect to experience some powerful withdrawal symptoms. Symptoms of nicotine withdrawal include a slowed heart rate, difficulty concentrating, difficulty thinking, irritability, anger, anxiety, restlessness, insomnia, tremors, headaches, dizziness, feeling "spaced out," tingling or numbness in the arms and legs, increased hunger (especially for sweets), increased coughing (as the cilia in the lungs regain their cleaning action and begin cleaning up the lungs), and a killer craving for a cigarette. Fortunately, these symptoms tend to be relatively short-lived, peaking at around 96 hours after you quit lighting up, and disappearing entirely before your one-month smoke-free anniversary rolls around. (Find out what else to expect and how to manage these symptoms by visiting the Lung Association's website at www.lung.ca/smoking.)

Get others in on the act. A recent study conducted at the University of Pittsburgh School of Public Health concluded that, from the standpoint of the developing baby, there's no appreciable difference between being exposed to second-hand smoke and having a mother who smokes.

Avoid second-hand smoke at all costs. Not only is smoking harmful to a pregnant woman and her baby—one study showed that exposure to second-hand smoke during pregnancy increases the baby's chances of developing certain types of childhood leukemia—it lowers a man's sperm count by 20 per cent. (So much for those manly Marlboro ads!) Exposure to second-hand smoke can even affect female fertility. A Bristol University study found that having a partner who smoked can reduce a woman's fertility by 34 per cent.

While you're on a roll, deal with your weight problem, too (if you have one). Research has shown that mothers who smoke during pregnancy are more likely to have overweight children. If those moms are overweight, too, the risk of their child becoming overweight was nearly twice as high. Whether it's nature, nurture, or a bit of both, there's no time like the present to start taking the best possible care of yourself (and your baby-to-be).

Note: If you're planning to use a nicotine patch or nicotine chewing gum to help you break your smoking habit, talk to your doctor. These products may be used during pregnancy, provided that you are under a physician's care.

Pass on that glass of wine

According to the Canadian Paediatric Society, there's no safe level of alcohol consumption during pregnancy. Women who drink large amounts of alcohol on a regular basis while they're pregnant risk giving birth to a baby with fetal alcohol spectrum disorder (FASD)—a term that describes a range of behavioural and learning disabilities that may affect people whose mothers drank while they were pregnant. FASD currently affects approximately 1 per cent of Canadians.

Your partner should also plan to abstain from alcohol while you're trying to conceive. Alcohol has been proven to contribute to ejaculatory dysfunction and depressed sperm counts and testosterone levels, and some studies have indicated that babies fathered by men who consume alcohol on a regular basis tend to be of lower birth weight.

If you need support and information about trying to kick your alcohol or drug problem, contact the Alcohol and Substance Abuse in Pregnancy Helpline at the Motherisk Clinic at the Hospital for Sick Children in Toronto: 1–877–327–4636. The Motherisk Clinic is also an excellent source of advice on drug or chemical exposure during pregnancy. If that's the type of information you're seeking, call 1–416–813–6780 instead.

Had a glass of wine at your office party before you even suspected you were pregnant? Forget about all the healthy meals you ate and all the times you worked out at the gym: it's the thought of yourself clinking wine glasses with your coworkers that's bound to flash into your head the moment the pregnancy test comes back positive.

As tempted as you might be to sign yourself up for a nine-month-long immersion class in mother guilt, you're not going to do yourself or your baby any good by obsessing about that single mistimed glass of wine for the next nine months. A better bet is to stop drinking now and decide to take the best possible care of yourself and your baby between now and delivery day. Besides, binge drinking—which is defined as having the equivalent of five glasses of wine on any single occasion—is thought to be more of a risk to the developing baby than a one-time glass of wine. Of course, it's always best to avoid exposing your baby to any alcohol while you're pregnant or even thinking of becoming pregnant, both because of the risk to the developing baby and because of the potential impact on your fertility.

Bottom line? While you should do your best to avoid consuming any alcoholic beverages while you're trying to conceive, don't spend your entire pregnancy beating yourself up if you drank a glass of wine at some point after you conceived. It's all water under the bridge now, so it's best to just forget about it and move on.

Just say no to drugs

Like alcohol, illicit drugs should be avoided when you're trying to conceive and after you become pregnant. The reason is obvious: illicit drugs have been proven to cause a smorgasbord of problems in the developing baby, including cleft palate, heart murmurs, eye defects, facial deformities, central nervous system problems, damage to major organs, and low birth weight. What's more, babies who become addicted to drugs while in the womb experience painful withdrawal effects after birth. Cocaine has been linked to both miscarriage and placental abruptions (the premature separation of the placenta from the uterine wall) and maternal death from cardiac overload, while marijuana is believed to be responsible for a variety of neurobehavioural abnormalities in the newborn.

The party lifestyle can also take its toll on the male reproductive system. Alcohol and cocaine can bring down sperm counts (in the case of cocaine, the impact lasts for up to two years), and marijuana makes it difficult for sperm to travel toward and penetrate the egg.

Kick your coffee habit

While you might find it hard to imagine starting your day without a steaming cup of coffee, most experts agree that caffeine use during pregnancy may pose some significant risks to the developing baby. Recent studies have linked caffeine to decreased fertility, an increased risk of miscarriage (in women who consume more than five cups per day), and lower birth weight.

Unfortunately, the one thing the experts can't seem to agree on is what constitutes a "safe" amount of caffeine during pregnancy. Until the jury comes back with a more definitive answer, it's probably best to err on the side of caution. If you can't kick your caffeine habit entirely, you should at least try to limit your intake to no more than one or two cups of coffee each day. (We're talking 175-millilitre (6-ounce) cups here—not those bowl-sized latte mugs!) Here are some more reasons to cut back on your caffeine consumption prior to pregnancy. Caffeine . . .

- acts as a diuretic, removing both fluid and calcium from your body;
- interferes with the absorption of iron—something that can contribute to anemia;
- heightens mood swings and causes insomnia—the last thing you need when you're trying to cope with the highs and lows of trying to conceive.

Don't douche

For the longest time, douching had all but disappeared, but it never quite managed to go the way of the dodo bird. And it's been enjoying a rather creepy resurgence lately, which brings to mind an army of Stepford-like women marching to the drugstore en masse to pick up the douche of the month.

If you're in the habit of douching, you'll definitely want to give the douche bottle the old heave-ho before you start trying to conceive. For one thing, douching significantly reduces your fertility: one study showed that women who douche on a regular basis are 30 per cent less likely to conceive in any given month than women who don't douche at all. Note: Anything that you insert into your vagina during or right after you have sex has the potential to kill sperm, whether it's a spermicide, a lubricant, or soap. So if you're in the habit of showering after sex, avoid washing around the vaginal area. Better yet, stay in bed and enjoy some extra cuddling. You can have a shower once those sperm have had a chance to head off on their journey.

And as if that weren't enough, women who douche are at increased risk of experiencing pelvic inflammatory disease (one of the leading causes of infertility) and ectopic pregnancy (in which the fertilized ovum implants somewhere other than inside the uterus, most often in the Fallopian tube).

Even if you're not into commercial douche products, don't make the mistake of assuming that it's safe to douche with water. Studies have shown that it's the mechanics of douching rather than what you douche with that's responsible for gynecological problems.

Keep your stress level down

Here's one of those bits of advice that belongs in the "easier said than done" category: it's a good idea to try to reduce your stress level if you're hoping to conceive in the near future. Here's why. Studies have shown that high levels of stress can disrupt ovulation and increase your odds of giving birth to a baby with a birth defect. While the effects of stress on ovulation have been demonstrated time and time again, the evidence concerning birth defects is a little more groundbreaking. A study conducted by the March of Dimes in the United States indicates that women who experience a very stressful event during the month prior to conception or during the first three months of pregnancy are more likely to give birth to a baby with a birth defect.

Now before you start feeling stressed about, well, *feeling stressed*, relax. This shouldn't be about minor, day-to-day stress—conflicts at work, arguments with your partner, the frustration of having to fill out the most annoying piece of paperwork ever, that kind of thing. We're talking about the big stuff.

If you find yourself experiencing this kind of high-level stress while you're trying to conceive or during pregnancy, or if your day-to-day stress is building to the point where you find it hard to cope, you may want to talk to your health-care provider about how you're feeling. He or she will be able to refer you to a counsellor who can help you to come up with strategies for managing the stress you are experiencing. If you are having difficulties with anxiety or depression, your health-care provider may discuss the pros and cons of taking medication when you're hoping to be pregnant in the near future. Your health-care provider will help you to weigh the risks and benefits that various types of medications may pose to you and your baby.

stay safe

It's important to let your health-care provider or some other trusted person know if you are being subjected to intimate partner violence (physical violence, psychological attacks, and other controlling behaviours that create fear and inflict harm). While research has indicated that between 6 and 8 per cent of Canadian women are abused by their partners, it is believed that the incidence of violence is even higher for pregnant women. Forty per cent of abused women report that the first incidence of abuse happened during pregnancy. Women who are subject to violence during pregnancy are more likely to be stressed, depressed, suicidal, and to experience pregnancy and labour complications (miscarriage, insufficient weight gain, premature rupture of membranes, premature labour and birth, placental abruption). They and their babies also face a higher risk of injury and death. The Peel Committee Against Woman Abuse has created a safety-planning guide (translated into a variety of languages) that describes practical steps a woman can take to try to stay safe. You can download a copy from www.pcawa.org.

Delegate the dirty work

Play the part of the pregnant diva by delegating the dirty work to someone else—or (if you must) by slipping on a pair of rubber gloves while you deal with the kitty litter. You're not really being a diva by steering clear of a litter box, by the way. Toxoplasmosis—a virus that can be transmitted via cat feces and that can be found in kitty litter and in garden soil—can lead to miscarriage, birth defects, and developmental disorders in the developing baby. However, your health-care provider will test for toxoplasmosis, and you may have immunity.

As for the other household chores that aren't recommended for pregnant women (for example, using paints, solvents, or pesticides; cleaning rodent cages or any messes created by wild mice; or retrieving any half-eaten dead bird that your cat left for you in the backyard): it's not your department—at least not for the next nine and a half months. Delegate!

Watch out for workplace hazards

We all like to joke about how work can be dangerous to the health (or at least the mental health), but sometimes it really *can* be—particularly if you're thinking of getting pregnant in the near future: metals, pesticides, and chemicals (such as paints, lacquers, gases, industrial or household solvents, wood-finishing products, darkroom chemicals, leaded glass, X-rays, anaesthetics, or nuclear *hair care*

Planning to conceive in the very near future? While the jury is still out on the dangers of dyeing, perming, or straightening your hair during pregnancy, this is one potential risk to your baby you can easily avoid. Either switch to a toxin-free type of hair product, or plan to postpone your visit to the hairdresser until after the first trimester. And make sure the salon is well ventilated so that you won't be breathing in as many product fumes.

medicine) are just a few of the workplace hazards that have been linked with miscarriage, premature labour, low birth weight, birth defects, and reduced fertility. Wondering whether it's dangerous to work with a particular product or substance while you're trying to conceive? Get the facts from the Motherisk Clinic at the Hospital for Sick Children in Toronto (1–416–813–6780).

Other on-the-job hazards that should be avoided include high noise levels (associated with preterm birth, fetal hearing loss, and a decrease in fetal birth weight), high heat (may cause increased risk of miscarriage, neural tube defects, and low birth weight; can also temporarily impair male fertility), and strenuous physical activity (can lead to preterm labour or maternal injury).

If you feel that your workplace environment could be harmful to you or the baby you hope to conceive, talk to your employer. A job modification may be necessary once you start trying to get pregnant.

Dad's the word:
More reproductive health issues for fathers-to-be

Smoking, alcohol, drugs, and workplace hazards aren't the only issues that should be of concern to fathers-to-be. Prospective fathers also need to think about

- avoiding injuries to the genital area, since such injuries can hamper the production of sperm, interfere with the transport of sperm, affect hormone levels, and/or lead to ejaculatory problems;
- steering clear of anabolic steroids, as they could jeopardize a man's chances of becoming a father (some men find that the drop in testosterone production and the shrinking of the testes that result from steroid use continue long after they've stopped using);
- not exposing the genitals to excessive heat, which can hamper the production of sperm;
- avoiding workplace exposures to such industrial solvents as benzene and ethylene glycol ethers, or wearing protective clothing to minimize exposure;

- avoiding exposure to toxic chemicals and radiation, which can destroy sperm production and/or damage a man's genetic material;
- achieving a healthy weight (men who are significantly overweight tend to have an abundance of the female sex hormone estrogen—something that can interfere with the transmission of messages between the testes and the pituitary gland);
- getting the doctor's okay about using herbal medicine products (some products—including St. John's wort, ginkgo biloba, and echinacea—are thought to damage sperm);
- talking to their doctor about which medications are (and aren't) recommended for couples who are trying to conceive. Miscarriages and fetal abnormalities are more common in women whose partners take the drug 6-mercaptopurine to treat inflammatory bowel disease. What's more, certain antibiotics, chemotherapeutic agents, and other drugs (such as cimetidine, an antacid) can reduce sperm counts; and certain types of blood pressure drugs can contribute to ejaculatory dysfunction. Note: If your partner will be having cancer-related surgery to his urogenital area in the near future, you may want to encourage him to consider making a sperm bank deposit before he checks in to the hospital. That way, he'll still be able to father any future children the two of you decide to have.

boxers vs. briefs

The latest round in the never-ending battle of boxers vs. briefs has ended in favour of the boxers (or the boxer-less). Researchers have concluded that wearing boxers—or no underwear at all—results in a lower scrotal temperature (and hence a more sperm-friendly environment) than wearing briefs. Some related findings from other recent studies are also worth noting: working with a laptop on your lap can be detrimental to sperm, as can wearing bicycle shorts and riding for more than two hours a day, six days a week; and hanging out in hot tubs and saunas. The take-home message is clear: keep it cool, dudes!

Your Pre-conception Checkup: The Insider's Guide

You've started making some important lifestyle changes because you're determined to get your body in the best possible shape for pregnancy. Now it's time to pay a visit to your doctor to get a clean bill of health. Here's what to expect during your pre-conception checkup.

Your doctor should . . .

- talk with you about your plans to start trying to conceive and answer any questions you may have about conception, pregnancy, and birth;
- evaluate your lifestyle habits and recommend any changes that will boost your odds of conceiving and giving birth to a healthy baby;
- review the list of medications you're currently taking (both over-the-counter and prescription drugs) and discuss any changes that should be made before you start trying to conceive (for example, if you're using the prescription acne medication Accutane, you'll need to discontinue use before you start trying to conceive because this medication can cause miscarriage and birth defects);
- inquire about your use of herbal products (to ensure that what you are taking is considered safe for use during pregnancy);
- do a rubella test (German measles test) to determine whether you're immune to the disease (if you're not, you'll need to postpone your plans to start trying to conceive until three months after your vaccination: rubella exposure during the first three months of pregnancy increases the risk of miscarriage or of giving birth to a baby with severe birth defects);
- check that your immunizations are up to date and screen for hepatitis B (a disease that can be passed on to the developing baby and that can result in liver disease and cancer during adulthood);
- ask you whether you've ever had chicken pox and, if you haven't, talk to you about the benefits of vaccination (you'd have to postpone becoming pregnant after obtaining the vaccine, and pay for the vaccination out of your own pocket, but you'd reduce the risks of pneumonia and other complications should you develop chicken pox during pregnancy);
- talk to you about whether you should get yourself to the next flu shot clinic (pregnancy is considered a high-risk condition for influenza, and women who expect to be pregnant during flu season—from November to April—should consider receiving the flu shot if they are otherwise good candidates for it);
- answer your questions about how any chronic health conditions including mental health conditions may affect your ability to conceive and/or to give birth to a healthy baby (see Table 2.3 for a list of questions to ask and Table 2.4 for a summary of the effects of certain chronic health conditions on pregnancy);
- give you a breast exam (pregnancy can change the shape and feel of your breasts, making it harder for you to detect the early signs of breast cancer during your monthly breast self-examination, so it's best to

| 2.3 | **Questions to Ask Your Doctor about Any Chronic Medical Condition** |

Will my medications need to be changed before I become pregnant? If so, how long should I wait after discontinuing/changing medications before I start trying to conceive? How will stopping or changing my medications affect my well-being?

How will pregnancy affect my medical condition? Can I expect my symptoms to improve, worsen, or stay the same?

How will my medical condition affect my pregnancy? Am I at increased risk of experiencing any pregnancy-related problems as a result of my medical condition?

Will my pregnancy automatically be classified as "high risk"?

Will my life be affected in any major ways? Will I be able to continue working? Will I need to go on bedrest?

Will additional testing be required during my pregnancy as a result of my medical condition? If so, which types of tests will be ordered and why?

---

have a breast exam prior to pregnancy), a pelvic exam, and Pap smear (to check for symptomless infections, ovarian cysts, and any gynecological conditions that could be difficult and/or risky to treat during pregnancy), as well as a general physical exam;

- discuss your family health history and your gynecological and/or obstetrical history (depending on what is revealed, your health-care provider may recommend pre-conception genetic counselling or other types of pre-conception/pregnancy care—for example, grief support if your first child died shortly after birth, or a referral to a psychiatrist who specializes in perinatal mood disorders if you had difficulty with prenatal depression or postpartum depression with your first baby. Your health-care provider may also make specific health recommendations, such as recommending an iron supplement if you're breastfeeding and planning another pregnancy);

- talk to you about whether or not any pregnancy-related complications that you experienced in previous pregnancies are likely to recur this time around;

- find out if your mother took a drug called diethylstilbestrol (DES) when she was pregnant with you. The drug was prescribed to millions of women between 1938 and 1971 to prevent miscarriage or premature birth, and 90 per cent of so-called DES daughters have experienced abnormalities of the cervix, vagina, and uterus that make it difficult for them to conceive and carry a baby to term. It's not just DES *daughters* who may experience fertility problems. The sons of women who took DES back in the 1950s and 1960s may also have genital abnormalities, including smaller-than-average testicles and penis, undescended testicles, low sperm counts, poor motility of sperm, cysts, and possibly even testicular and prostate cancer.

- do a blood test to determine whether you're anemic and whether you've been infected with any sexually transmitted infections (undiagnosed genital herpes can be harmful—even fatal—to your baby; gonorrhea and chlamydia can scar your Fallopian tubes and make it difficult to conceive, or can increase your chances of experiencing an ectopic pregnancy; syphilis, if uncured, can cause birth defects; and your pregnancy will have to be carefully managed to reduce the risk of infecting your baby if you're HIV-positive or have AIDS);

- do a urine test to screen for such conditions as diabetes, urinary tract infections, and kidney infections;

- talk about whether you're a good candidate for genetic counselling (something that's generally recommended if you have a family history of intellectual disabilities, cerebral palsy, muscular dystrophy, cystic fibrosis, hemophilia, or spina bifida; if your ethnic background puts you at increased risk of giving birth to a baby with Tay-Sachs disease, thalassemia, or sickle-cell anemia; if you're over 35; or if you feel quite strongly that you'd like to know ahead of time what your risks may be of giving birth to a baby with a genetic problem);

- warn you about any hazards you may face on the job that should be avoided during pregnancy (for example, exposure to X-rays, toxins such as paints and solvents, and other substances like gases that could be harmful to the developing baby) as well as any job modifications that may be necessary (such as no heavy lifting);

- provide your partner with information on his role in giving your future baby the healthiest possible start in life (for example, not drinking when you're trying to conceive, quitting smoking so that you and the baby won't be exposed to second-hand smoke, and avoiding exposure to substances that may be harmful to sperm).

As you can see, there's a lot to think about before you start trying to conceive: your overall health, your gynecological history, your current lifestyle, and much more. And, as you've seen from our discussion, preparing for pregnancy isn't just a "woman's problem." Fathers-to-be also need to take steps to ensure that the sperm they contribute to Project Baby is every bit as healthy as possible. Baby making is, after all, a team sport.

2.4 Chronic Health Conditions and Pregnancy

Condition	Effect During Pregnancy
Adrenal Gland Disorders	
Addison's disease (a disease characterized by inadequate adrenal production)	You may experience life-threatening infections and other health complications during pregnancy.
Cushing's syndrome (a disorder caused by the body's exposure to too much cortisone)	There is increased risk that your baby will be stillborn or born premature.
Autoimmune Disorders	
Lupus (an autoimmune disease that primarily affects the skin and joints, but that can also affect the heart, kidneys, and nervous system)	You face a 25 per cent chance of experiencing a miscarriage or stillbirth, a 25 per cent chance of going into premature labour, a 20 per cent chance of developing pre-eclampsia, and a 3 per cent chance of giving birth to a baby with neonatal lupus (a form of lupus that lasts for the first six months of life and that can leave an affected baby with a permanent heart abnormality). Women with heart, kidney, or other internal organ involvement are generally advised to avoid pregnancy.
Myasthenia gravis (an autoimmune disease that causes the skeletal muscles to weaken and that contributes to fatigue)	There's a 40 per cent chance that your condition will worsen during pregnancy, a 25 per cent risk of giving birth to a preterm baby, and a 10 to 20 per cent chance that your baby will be born with a temporary form of myasthenia gravis.
Scleroderma (a progressive connective tissue disorder that can cause lung, heart, kidney, and other organ damage, and that's characterized by joint inflammation and decreased mobility)	There is a 40 per cent chance that your condition will worsen during pregnancy.

continued

2.4 Chronic Health Conditions and Pregnancy (continued)

Condition	Effect During Pregnancy
Blood Disorders	
Anemia (a condition characterized by a deficiency of iron in the body)	You may experience fatigue, weakness, shortness of breath, and dizziness; tingling in the hands and feet; a lack of balance and coordination; a loss of colour in the skin, gums, and fingernails; jaundice of the skin and eyes; and—in severe cases—heart failure. Severe anemia can contribute to fetal growth restriction and prematurity, and may make it more difficult for the baby to tolerate labour. Anemia also increases your odds of needing a blood transfusion during or after childbirth.
Sickle-cell anemia (a genetic blood disorder in which the body makes sickle- or crescent-shaped blood cells that block blood vessels, causing pain and organ damage)	There is a 25 per cent chance of miscarriage, an 8 to 10 per cent chance of stillbirth, a 15 per cent chance of neonatal death (death during the first 30 days after birth), and a 33 per cent chance the mother will develop high blood pressure problems and toxemia. You may also experience urinary tract infections, pneumonia, and lung tissue damage. You are more susceptible to sickle-cell crises during pregnancy. You can pass the disease along to your baby if your partner also carries the gene for this disease.
Thalassemia (a genetic blood disease; people with thalassemia are unable to manufacture hemoglobin, which is needed to produce healthy red blood cells)	You may develop severe anemia and congestive heart failure requiring a transfusion. If you have thalassemia minor (a less severe form of thalassemia), you may require blood transfusions during pregnancy, and run the risk of passing the disease along to the baby if your partner also carries the gene for thalassemia.
Thrombocytopenia (a blood platelet deficiency)	There is an increased chance you will need a Caesarean section. Babies born to mothers with severe forms of this condition may have increased platelet counts and problems with hemorrhaging—especially around the brain.
Von Willebrand's disease (an inherited bleeding disorder)	You may need to be treated with intravenous clotting factors to prevent severe blood loss during the delivery.
Brain Disorders	
History of strokes, hemorrhages, or blood clots	Pregnancy may not be advisable, depending on the severity of your condition.

Cancer

Cancer (malignant diseases)	Avoid conceiving until you and your doctor feel confident that the condition won't recur while you're pregnant. Otherwise, you could find yourself faced with the heart-wrenching decision to terminate your pregnancy in order to save your own life. Pregnancy can speed the growth of estrogen-dependent cancers. Radiation used in the diagnosis and treatment of cancer can be harmful—even fatal—to the developing fetus. Chemotherapy can also be harmful to the developing baby. Both chemotherapy and radiation may affect your future fertility. Surgery is the least hazardous option for cancer treatment during pregnancy.

Diabetes

Diabetes	You will face an increased risk of fertility problems, miscarriage, stillbirth, toxemia, birth-related trauma, and neonatal death. You will also risk requiring a Caesarean section, giving birth to a very large baby, and giving birth to a baby with heart, kidney, or spinal defects. These risks can be reduced by consuming large quantities of folic acid prior to pregnancy and by keeping your blood sugar levels down in the 4 to 7 millimoles per litre (72 to 126 milligrams per decilitre) range prior to pregnancy, and averaging 4.5 to 5 millimoles per litre (81 to 90 milligrams per decilitre) during pregnancy. Women whose diabetes is poorly controlled have seven times the risk of giving birth to a baby with severe fetal anomalies and a 32 per cent chance of miscarrying, as compared to women whose diabetes is well controlled. Note: The nausea and vomiting of pregnancy can upset your blood sugar levels. So can infections. Get in touch with your doctor right away if you experience nausea and vomiting or an infection during your pregnancy.

Gastrointestinal Disorders

Crohn's disease (an inflammatory bowel disease)	There is a 50 per cent chance of miscarriage if your condition is active when you conceive.
Peptic ulcers (chronic sores that protrude through the lining of the gastrointestinal tract and that can penetrate the muscle tissue of the duodenum, stomach, or esophagus)	There is a 12 per cent chance that your symptoms will worsen during pregnancy.

continued

2.4 Chronic Health Conditions and Pregnancy (continued)

Condition	Effect During Pregnancy
Gastrointestinal Disorders (continued)	
Ulcerative colitis (an inflammatory disease of colon and rectum)	There is a small chance that emergency surgery may be required if your disease is active during pregnancy—something that could increase your chances of requiring a premature delivery or a Caesarean section.
Heart Disease	
Congenital heart problems (heart defects that are present at birth)	There are no significant risks to you or your baby if you have a minor congenital heart condition (such as mitral valve prolapse), but you could face some significant risks if you have a serious congenital heart problem (such as Eisenmenger syndrome). You may wish to have your baby screened for heart problems prenatally, since certain types of congenital heart problems are genetic. There's a 4 per cent risk of congenital heart disease in children of affected mothers, although the incidence of certain types of congenital heart disease can be even higher. Note: If you have a mitral valve prolapse, your doctor will likely order a dose of antibiotics during delivery to minimize the risk of infection.
Coronary artery disease (angina, heart attacks)	You will face a significant risk of heart attack and death during pregnancy if your disease is unstable, since pregnancy increases the heart's workload. There's also a significant risk that you might not live long enough to see your child reach adulthood.
Rheumatic heart disease (an autoimmune response to an infection that results in damage to the heart valve)	You will require intensive monitoring during your pregnancy and you will require multiple cardiac drugs during labour. There's a high maternal mortality rate for pregnant women with this condition. The risks are much greater for women who have sustained a lot of damage to their heart.
High Blood Pressure	
High blood pressure (hypertension)	Your doctor may want to assess the functioning of your heart and kidneys throughout your pregnancy. It may be necessary to change your blood pressure medications before you start trying to conceive. Most women with mild high blood pressure deliver healthy babies, but they still require more frequent prenatal checkups, and face an increased risk of premature delivery. If your condition is severe (your blood pressure is over 160/105 or your condition is complicated by either heart or kidney disease), you face a 50 per cent chance of developing pre-eclampsia or of requiring a Caesarean section, and a 10 per cent chance of experiencing a placental abruption (premature separation of the placenta from the uterine wall). There is also an increased risk that your baby will develop intrauterine growth restriction or experience problems with renal failure or congestive heart failure.

Other risk factors include age (if you're under 16 or over 40), a long history of blood pressure problems (for more than 15 years), previous clot-related problems, and past experience with pre-eclampsia early on in a previous pregnancy or a placental abruption in a previous pregnancy.

Kidney Disease

Kidney disease	One-third of women with kidney disease find that their disease worsens during pregnancy. Your doctor will want to monitor you carefully for urinary tract infections, as they frequently progress into kidney infections. Women with severe kidney disease often experience fertility problems, since ovulation is frequently disrupted. Those who become pregnant face a higher-than-average risk of developing pyelonephritis (an acute kidney infection that can result in permanent damage), of experiencing a premature delivery, and/or (if women have a severe form of kidney disease) of having their baby experience intrauterine growth restriction. There's a 50 per cent chance of developing severe hypertension during pregnancy if you've got both chronic kidney disease and high blood pressure. If you were already on dialysis treatments prior to pregnancy, you'll require them more frequently during pregnancy. If you've had a kidney transplant and are on anti-rejection medications, you'll need to continue taking your medications during pregnancy. Note: Most doctors recommend that you wait for two to five years after a transplant before attempting a pregnancy.

Liver Disorders

Hepatitis B (a virus transmitted via blood and other body fluids that can lead to cirrhosis and liver cancer)	You have a 10 to 20 per cent chance of passing the hepatitis B virus on to your baby if you don't receive any preventative treatment. Women who become infected with hepatitis B during the third trimester have a 90 per cent chance of passing the disease on to their babies if no preventative treatment is provided.
Hepatitis C (a virus transmitted via blood products that results in cirrhosis and liver cancer)	Approximately 7 per cent of women carrying the hepatitis C virus transmit it to their babies during pregnancy or at the time of birth. There is no known way of preventing transmittal of the virus from mother to baby. The risk of transmittal is higher if the mother also has AIDS.

Lung/Respiratory Diseases

Asthma	Asthma affects approximately 2 to 4 per cent of pregnant women. Most of them report either no change or a lessening of symptoms during pregnancy. When symptoms occur, they are most likely to occur between 24 and 36 weeks of pregnancy. The key to managing asthma during your pregnancy is to have your symptoms under

continued

2.4 Chronic Health Conditions and Pregnancy (continued)

Condition	Effect During Pregnancy
Lung/Respiratory Diseases *(continued)*	
	control before you conceive (meaning that you have your best possible lung function, you can sleep through the night without asthma symptoms, and you can be active without asthma symptoms) and to stay as healthy as possible during pregnancy. You should try to avoid exposing yourself to the types of substances that tend to trigger your asthma; to avoid the flu, colds, and respiratory infections; to consider having a flu shot; to continue taking your allergy shots; to continue to use your asthma medications (with your doctor's approval); and to be sure to treat asthma attacks immediately to avoid depriving your baby of oxygen. Note: 1 per cent of women who've never had trouble with asthma before will develop the disease as a complication of pregnancy. When asthma does occur, it's important to get it under control quickly. Uncontrolled asthma can lead to pregnancy-induced high blood pressure, preterm birth, low birth weight, and infant health complications.
Cystic fibrosis (a multi-organ disease that primarily affects the lungs and digestive system)	In women with mild cases of cystic fibrosis, pregnancy is generally considered safe. In women with moderate to severe cases, there is an increased risk of maternal complications and premature birth.
Primary pulmonary hypertension (a rare lung disorder in which blood pressure in the pulmonary artery—the artery that carries oxygen-poor blood away from the heart to the lungs—is elevated, putting a strain on the heart)	Pregnancy is risky. The maternal mortality rate is 50 per cent and the fetal mortality rate is 40 per cent.
Sarcoidosis (a lung disease caused by non-cancerous tumours called tubercles)	No special monitoring is required during pregnancy. Pregnancy is risky only if your lungs are badly scarred, in which case right-sided heart failure may result.
Tuberculosis (a bacterial disease that attacks the lungs)	No special monitoring is required during pregnancy. Some drugs used to treat this disorder, however, are not safe for use during pregnancy.

Metabolic Disorders

Phenylketonuria (PKU) (a genetically transmitted metabolic disorder that results in elevated levels of the amino acid phenylalanine in your blood)

You will face an increased risk of miscarriage and of giving birth to a baby with microcephaly or congenital heart defects, with intellectual disabilities, or who suffers from intrauterine growth restriction and/or low birth weight. Decreasing your intake of foods that are high in phenylalanine content (such as red meats and soy products) both prior to conception and during the first trimester of pregnancy can help to reduce these risks.

Neurological Disorders

Epilepsy and other seizure disorders

Approximately 90 per cent of women with epilepsy have normal pregnancies and end up giving birth to healthy babies. About one-third of women have more seizures when they are pregnant and one-third have fewer seizures. Studies have shown, however, that you can dramatically increase your chances of giving birth to a healthy baby by taking your medications as directed and by taking a higher-than-average dose of folic acid prior to and during pregnancy. Note: Your seizures must be well under control before you start trying to conceive. In some cases, doctors will discontinue anti-epileptic medications on a trial basis if you have not had any epileptic episodes for more than two years. In other cases, doctors will try to prescribe a single anti-convulsant at the lowest possible dose. This is because the risk of birth defects in the baby increases with the number of drugs you're taking. Some women with epilepsy stop taking their drugs out of concern about the possible effects of the medications on their baby. The current research seems to indicate that maternal seizures are more harmful to the developing baby than having a mother on anti-epileptic drugs. Regardless of whether you're on medication or not, your pregnancy will also have to be carefully monitored because you'll face a high risk of having seizures if you develop pre-eclampsia (a potentially life-threatening condition characterized by high blood pressure).

Multiple sclerosis

You are likely to experience fewer relapses during pregnancy, particularly during the third trimester, but an increase in relapses during the first three months postpartum. There's a small risk (1 to 5 per cent) that your baby will be born with multiple sclerosis. If you haven't got any sensation in your lower body, you'll need to be monitored carefully during the final weeks of pregnancy in case you're unable to detect the onset of labour. Since multiple sclerosis can affect your ability to push, you may require a forceps or vacuum-assisted delivery or a Caesarean section. Note: You should contemplate a pregnancy only if you haven't had any recent relapses.

continued

2.4   Chronic Health Conditions and Pregnancy (continued)

Condition	Effect During Pregnancy
Parathyroid Disorders	
Hyperparathyroidism (too much parathyroid hormone in the body)	You will face an increased risk of stillbirth, neonatal death, or of giving birth to a baby with tetany (severe muscle spasms and paralysis caused by inadequate levels of calcium).
Hypoparathyroidism (too little parathyroid hormone in the body)	Your doctor will likely prescribe calcium and vitamin D to reduce the likelihood that your baby will develop a bone-weakening disorder.
Pituitary Disorders	
Diabetes insipidus (a rare condition caused by a deficiency of an antidiuretic hormone manufactured by the pituitary gland)	You may require special monitoring or treatment during your pregnancy.
Pituitary insufficiency	You may require special monitoring or treatment during your pregnancy.
Pituitary tumours	You may require special monitoring or treatment during your pregnancy
Psychiatric Disorders	
Depression, anxiety (panic, obsessive / compulsive disorders, post-traumatic stress disorder), bipolar disorder	It's important to plan your pregnancy, particularly if you're taking medication. Your doctor will want to evaluate your medications and consider the types and doses of medications you are taking. If the decision is made to keep you on your medication(s), your doctor will try, as much as possible, to limit the number of medications that are being prescribed (the fewer medications you are on, the less risk to the baby) and to minimize your dose. Your doctor will also choose the medications that are considered to be least harmful to the developing baby, wherever possible. Note: It's important to let your doctor know if your symptoms begin to worsen at any point during pregnancy or postpartum, and to have a plan for dealing with your illness. It's a good idea to have a circle of friends and family members who are also available to lend their support.
Sexually Transmitted Infections and Other Infections	
Bacterial vaginosis (a vaginal infection sometimes associated with a thin, milky discharge and fishy odour)	You will face an increased risk of preterm labour, premature rupture of membranes, and/or a preterm delivery.

Chlamydia (a sexually transmitted infection that can result in pelvic inflammatory disease; it is often symptomless)	You will face a greater risk of ectopic pregnancy and infertility.
Gonorrhea (a sexually transmitted disease that can result in pelvic inflammatory disease)	You will face a greater risk of ectopic pregnancy and infertility.
Hepatitis B	Treatment is required to reduce the chances that you will transmit the hepatitis B virus to your baby. (Your baby will be given the hepatitis B vaccine and immune globulin within 12 hours of birth and then again at one month and six months of age.)
Herpes	Treatment is required to prevent the disease from being transmitted from mother to baby. Herpes can be fatal to the developing baby. A Caesarean delivery will be required if the disease is active at the time of delivery or near term.
HIV	Treatment with the drug AZT is required to reduce your chances of passing on HIV to your baby. (The risk of passing on HIV to your baby without treatment is 20 to 32 per cent. The risk with treatment is less than 1 per cent.) Note: The risk of transmission is further reduced if the baby is delivered by Caesarean section and you do not breastfeed. The Motherisk Clinic at the Hospital for Sick Children in Toronto offers confidential counselling to Canadian women and their families about the risk of HIV and HIV treatment during pregnancy. Call the HIV Healthline at 1–888–246–5840.
Syphilis	Untreated syphilis can cause birth defects in the developing baby.
Thyroid Disorders	
Graves' disease (an immunological form of thyroid disease)	Can affect the fetal thyroid even if maternal thyroid levels have been brought under control.
Hyperthyroidism (an overactive thyroid)	Hyperthyroidism can interfere with ovulation, making it difficult to conceive. Pregnant women with hyperthyroidism are at risk of developing thyroid storm—a severe form of hyperthyroidism that is associated with an increased risk of premature delivery and low birth weight, and that can put the mother's life at risk.
Hypothyroidism (an underactive thyroid)	There are no special risks during pregnancy as long as you continue to take your prescribed thyroid medication. Women with untreated hypothyroidism are at increased risk of experiencing infertility, miscarriage, and of giving birth to a baby with growth or developmental abnormalities.

CHAPTER 3

Sperm, Meet Egg

"When I sometimes consider how small a window exists for conditions to be ripe for conception, it's a miracle that the world is as populated as it is."

—ROSA, 34, MOTHER OF TWO YOUNG CHILDREN

After years of panicking about missed birth control pills and broken condoms, it may feel more than a little strange to be consciously trying to arrange a meeting between sperm and egg. It can be tremendously liberating: you don't have to pause at the most passionate point in a romantic interlude to search for the appropriate birth control paraphernalia. At the same time, you may find yourself feeling slightly in awe of this entire process. It's amazing what has to happen from a biological standpoint in order for a pregnancy to occur. That series of biological miracles is the science of pregnancy. But there's also an art to this pregnancy thing, and understanding that can help you to boost your chances of conceiving quickly. (Despite what those scary grade six health films like to claim, you might not automatically get pregnant the very first time you "do it" without birth control.)

The Numbers Game

While many couples naively assume that getting pregnant is simply a matter of losing the birth control for a month, some find out the hard way that it's not always quite that simple. Since even couples at their peak of fertility have, at best, one-in-four odds of conceiving during any given cycle (see Table 3.1), it's hardly surprising that the vast majority of couples don't end up winning at baby roulette the first time around.

3.1 The Odds of Conceiving in Any Given Cycle or Year for Women of Various Ages			
Age	**Odds That You'll Conceive in Any Given Month**	**Average Number of Months It Takes to Conceive**	**Probability That You'll Be Pregnant Within One Year**
Early 20s	20% to 25%	4 to 5 months	93% to 97%
Late 20s	15% to 20%	5 to 6.7 months	86% to 93%
Early 30s	10% to 15%	6.7 to 10 months	72% to 86%
Late 30s	8.3% to 10%	10 to 12 months	65% to 72%

Adapted from a similar chart in *How to Get Pregnant* by Sherman J. Silber, MD, (New York: Warner Books, 1980).

Note: The data reported by Silber is supported by more recent data from the National Center for Health Statistics in the United States, which reports that a couple under the age of 25 has a 96 per cent chance of conceiving within one year; a couple between the ages of 25 and 34 has an 86 per cent chance of conceiving within a year; and a couple between the ages of 35 and 44 has a 78 per cent chance of conceiving within one year.

While the odds that you'll end up conceiving this month may be discouragingly low, it's important to take a look at the big picture. As Table 3.1 indicates, a couple in their late twenties has an 86 to 93 per cent chance of conceiving within one year of actively trying (for example, having intercourse daily or every other day during the woman's most fertile period). That's not to say you have to aim to have intercourse every day; in fact, most fertility experts agree that every other day is plenty.

The Science of Conception

While you might think you paid enough attention in grade six health class to pick up the necessary facts about human reproduction, chances are you acquired at least a few pieces of misinformation along the way. Studies have shown that there are still a surprising number of conception misconceptions kicking around. Consider these facts.

Researchers have found that many couples wrongly assume they can become pregnant by timing intercourse to occur during the day or two following ovulation, when quite the opposite is true. It's only possible if there are sperm waiting to fertilize an egg at the time of ovulation (the point in a woman's menstrual cycle when the egg is released from the ovary) or shortly thereafter. Once ovulation has occurred, the window of opportunity for conceiving during that cycle slams shut within about 12 to 24 hours.

why it's not always easy

Wondering why conception doesn't happen each and every time a woman has sex? Because a typical woman would end up with 3,000 children, that's why! According to Robin Baker and Elizabeth Oram, authors of *Baby Wars*, that's how often a typical woman has sex over her lifetime. And since that size of family would put even the Old Woman Who Lived in a Shoe to shame, in humans, the female reproductive system is designed for just a few hits and a whole lot of misses.

A female honeybee's reproductive system works in an entirely different fashion, however. Instead of having sex far more often than is necessary to achieve a pregnancy, as is the case with humans, she can conceive millions of offspring over a period of years from a single episode of intercourse. Her secret? She stores the sperm in her body so that it'll be there whenever she's ready to get pregnant again.

Other studies have indicated that many couples who show up for an infertility assessment don't have fertility problems, they have timing problems. There's a common misconception that a woman ovulates two weeks after the first day of her last period when, in fact, she actually ovulates 14 days before the first day of her next period. It's a moot point if you have a textbook 28-day menstrual cycle, but it can throw your baby-making efforts off by an entire week if your cycles tend to be 35 days long. After all, even the hardiest and most determined of sperm can't camp out indefinitely in the Fallopian tube, hoping that some egg will come strolling by. The life cycle of a sperm cell is, after all, short and sweet: even Canada Grade A sperm can't live for much longer than five days.

Because it's so important to have your facts straight when you're trying to conceive, we're going to take a few more minutes to talk about how the whole reproductive process works—and clear up a lot of conception misconceptions along the way.

Here goes.

A tale of two phases

A woman's menstrual cycle is divided into two distinct phases: the follicular (or proliferative) phase, which precedes ovulation; and the luteal (or secretory) phase, which follows it.

how to boost your odds of conceiving

Trying to time intercourse to coincide with a 12- to 24-hour window of opportunity for conception is a bit like spinning the reproductive roulette wheel. You have to be really, really lucky. A better strategy is to have sperm waiting for the egg. This is because sperm have a much longer shelf life than eggs. They can survive for three to five days in the female reproductive tract. So what does this mean in practical terms? Having sex every other day from the ninth or tenth day of your cycle (assuming you have a "classic" 28-day cycle) or approximately five days before you think you are due to ovulate is your reproductive best bet if you want to maximize your chances of conceiving in any given cycle.

And what about that once much-lauded strategy of trying to "conserve" sperm: abstaining from sex—or any form of ejaculation—in the days leading up to ovulation? Forget about it. Rather than recruiting a large number of healthy, well-rested sperm for Operation Fertilization, you'll end up with aged, unhealthy, and even dead recruits—not exactly the best way to embark on a successful reproductive mission.

Can you get too much of a good thing (that good thing being sex)? You betcha. Having sex every day can be overkill, particularly if you're trying to minimize the stress of conceiving. (Of course, if you're at the stage of baby-making when having sex more frequently is fun, you can take this information under advisement. There are times when your sex life gets to trump the reproductive "rules.")

During the follicular phase, your body has one mission and one mission only: to prepare itself for ovulation. Inside your ovaries, approximately 1,000 eggs begin to mature. Of these, just 20 eggs (or ova) respond to the release of follicle-stimulating hormone (FSH) by the pituitary gland in the brain and begin to ripen and to occupy fluid-filled sacs known as follicles.

Since you couldn't possibly conceive and carry 20 babies to term (nor would you want to—just think of the stretch marks!), your body is just hedging its bets. It hopes that by entering 20 candidates in the Ms. Follicle contest, at least one will end up making the glorious trip down that runway known as the Fallopian tube. (To qualify for the Fallopian-runway stroll, the follicle doesn't need a slinky ball gown or a flashy tiara à la Miss America: it simply needs to be the dominant follicle—the one that gets chosen to rupture. Yes, ladies, this is one contest where the skinnier contestants get left behind: for once, bigger is better!) Sometimes two or more follicles will end up rupturing in the same cycle, in which case a multiple pregnancy may result; at other times, none of the 20 follicles manage to mature enough to rupture, in which case an anovulatory cycle (a cycle without ovulation) is said to have occurred. (Believe it or not, even the most fertile women in the world have anovulatory cycles on a regular basis. Scientists estimate that one in five cycles does not result in the release of an egg.)

A lot of people believe that the two ovaries share egg-releasing duties on some predetermined schedule—that they alternate from month to month. This is simply not the case. Researchers have discovered that it's purely a matter of chance which ovary ends up releasing the egg—although, of course, if you have only one functioning ovary, it'll win the draw by default. This is Mother Nature's way of maximizing your childbearing potential: equipping you with a "spare" ovary.

At the same time, the level of estrogen in your body begins to rise. This causes the endometrial lining of your uterus to thicken significantly (from 1.02 millimetres to 4.32 millimetres (0.04 inches to 0.17 inches)) and prepares it for the possible implantation of a fertilized egg. The rising levels of estrogen also change the quantity and quality of your cervical mucus. Scant and sticky during the early part of your cycle, the mucus becomes increasingly abundant and slippery—like egg white—as ovulation approaches. This "egg white" cervical mucus is designed to help transport the sperm into the uterus and to protect it from the harsh vaginal environment. (Believe it or not, a healthy vagina has the same acidity level as a glass of red wine.)

---

a numbers game

The old expression "waste not, want not" seems to go out the window as far as the female reproductive system is concerned. While the ovaries of a female fetus contain 6 to 7 million eggs by the time she reaches 20 weeks of gestation, at birth, her supply will have dwindled to just 2 to 3 million eggs. And by the time she reaches puberty, just 400,000 of those eggs will be left. During her reproductive years, she'll use fewer than 500 of them and, in the end, she may give birth to, at most, a handful of children. (Not exactly a model of efficiency, now is it?)

The hormonal changes that occur as ovulation approaches also trigger some noteworthy behavioural changes. You may find yourself feeling increasingly interested in sex and more susceptible to the charms of the male species. Here's why:

Studies have shown that a woman's vision and sense of smell become more acute around the time of ovulation. Scientists theorize that this may be Mother Nature's way of encouraging her to give more notice to members of the opposite sex. After all, if the man in your life starts looking more appealing and starts smelling irresistible, you're more likely to hop in the sack with him. There's just one disturbing footnote to this research: apparently the one scent that we find truly irresistible as ovulation approaches is the smell of male armpit sweat. I don't know about you, but I'd take a truckload of Old Spice in place of Eau de Sweat any day. (Or at least I think I would. Perhaps my subconscious mind doesn't agree . . .) Here's another interesting finding related to the science of attraction. Researchers in Switzerland have discovered that women tend to be most attracted to those men who smell the least like themselves. There's just one small but noteworthy exception: women who are taking birth control pills tend to gravitate toward those men who smell the most like themselves.

We're programmed to act more provocatively as ovulation approaches. Researchers have found that the skimpier the clothing a woman wears to a nightclub, the more likely she is to be ovulating.

Our criteria for the ideal man changes as ovulation approaches. While we generally tend to prefer men with slightly more feminine facial features (we tend to link these features with more positive personality traits, apparently), according to researchers at the University of St Andrews in Scotland, we're drawn to men with more masculine features during the days when we're most likely to conceive. So next time you find yourself adding the entire Eastwood and Schwarzenegger catalogues to your Netflix queue, reach for your calendar. Perhaps the moment of truth has arrived again.

Hormonal changes are also responsible for triggering the big event around which the entire female menstrual cycle is centred: ovulation. Just prior to ovulation, rising levels of estrogen prompt the pituitary gland to trigger a brief but intense surge of luteinizing hormone (LH). This causes the dominant follicle to rupture and release its egg 36 to 42 hours later. Some women experience pain in the lower abdomen as ovulation occurs—a sensation that the Germans call *mittelschmerz* or "pain in the middle." Some scientists theorize that mittelschmerz may be caused by the irritation of the lining of the body cavity by blood or other fluid that escapes from the ovary at the time of ovulation.

Once the egg has been released, it needs to find its way to the Fallopian tube. (Contrary to what most people believe, the ovaries aren't actually attached to the Fallopian tubes. They just happen to live in the same neighbourhood.) Fortunately, Mother Nature—amazing designer that she is—put some thought into this whole process as well. Cilia (tiny hairs that line the inside of the Fallopian tubes) create a suction-like effect that's designed to draw the egg into the Fallopian tube. Once the egg gets inside, the cilia move the egg in conveyer-belt fashion to the inner portion of the Fallopian tube (the isthmus)—the zone where the egg can be fertilized. (There's only about a six- to twelve-hour window when fertilization can occur or else the egg shall become overripe and die, so time is of the essence.) Once the egg has been fertilized, it spends the next 80 hours making its way through the tube at a speed of about 1 millimetre (0.04 inches) per hour before finally reaching the uterus. Timing is critical here. If the egg arrives too soon, the uterine lining won't yet be thick enough to promote a healthy implantation. If it takes too long to pass through the tube (which measures 3.56 millimetres (0.14 inches) at its widest point and 0.25 millimetres (0.01 inches) at its narrowest point), the egg will implant in the tube instead, resulting in an ectopic (tubal) pregnancy.

Having accomplished Mission Ovulation, your body now switches gears, focusing its energies on creating an egg-friendly uterine environment. The ruptured ovarian follicle (now known as the corpus luteum, or "yellow body," because of its colour) begins manufacturing progesterone. The progesterone causes the uterine lining to thicken so that it can receive a fertilized egg. It also causes your cervical mucus to become sticky and impermeable to sperm. (Hey, at this stage of the game, any sperm showing up would just be crashing the party. If a pregnancy is going to be achieved, it's already happened thanks to some earlier recruits to the Sperm Battalion.)

If conception has occurred, the corpus luteum continues to produce progesterone until the placenta takes over the manufacturing duties approximately three months down the road. If conception has not occurred, the corpus luteum begins to deteriorate, progesterone levels drop, your uterus begins to shed the endometrial layer it has built up, and your menstrual period begins.

Dr. Jekyll and Ms. Hyde

Wondering why you sometimes feel like two different people—Dr. Jekyll and Ms. Hyde? It's because, for all intents and purposes, you are two entirely different people, depending on which phase of your menstrual cycle you're in. The hormonal cocktail that affects how you feel changes dramatically over the course of your menstrual cycle. During the first half of your cycle (the so-called follicular or proliferative phase), your hormones are focusing on preparing for ovulation; and during the second half of your cycle (the so-called luteal or secretory phase), your hormones are hard at work trying to prepare your uterus to sustain any pregnancy that may have occurred. Since the recipes for these two cocktails— the follicular cocktail and the luteal cocktail—are dramatically different, you may experience some powerful physical and emotional changes over the course of your menstrual cycle.

The sperm connection

Until now, we've been ignoring the role that sperm has to play in the whole reproductive equation. Well, it's time to right that wrong!

We've already talked about how wasteful the female reproductive system is: 1,000 follicles begin to ripen each month, but usually only one ends up rupturing. Well, the female reproductive system looks like a model of conservation compared to the male reproductive system. Here's why. When a man ejaculates, he deposits approximately 250 million sperm in his partner's vagina. Of these, just 200,000 will make it beyond the vagina (one out of every thousand) and just 50 to 100 will make it into the Fallopian tube. It isn't hard to figure out what's responsible for the loss of so many sperm. Despite the fact that the semen that carries the sperm is alkaline (Mother Nature's way of providing a barrier between the sperm and the harsh vaginal environment), the vast majority of sperm are unable to survive in the acidity of the vagina. (Remember, the poor little sperm are being asked to swim through the pH equivalent of a glass of red wine.) And if you happen to have BV—bacterial vaginosis (a common type of vaginal infection)—the sperm may have a particularly tough time going about their business.

Those sperm that do end up surviving are the ones that manage to make their way into the cervical mucus as quickly as possible. (Like the semen, the cervical mucus is alkaline and designed to help to protect the sperm.) Once they've reached this safe haven, they start making their way to the Fallopian tube.

While we may have visions of all the sperm setting course for the Fallopian tube in flotilla-like formation, medical science has proven that theory wrong. As it turns out, only a few sperm actually set out for their destination right away, arriving within an hour of ejaculation. Some choose to make a stopover at the lower end of the Fallopian tube, below the fertilization zone, while others remain in storage sites within the cervix, gradually heading northward over the next five days. Consequently, rather than arriving all at once, there's a steady migration of sperm through the fertilization zone over a five-day period. Since sperm remain fertile for up to five days, this helps to maximize the chance that some sperm will be on hand whenever the egg decides to show up for a Fallopian rendezvous.

Scientists have also figured out what guides sperm to their destination. No, it's not some intrauterine road map. Sperm follow their noses—or at least a primitive type of nose that allows them to sniff out the egg and start swimming toward it.

While it technically takes just one sperm to fertilize the egg, it takes many more than that to ensure conception will take place. Scientists have discovered that it takes hundreds of sperm working as a team in order to penetrate the membrane of the egg. Once the first sperm has managed to penetrate the egg membrane, no other sperm can pass through. (As Robin Baker puts it in *Sperm Wars*, "If you are a human sperm, there is no prize for second place.")

Wondering what is required to make healthy sperm? The recipe for healthy sperm includes the following ingredients:

Good nutrition. Your partner should consider taking a daily multivitamin if his diet is less than healthy. Sperm need selenium, zinc, and folic acid to thrive. What's more, recent studies have indicated that antioxidants (vitamins A, C, E, beta carotene, and selenium) may help to protect sperm against the harmful effects of free radicals, which can damage DNA and affect the quality and number of sperm. The following foods are naturally rich in antioxidants: blackberries, blueberries, strawberries, kale, Brussels sprouts, plums, alfalfa sprouts, broccoli, and red peppers.

Less stress. Stress can interfere with the hormones involved in the manufacturing of sperm as well as with sexual function.

Regular exercise. A fit body is a reproductively healthy body. Having too much or too little body fat can interfere with the production of reproductive hormones, which can reduce sperm count and increase the percentage of abnormal sperm. Aim for a BMI in the 18.5 to 24.9 range for optimal fertility. Just one thing to bear in mind on the exercise front: cycling for more than 30 minutes at a time can raise a man's scrotal temperature. To make matters worse,

---

the wet spot demystified

Worried that the wet spot on the bed means that all the sperm have dripped out? Relax! Mother Nature's got you covered. The coagulation that occurs after ejaculation helps to minimize the amount of ejaculate that is lost. The ejaculate thickens and sticks to the area where it's been deposited—ideally the upper vagina and cervical area, if you're trying for a baby. The fluid that drips out of your vagina after intercourse tends to be made up of cervical mucus, seminal fluid, and sperm that are too old or too damaged to penetrate the cervical mucus. In other words, what you're losing are the waste products of intercourse—not the sperm itself.

the bouncing and jarring associated with riding on a hard, narrow bicycle seat can lead to genital numbness and damage nerves and arteries. The word on the daddy cycle circuit? Wide saddles, padded shorts, and short runs are in.

Cool temperatures. After that workout, skip the sauna, the steam room, and the hot tub: heat is the enemy, if you're a sperm. (This explains why men's sperm counts are lower in the summer than in the winter.) Men should also take frequent breaks if they have a sedentary job. Spending too much time sitting at a desk or behind the wheel of a car increases the temperature in the scrotum, which can impair sperm production.When your guy is strutting around naked, the external temperature of the scrotum is a cool 32.5°C to 33.0°C (90.5°F to 91.4°F). Once he puts on clothes, things heat up by 0.5°C to 1.0°C (0.9°F to 1.8°F). (The temperature of his testicles is between 0.1°C and 0.6°C (0.2°F and 1.1°F) higher than the external temperature of his scrotum.) His scrotal temperature can even vary by about 1°C (1.8°F) depending on whether he's sitting with his thighs together (temperature increase) or apart (temperature decrease).

Of course, having enough players on the team is only one of the keys to reproductive success. You also want to ensure that those guys are healthy and able to move well. This is where the sperm morphology and sperm motility measures on the sperm analysis lab results figure in, if you go for fertility testing and your partner is asked to provide a sperm sample. See Chapter 4 for some help in interpreting those semen analysis results.

Now that we've completed this refresher course in human reproduction, let's get down to the real nitty-gritty.

What You Can Do to Increase Your Odds of Conceiving Quickly

Some couples like to take a completely relaxed approach to conception, simply abandoning the birth control and deciding to let nature take its course. Others, however, are card-carrying Type As. Having made up their minds that they want a baby, they want to be pregnant now.

Which camp you end up falling into will be determined by a number of factors, including

- your age (if the alarm of your biological clock is about to go off, you'll be eager to get down to business right away);

- whether you are dealing with health issues and other life circumstances that make having a baby now (as opposed to five years from now) a good idea;
- your eagerness to start a family (if it's important to you to conceive this month rather than next year, you may want to ensure that you're maximizing your chances of conceiving);
- your personality (if you have control-freak tendencies, you may find it impossible to take the more laid-back Type B approach to baby making);
- the likelihood that you or your partner might have an underlying fertility problem (if there's any reason to suspect that you might have trouble conceiving, you'll want to do whatever you can to help Mother Nature along).

While there's no magic set of instructions I can give you to ensure this will be your lucky month—the month in which you conceive little Wayne or Shania—there are some things you can do to increase your odds of winning at baby roulette. Here's what you need to know.

Know thy cycle

One of the best things you can do to increase your chances of conceiving is to get to know your menstrual cycle so that you can begin to pinpoint your most fertile days. Start out by identifying the length of your menstrual cycles—something that's easier said than done if your cycles tend to be a bit irregular. You may find it helpful to keep a menstrual calendar, noting the day on which your period starts, the day on which it ends, any pre-ovulatory symptoms you notice (changes to the quantity and texture of your cervical mucus, for example), and so on. This can be helpful in deciding when it's time to start trying to get pregnant, and can be a useful diagnostic tool for your doctor if you end up having any difficulty conceiving.

While it's common knowledge that there's no such thing as a "one size fits all" menstrual cycle, what some women forget is how this simple fact can affect the timing of ovulation. While women who have 28-day cycles tend to ovulate on or around day 14, women who have shorter or longer cycles ovulate earlier or later than that. There's also no absolute guarantee, by the way, that you'll automatically ovulate on day 14 if you have a 28-day cycle. Every woman's cycle is unique in this regard. What's more, things like stress or illness can delay ovulation or cause you to experience an anovulatory cycle (a cycle in which ovulation does not occur). Note: If your menstrual cycle is overly short (fewer than 21 days) or overly long (more than 35 days), it's possible that you have a fertility problem. Overly short or overly long menstrual cycles can be indicative of a hormonal issue that may be interfering with your efforts to conceive. Fortunately, these types of problems can often be resolved through treatment, so you should discuss them with your doctor during your pre-conception visit.

In addition to paying attention to the length of your menstrual cycles, you'll also want to learn how to predict your most fertile days. That means learning how to monitor your three key fertility signals: the quantity and quality of your cervical mucus, the position and feel of your cervix, and fluctuations in your basal body temperature.

The quality and quantity of your cervical mucus. The quality and quantity of your cervical mucus changes dramatically over the course of your menstrual cycle. During the early part of your cycle the mucus tends to be sticky and opaque. (Its job at this stage is, after all, to plug the cervix and make it difficult for sperm to enter your uterus and Fallopian tubes.) Then, as ovulation approaches, your mucus becomes increasingly wet, slippery, and abundant, and—on your most fertile days—it may actually resemble egg white. (The function of this sperm-friendly "egg white" mucus is to help transport the sperm through the uterus and into the Fallopian tubes.) Once ovulation has occurred, your cervical mucus changes again, going back to its usual sticky and opaque texture. (It's not needed to transport sperm any more so it reverts to its non-fertile state.) Monitoring this particular fertility sign is relatively easy: you simply keep track of the quantity and quality of the cervical mucus that you find on the toilet tissue each time you go to the bathroom. (If you're really obsessive, you can insert your fingers into your vagina to obtain a sample of cervical mucus, but this really isn't necessary.) You can then record your results on the chart on page 67 (Table 3.2).

The position and feel of your cervix. Your cervical mucus isn't the only thing that changes over the course of your menstrual cycle; the position and feel of your cervix changes as well. During the non-fertile parts of your cycle, your cervix is low, hard, and closed; by mid-cycle it is high, soft, and open. (The rise doesn't just happen by chance. It's designed to make it easier for sperm to make their way through the cervix.) You can monitor the changes in your cervix by checking it at the same time each day and noting its position, feel, and the size of the os (the opening in the cervix) (for example, can you insert the tip of your finger into it?). While it's challenging to monitor changes in your cervix—some obstetricians swear that even they can't get the knack of it—basically you're trying to decide whether your cervix feels soft and mushy (like your lips) or firm (like the tip of your nose). If it's high, soft, and open, you're probably fertile right now—information that you can record on the chart.

Fluctuations in your basal body temperature. The term "basal body temperature" refers to the temperature of your body first thing in the morning, before you even get out of bed. It can be used to predict your most fertile periods because it will show a distinct shift after ovulation occurs. (If there's no such shift, chances are you're not ovulating.) This shift occurs when the corpus luteum starts producing large quantities of progesterone, a hormone that causes your temperature to zoom upward. Typically, right before ovulation, your temperature will dip slightly, dropping below its usual pre-ovulatory range of 36.1°C to 36.4°C (97.0°F to 97.5°F), and then shooting up to the post-ovulatory 36.4°C to 36.6°C (97.6°F to 97.8°F). (Don't panic if you don't experience the brief temperature dip. Not everyone does.) You can monitor this fertility signal by taking your temperature before you get out of bed each morning and then plotting your results on the temperature chart in Table 3.2. Basal thermometers—ultra-sensitive thermometers that track even the slightest shift in your body's basal body temperature—are available at the drugstore.

While your BBT chart can't tell you when to have intercourse (by the time your temperature graph registers the upward shift in your temperature, the window of opportunity for baby making will have already slammed shut), your chart can still provide you with a lot of valuable information about your reproductive system. It can tell you

- whether or not you're ovulating (if you don't experience that classic temperature shift at ovulation, you're *probably* not ovulating. Note: Five per cent of women who ovulate don't experience this classic temperature shift);
- whether your luteal phase (the last half of your menstrual cycle) is long enough to allow for implantation and the early development of the fertilized egg;
- whether your progesterone levels are sufficiently high to support a pregnancy (if your temperature levels are roughly the same both before and after ovulation, it's possible that your body isn't manufacturing sufficient quantities of progesterone, which can lead to miscarriage);
- whether or not you're pregnant (if your temperature remains elevated for at least 18 days after ovulation—or for at least three days longer

than your longest-ever non-pregnant luteal phase—you're probably pregnant);

- if you've miscarried (if your temperature remains elevated for at least 18 days and then begins to drop, you may have experienced a miscarriage);
- when your most fertile days are likely to occur—assuming, of course, that you've been blessed with relatively regular menstrual cycles (if you go back and analyze a couple of months' worth of temperature charts, you'll likely begin to see some patterns to your cycles. This can help you to time future baby-making efforts more precisely).

So is temperature charting for everyone? Absolutely not. Some couples find that charting creates more problems than it solves, eliminating the spontaneity from sex and making intercourse feel like some sort of clinical procedure. It can also have a rather dampening effect on the male libido. Many guys find that their urge to make love disappears the moment they're confronted by a woman who's frantically waving a temperature chart and gesturing toward the bedroom. The pressure to perform can be simply too daunting. The moral of the story? If you do decide to go the temperature chart route but you're worried about the effect that too much information will have on your guy, simply keep your lips sealed until after the deed's been done.

"We tried to get pregnant for about six months before it happened. It's a joke now, but at the time whenever I suspected I was going to ovulate, David was required to perform, whether he liked it or not! The poor guy. His friends envied the amount of sex he was getting—I gave myself a 16-day window for baby making!—but David was actually dreading each passing month. He was relieved he could abandon his rigorous sex routine when I finally got pregnant."

—TRACEY, 31, MOTHER OF ONE

There's another way to predict ovulation—a method we haven't discussed until now. What I'm talking about are ovulation predictor kits: those pricey, high-tech kits that are always conveniently situated next to the pregnancy kits on the drugstore shelves. (When I say pricey, by the way, I'm not kidding. These things cost about $40 a pop and you may need more than one per cycle. Given that it takes a "typical" couple around six months to conceive, you could easily end up spending a couple hundred dollars or more before you manage to get pregnant.)

Just in case you haven't had occasion to use one of these gizmos, let me explain how they work. Basically, they're designed to predict the LH surge that typically occurs anywhere from 24 to 36 hours before a woman ovulates—information that you can't pick up from your temperature chart alone. In most cases, that handy bulletin can help you ensure that an ample supply of sperm is waiting to greet the egg by the time it makes its way into the Fallopian tube.

Sound great, don't they? And for many couples, they are. Unfortunately, they aren't necessarily the amazing crystal balls the drug companies would have you believe. They suffer from a few key drawbacks: they can't tell you whether a particular LH surge is the real thing (some women have a couple of false starts before the real one occurs) and they can't tell you whether you're actually ovulating (it's possible to have an LH surge without ovulating). What's more, they don't work for everyone: some women have such low levels of LH that the kit never tests positive, while others have a base level that's above the threshold, so the test results are inaccurate.

---

reproductive red flags

The following body signs and symptoms are worth discussing with your doctor if you're trying to conceive. Treat them as reproductive red flags—a sign that something is out of whack and/or warrants treatment or attention.

- Your menstrual cycle is shorter or longer than usual: this could be a sign of a hormonal imbalance—or it could be that you've been ill or under a lot of stress lately. Sometimes our cycles miss a beat.
- Your periods are lighter, heavier, or otherwise "different" (for example, you experience mid-cycle bleeding, bleeding or spotting after intercourse, or some other sort of vaginal discharge).
- You are no longer breastfeeding, but you're getting a discharge from your breasts: this can be a symptom of a hormonal imbalance or of breast-related problems.

Still, despite these obvious drawbacks, some couples swear by them. Consider what Tracey, a 31-year-old mother of one, has to say: "The kit showed me that I was completely wrong about the time I thought I was ovulating. When I discovered the correct time, we were able to get pregnant that month."

Make love on the right days

This may seem like a no-brainer, but it's at the root of more fertility problems than you might think. Studies have shown that there's a fairly limited window

3.2 Basal Body Temperature (BBT) Chart

Date																																			
Time																																			
Intercourse																																			
Cervical mucus / cervical position																																			
Menstruation																																			
Cycle day	1	2	3	4	5	6	7	8	9	10	11	12	13	14	15	16	17	18	19	20	21	22	23	24	25	26	27	28	29	30	31	32	33	34	35
37.2°C / 99.0°F																																			
37.1°C / 98.8°F																																			
37.0°C / 98.6°F																																			
36.9°C / 98.4°F																																			
36.8°C / 98.2°F																																			
36.7°C / 98.1°F																																			
36.6°C / 97.9°F																																			
36.5°C / 97.7°F																																			
36.4°C / 97.5°F																																			
36.3°C / 97.3°F																																			
36.2°C / 97.2°F																																			
36.1°C / 97.0°F																																			
36.0°C / 96.8°F																																			
35.9°C / 96.6°F																																			
35.8°C / 96.4°F																																			

INSTRUCTIONS:

Start a new chart on the first day of each menstrual cycle (the day on which your period begins).

Keep the chart, the thermometer, and a pencil on the night table beside your bed. (If you have to hop out of bed to find all this paraphernalia, your temperature reading won't be accurate.)

Place the thermometer in your mouth each morning as soon as you wake up. Record your temperature on the chart provided in Table 3.2 by drawing a dot in the centre of the appropriate box and then connecting the dot to the previous day's dot. (This will help to give you a feel for the pattern of your temperature readings.) If you had less than four hours' sleep, be sure to note this on your chart because it can affect your temperature reading.

Note the days when you have menstrual bleeding or spotting by placing a checkmark in the boxes for those days. (If you're really into charting, you can differentiate between bleeding and spotting by writing a "B" or an "S" in the appropriate place on the chart.)

Record your baby-making efforts by placing a checkmark in the "intercourse" section of the chart for the appropriate days.

If you're also monitoring your cervical mucus and your cervical position, there's room on the chart for these observations, too. You'll probably want to come up with some form of shorthand for this: perhaps a "+" or "−" to indicate changes in the quantity of cervical mucus, an "s" to describe sticky mucus, a "c" to describe creamy mucus, and an "e" to describe egg-white mucus; an "h" for high and an "l" for low to describe the position of your cervix, and an "f" for firm and "m" for mushy to describe how your cervix feels. How you use this part of the chart is up to you.

Take note of anything else that may have thrown your temperature reading off on a particular day (such as illness, insomnia, taking your temperature earlier or later than usual, or the fact that you consumed a lot of alcohol the night before). Be sure to make note of the date and/or the cycle day in each comment.

of opportunity for conception. A woman can only conceive as a result of having had intercourse during the five days preceding ovulation. (While she has just a 5 per cent chance of conceiving on the fifth day prior to ovulation or on the day of ovulation itself, she has one-in-three odds of conceiving two days before ovulation—the reproductive world's equivalent of hitting the jackpot.) So you and your partner really need to make hay during your most fertile period.

Does this mean that you should make love every day? It's up to you, but it's probably not necessary. As I mentioned earlier, sperm are capable of surviving inside the female reproductive tract for up to five days (unlike eggs, which have an incredibly short "best-before date").

Have unbelievably great sex

This is one bit of baby-making advice that shouldn't be too hard to swallow! Believe it or not, some researchers maintain that one of the keys to conceiving on your fertile days is to have unbelievably great sex. And if you're looking for a way to relieve the stress of trying to conceive? An orgasm could be just what the doctor ordered. Studies have shown that a typical orgasm is 22 times as relaxing as a typical tranquilizer.

Now no one is suggesting that you try any outlandish positions. After all, the missionary position is about the most conception-friendly position around. What the experts are saying, however, is that pleasure and procreation aren't mutually exclusive. These experts argue that there's a biological reason why having an orgasm may increase your odds of conceiving. They note that a suction effect is created when the female partner reaches orgasm, causing the cervix to draw up high in the vagina, pulling sperm into the uterus. Since this can help to transport sperm out of the acidic vaginal environment as quickly as possible, it may help to ensure that a greater number of sperm make it across the great divide (a.k.a. the cervix). So don't assume you have to sacrifice pleasure for reproduction. You can have it both ways.

Don't get too much of a good thing

If some sex is good, more sex must be better, right? Not necessarily. Not only can attempting to make love every single day be physically and mentally exhausting (particularly if you start your monthly baby-making routine too early on in your cycle), it doesn't do much to boost your odds of conceiving. Consider the facts: researchers at the National Institute of Environmental Health Sciences in the United States have concluded that couples who have intercourse every other day during their most fertile period are only slightly less likely to conceive in any given cycle than couples who have intercourse daily.

There are some couples who should definitely plan to cancel the daily romantic rendezvous: daily sex is not recommended when the male partner is subfertile as a result of a lower-than-average sperm count. Fertility specialists advise such couples to stick with an "every other day" baby-making regime during their most fertile period and to conserve sperm by refraining from ejaculating at all during the couple of days leading up to this period.

Abstaining from intercourse in order to conserve sperm isn't a good strategy for all couples, however. Studies have shown that sperm counts begin to decline if a man doesn't ejaculate for more than seven days. (Researchers have found that any gain in sperm count resulting from this temporary abstinence is more than offset by the buildup of aged sperm cells that have lower fertilization potential.) Even worse, if you accidentally miscalculate the timing of your fertile period, you could drastically reduce your chances of conceiving in any given cycle: studies have shown that couples who have intercourse only once during their fertile period have just a 10 per cent chance of conceiving.

Create a "sperm-friendly" vaginal environment

We've already talked about the importance of not douching. What you might not realize is that other personal hygiene habits are also decidedly unfriendly to sperm. While you're trying to conceive, you should make a point to avoid vaginal sprays and scented tampons, both of which can cause a pH imbalance in your vagina, as well as douches, artificial lubricants, vegetable oils, glycerin, and natural lubricants such as saliva, all of which kill off sperm.

You can naturally boost the amount of lubricant your body produces by drinking plenty of water; eating foods that are rich in B vitamins (such as spinach, broccoli, romaine, and lentils for folic acid; peppers and spinach for B6; and chicken and beef for B12); maximizing sexual arousal; avoiding perfumed toilet paper, tampons, and fabric softeners, which can interfere with natural vaginal secretions; and avoiding second-hand cigarette smoke (smoking alters the way that the body metabolizes estrogen).

You might also want to ask your doctor or pharmacist if you are currently taking any medications (either prescription or over-the-counter) that could be interfering with the production of cervical mucus: for example, medications that dry out, thicken, or decrease mucus in the body.

One final thought: you may want to treat the absence of vaginal lubrication like the proverbial canary in the coal mine—as a sign of possible underlying sexual or reproductive difficulty. If you're having trouble becoming lubricated enough to have sex (or enough to provide the kind of lubricant that allows sperm to thrive), you should mention it to your doctor. This could be a sign of an underlying hormonal imbalance that could ultimately interfere with your plans to conceive.

pink or blue?

You've no doubt heard whispers about all the things you should and shouldn't do to increase your odds of giving birth to a baby of a particular sex. Here is a selection:

- According to the Shettles Method, if you want to conceive a baby boy you should time intercourse so that it occurs as close to ovulation as possible. (Shettles makes the case that sperm cells that result in the conception of a male move more quickly but don't last as long.)

- According to the Whelan Method, if you want to conceive a male baby, you should have sex as early in your fertile period as possible—four to five days prior to ovulation. (Whelan argues that biochemical conditions in a woman's body become less favourable to male sperm as ovulation approaches.)

- According to an article in the British journal *Nature*, the age of your mate may help to determine the sex of your child. A recent study showed that women with partners at least five years older than they are were twice as likely to give birth to sons, while women who married younger men produced twice as many daughters as sons.

- Another study indicates that climate has an effect on the sex of your baby. Researchers at the University of Malta Medical School found that warmer countries record higher numbers of male births than do colder and more northerly countries like ours.

- Researchers in North Carolina have uncovered a link between the length of the follicular (pre-ovulatory) phase of a woman's menstrual cycle and the sex of the baby subsequently conceived. The researchers found that conception cycles with short follicular phases and early ovulation are more likely to produce boys, while cycles with long follicular phases and later ovulation tend to produce girls.

While it's fun to think you can determine the sex of a baby by taking these factors into account, most medical experts will pooh-pooh your chances of succeeding. A 1995 study conducted by the National Institute of Environmental Health Sciences in the United States, for example, concluded in no uncertain terms that there's no connection between the timing of intercourse and the ability to conceive a baby of a particular sex. (Hey, even the best sperm separation clinics aren't able to offer couples much better than 75–25 odds.) And websites that offer gender prediction for an exorbitant rate haven't been scientifically validated—nor do they offer money-back guarantees.

Bottom line? Go ahead and have fun with these sex-selection theories, but don't take any of them too seriously. And hold off painting the nursery pink or blue until you're sure about the sex of your baby.

CHAPTER 4

Winning at Baby Roulette

The more things change, the more they stay the same. Four thousand years ago, a woman who was wondering if she was going to have a baby mixed barley seed into her urine to test for pregnancy. If the barley grew more quickly than normal, thanks to the high levels of estrogen in her urine, chances were she was pregnant.

The two weeks after ovulation are the pregnancy world's equivalent of purgatory. You're desperate to find out whether you've conceived, but it's too soon to start loading up on home pregnancy tests. So instead you spend hours obsessing over every little symptom and twinge, trying to decide if your tender breasts or the bloating in your belly are pregnancy-related or a sign that you're about to get your period.

A Little Bit Pregnant

You can always tell when the heroine in a Really Bad Movie is pregnant (and, invariably, before the heroine clues in herself). The impeccable makeup and hair get sacrificed in favour of a bit of extra sleep and the script suddenly calls for her to be exposed to horrendous odours and stomach-churning foods—anything that might reasonably cause her to sprint to the nearest washroom.

Off-camera, pregnancy symptoms aren't always quite so clear-cut. You might experience some telltale early pregnancy symptoms (see Table 4.1)—or you could be so symptom-free that, if the test comes back positive, you may find yourself staring at the result for a surprisingly long time, waiting for the news to sink in.

Early pregnancy symptoms

You may be experiencing many of the symptoms listed below or you might not be experiencing any at all. There's no such thing as a "typical" early pregnancy experience. Every pregnancy is unique—an important point to keep in mind if you've been pregnant before and your early pregnancy symptoms this time around are very different from the symptoms you experienced during your previous pregnancy—or if your early pregnancy symptoms seem very different from those of a friend who is newly pregnant, too.

Testing, one, two, three . . .

Second-guessing the results of the pregnancy test is an almost universal pregnancy rite of passage. And if you happen to feel confident in that test result, someone else in your life (your partner? your mother? your so-called best friend?) is likely to come along and start questioning it for you. If you've got your pregnancy testing protocol down to an art, there'll be less second-guessing (and re-testing) on everyone's part. Here's what you need to know to keep the naysayers at bay.

- Use your first morning urine. The concentration of hCG is greatest at that time of day.
- Check the expiry date. If the test is past that all-important "best-before" date, chuck it. The test results can no longer be relied upon, so there's really no point in using the test.
- Follow the testing instructions to the letter. Pay particular attention to *how long you have to wait before you read the test results* and *at what point the test results are no longer valid*. (Some tests will eventually turn positive, even if they initially provided a negative result. This doesn't mean the test result has changed; it means it's time to stop pulling the pregnancy test out of the garbage can to recheck the results!)
- If you initially test positive on a pregnancy test, but re-test a week later and get a negative result, chances are you've experienced an early

4.1   Early Pregnancy Symptoms

Symptom	What Causes It to Occur During Pregnancy	Other Possible Causes
Menstrual Changes		
A missed period	Rising levels of progesterone fully suppress your menstrual period.	Jet lag, extreme weight loss or gain, a change in climate, a chronic disease such as diabetes or tuberculosis, severe illness, surgery, shock, bereavement, or other sources of stress (including the stress of trying to conceive). Taking birth control pills can also cause you to miss a period.
A lighter-than-average period	Your progesterone levels are rising, but not enough to fully suppress your menstrual period. This can make it difficult for your doctor or midwife to estimate your due date.	Can be experienced by users of birth control pills.
A small amount of spotting	May occur when the fertilized egg implants in the uterine wall—about a week after conception has occurred.	Can be experienced by users of birth control pills and women with fibroids or infections. What's more, some women routinely experience some mid-cycle spotting.
Breast Changes		
Breast tenderness and enlargement (You may also notice some related physical changes. The areola (the flat area around the nipple) may begin to darken and the tiny glands on the areola may begin to enlarge.)	Hormonal changes of early pregnancy.	Premenstrual syndrome (PMS), excessive caffeine intake, or fibrocystic breast disease.
Bloating, Cramping, and Nausea		
Abdominal bloating	Pregnancy-related weight gain.	PMS, excessive salt intake, irritable bowel syndrome, or normal weight gain.
Abdominal cramping (period-like cramping in the lower abdomen and pelvis and/or bloating and gassiness)	Hormonal changes of early pregnancy.	PMS, constipation, irritable bowel syndrome.

Symptom	Possible cause	Other causes
Morning sickness or nausea and vomiting (a catch-all term used to describe everything from mild nausea to vomiting to the point of dehydration)	High levels of progesterone. (Note: Can occur at any time of day, but tends to be worse first thing in the morning, when your blood sugar is at its lowest.)	Flu, food poisoning, or other illnesses.

Increased Need to Urinate and/or Constipation

Symptom	Possible cause	Other causes
Increased need to urinate	Increased blood flow to the pelvic area, triggered by the production of human chorionic gonadotropin (hCG) during early pregnancy.	A urinary tract infection, uterine fibroids, or excessive caffeine intake.
Constipation	Progesterone relaxes the intestinal muscles, resulting in varying degrees of constipation.	Inadequate intake of high-fibre foods or inadequate consumption of fluids.

Food Aversions and Cravings and/or Heightened Sense of Smell

Symptom	Possible cause	Other causes
Food aversions and cravings (e.g., a metallic taste in the mouth and/or a craving for certain foods)	Hormonal changes of early pregnancy.	Poor diet, stress, or PMS.
Heightened sense of smell (e.g., a sudden dislike of the smell of coffee, perfume, strong-smelling foods like onions, and/or cigarette smoke)	Hormonal changes of early pregnancy.	Illness.

Decreased Energy Level

Symptom	Possible cause	Other causes
Fatigue	Increased production of progesterone (which acts as a natural sedative) and an increase in your metabolic rate (your body's way of ensuring it will be able to support the needs of you and your developing baby).	Not getting enough sleep, not eating properly, flu, illness, or some other medical condition.

Changes to the Reproductive Organs

Symptom	Possible cause	Other causes
Changes to the cervix and the uterus (the cervix will take on a slightly purplish hue and both the cervix and uterus will begin to soften)	Hormonal changes of early pregnancy. These types of changes can be detected by your doctor or midwife during a pelvic examination.	A delayed menstrual period.

miscarriage. (Some people refer to this early pregnancy and subsequent miscarriage as a "chemical pregnancy," but many women who experience this type of loss find the term quite insensitive. I'm only introducing the term here so you'll know what people are talking about if they use it.) If you experience an early miscarriage, get in touch with your doctor or midwife right away. He or she may want to order an hCG test to confirm that you were, in fact, pregnant (as opposed to experiencing a longer-than-average menstrual cycle) and to determine that your hCG level was normal—information that could prove invaluable if you start trying to conceive again. (You'll find a detailed discussion of miscarriage in Chapter 9.)

- You can also obtain an inaccurate pregnancy test result if the urine and the home pregnancy test weren't at room temperature when the test was conducted; or if you had traces of blood or protein in your urine, had an active urinary tract infection, or are perimenopausal.

what your temperature chart can tell you	If you've been charting your temperature, your chart may be able to save you enough money on pregnancy tests to treat yourself to an early pregnancy massage. All you have to do is count the number of days your temperature has remained elevated since ovulation. If you've had 18 consecutive high temperatures (or at least three more high temperatures than you've experienced in any previous luteal phase to date), it's probably time to crack open the non-alcoholic champagne.

How you may feel about being pregnant

So the pregnancy test has come back positive. Time to hop on board the emotional roller-coaster—the one you'll be riding for the next eight and a half months or so. Depending on whether the news was welcome or unwelcome, expected or a complete shock, you may find yourself feeling one or more of the following ways as things begin to sink in.

- **Elated.** You may feel as if you're going to burst with excitement and that you've got to tell somebody—anybody!—about your news. Jane, a 33-year-old mother of two, remembers how she felt when she found out she was expecting her first baby: "I was elated! It was a snowy day, and

I actually called into work and said I couldn't make it in. I then spent the day celebrating being pregnant. I stopped by my husband's office on the way home from my doctor's appointment to tell him. We hugged in the falling snow."

- **Awestruck.** It's one thing to want to be pregnant, and quite another to discover that the deed has actually been done. Some women find themselves feeling positively wonderstruck at the realization that there's a baby growing inside their body. In fact, it may be all they can think about at first. Jennifer, 26, who is midway through her first pregnancy, describes how she continues to feel about being pregnant: "I still sometimes just sit back and shake my head at how overwhelmed I feel about carrying a child that's half me and half this man that I love more than anything in the world. I hope every day that the baby is happy and cozy inside of me, and that he or she is growing strong and healthy. I'm still very emotional about this awesome adventure."

- **Proud.** If becoming pregnant has been a goal of yours for some time, you may feel a tremendous sense of accomplishment when you discover you've actually managed to conceive. "I remember feeling as if I'd made this momentous step forward—that an entirely new chapter had opened in my life," says Marie, a 36-year-old mother of three. "And, in fact, it had."

- **Shocked.** Finding out that you're really and truly 100 per cent pregnant can be unnerving, even if you've been consciously trying to have a baby. "I was initially quite shocked and somewhat panicked," recalls 32-year-old Janet, who recently gave birth to her first baby. "I had expected it to take much longer. My husband was asleep when I did the test and I woke him up to tell him the news. I don't think either of us got very much sleep that night. It took us both a few weeks to get used to the idea and then we were both very happy about it."

- **Overwhelmed.** It's not unusual to feel completely overwhelmed and possibly even slightly panicked when you realize that you're going to become a mother. "Up until that point, it had all seemed like a game," recalls Maria, a 31-year-old mother of two young children. "Then I was thinking, 'What have we done?'"

- **Unenthused.** Some women find that the symptoms of early pregnancy leave them feeling less than thrilled about the situation. That was certainly the case for 31-year-old Debbie, who is currently pregnant with her first child: "I've found that people expect me to always be in a state of ecstasy. Even throughout the morning sickness and weeks of physical exhaustion, it felt like I was disappointing people if I wasn't skipping around talking about baby names, et cetera. It made me wonder how many women cover up their real feelings, especially in early pregnancy." Note: Persistent feelings of sadness may be a symptom of prenatal depression. Be sure to talk about how you're feeling with your doctor or midwife. See Chapter 5 for more about perinatal mood disorders.

- **Dismayed.** If your pregnancy was unplanned, you may need a little time to get used to the idea of having a baby. "I conceived in the blink of an eye—or perhaps even faster than that!" admits LeeAnne, a 29-year-old mother of three. "This made for a bit of a mental adjustment with each pregnancy, as we weren't really planning and trying to conceive."
- **Worried.** If you've experienced miscarriage, stillbirth, or the death of a baby, you may feel extremely anxious about being pregnant again. You may wonder if something will go wrong this time, too—whether daring to dream about ending up with a healthy baby in your arms will somehow prevent that dream from coming true. Note: You'll find a detailed discussion of the challenges of pregnancy after a loss in Chapter 9, and also in *Trying Again: A Guide to Pregnancy After Miscarriage, Stillbirth, or Infant Loss* by Ann Douglas and John R. Sussman, MD.

By the way, if you're expecting your partner to play the part of the euphoric father-to-be you see in the television commercials—he's supposed to pick you up and swing you in circles while declaring his undying love for you and the baby—you could be in for a bit of a disappointment. Not everyone reacts with quite that much enthusiasm: "My husband said, 'Oh, that's good' and kept watching the hockey game because he was in shock," recalls Darci, a 29-year-old mother of one. "Darin was a little more cautious than me," said Julie, 29, who is currently pregnant with her second child. "He looked at the pregnancy test and said, 'The line's not very dark.' I wanted to hit him!"

Of course, some women find that their partners are even more excited than they are. This was certainly the case for Marinda, a 30-year-old mother of two, who was initially shocked to discover she was unexpectedly pregnant with baby number two: "It took me about two weeks to come to terms with being pregnant and to start looking forward to having another baby. My husband, on the other hand, was happy right away."

Sharing your news with the world

One of the first decisions you and your partner will face as a newly pregnant couple is when to share your exciting news with the rest of the world. You may decide to tell everyone at once, or to be a bit more selective about whom you tell and when.

Marguerite, a 36-year-old mother of two, took the first approach: "I phoned everyone right away—as soon as I found out I was pregnant. I couldn't contain myself." Although she knew that spreading her news early on meant she might have to share some sad news if she ended up miscarrying, Marguerite felt that it made more sense to announce her pregnancy right away. "David and I decided not to wait until the pregnancy was further along because as soon as the pregnancy was confirmed, we were strongly attached to the presence of the baby in our lives. We felt that if any unforeseen problems arose it would affect us significantly and we'd therefore want and need the support of the people around us."

Anne, a 29-year-old mother of one, decided to wait to share the news with everyone until she'd passed the peak risk period for miscarriage (the first trimester): "We told our parents early on but we held off telling other family members and friends until we were about three months along. I felt that our parents would be there to help us through a miscarriage, but I couldn't cope with having to tell all our family members and friends if we were to miscarry."

Sometimes special circumstances force you to spill the beans about your pregnancy a little sooner than you might normally have planned. Jenna, a 25-year-old mother of one, had a particular reason for choosing to announce her pregnancy sooner rather than later: "My grandfather was very sick and I wanted him to know about his great-grandchild," she explains.

Just one quick word of caution: once you decide to share the news with one member of your extended family, you'd better plan to get on the phone to the rest of the clan as soon as possible. The family grapevine is never more

"I told my dad about my pregnancy over the phone because I didn't want to confront him in person. To my surprise, I heard a choke in his words and I thought he might be crying. I just didn't know if it was for joy or because he was upset that I was pregnant but not yet married. About an hour later, an absolutely huge bouquet of flowers arrived at my office door. It was from my dad. My question was answered and I was happy."

–TRACEY, 31, MOTHER OF ONE

effective than when there's news of a pregnancy to spread, and you don't want the grandparents-to-be (particularly first-time grandparents-to-be!) to hear your exciting news from someone else.

Sharing your news at work

You kicked your coffee habit weeks ago, but for some reason your boss still hasn't clued into the fact that you're pregnant. Now you're wondering how—and when—to announce your pregnancy at work. While there's no magic right time to make your big announcement, you're more likely to meet with a positive reaction if you plan that announcement carefully. Here are a few tips:

- **Put safety first.** If you work in a hazardous type of environment—you work with solvents that could be harmful to your baby, for example—you may need to announce your pregnancy sooner rather than later so that you can be reassigned to a different type of work for the duration of your pregnancy. Every province and territory has its own occupational health and safety legislation, and approximately 10 per cent of Canadian workers fall under federal jurisdiction. That means you'll need to make a few phone calls to find out what specific rights you have as a pregnant employee. If you are routinely exposed to infectious diseases, heavy metals, toxic chemicals, oil-based paints, radiation, anaesthetic gases, tobacco smoke, excessive heat or noise, or other harmful substances at work (check out Material Safety Data Sheets—consult www.msdsonline.com for help making sense of the information you find on the Material Safety Data Sheets in your workplace, or www.motherisk.org for questions about exposure to particular substances in the workplace); your job is highly strenuous or physically demanding; you have to stand for more than three hours per day at work or you have to do a lot of bending, stooping, stair or ladder climbing, or heavy lifting; you work in an extremely hot, cold, or noisy environment; or you work long hours or rotating shifts, you should plan to meet with your employer to discuss job modifications right away.
- **Keep the news under your hat a little longer if you can.** If your job doesn't pose any risks to your baby, and you're coping just fine with the day-to-day demands, you might want to consider keeping the news to yourself until you've passed through the highest-risk period for pregnancy loss. (Of course, if you're experiencing severe morning sickness or other pregnancy-related complications, you may have little choice but to spill the beans right away.)

- **Time your announcement carefully.** If you're expecting a performance review or a raise in the near future, keep your pregnancy to yourself for now. That way, if the news is less than what you'd hoped for, you won't have to wonder whether your poor review or less-than-spectacular raise is due to your performance or your pregnancy. It's also a good idea to time your announcement to coincide with a major achievement at work: that way, you can reassure your boss with actions as well as words that you're still as productive and committed to your job as ever.

- **Make sure your boss hears the news from you first.** If you feel the need to explain to a few trusted co-workers why you can no longer stand the smell of coffee or why you've suddenly morphed from your usual high-energy self into someone who has to take a quick catnap at her desk every afternoon, make sure you swear them to secrecy until you have the chance to deliver the news to your boss first-hand. And don't delay that meeting for too long, by the way. The office grapevine has a tendency to take on a life of its own.

- **Postpone your announcement if your boss is having a particularly bad day.** You're less likely to be met with a positive reaction if your boss is in the middle of dealing with a major computer problem or if she's spent the entire morning trying to placate the Customer from You-Know-Where.

- **Be prepared for a lukewarm reaction—and try not to take your boss's lack of enthusiasm personally.** As happy as your employer may be for you, you've just dropped a major staffing challenge in her lap! If this is the first time she's ever had to deal with a pregnant employee, she may be particularly apprehensive about what your pregnancy may mean for both her and the company.

- **Ask for other workplace accommodations, if you need them.** If you work for a company where employees rarely take breaks because things are so crazy on the job, you may worry about getting heat from co-workers if you have to wave the proverbial white flag. Don't let that stop you from taking proper care of yourself and your baby. Remind yourself that everyone needs some slack eventually, whether it's because they're pregnant, caring for an aging relative, or dealing with an injury or illness themselves, and that you'll be just as understanding when it's their turn to start waving the flag.

- **Don't make promises you may not be able to keep.** Rather than trying to reassure your boss that you'll work right until the bitter end of your pregnancy and that you'll return to work as soon as possible after your baby is born—commitments you might not be willing or able to keep in the end—simply agree to discuss your plans when your pregnancy is further along and you're better able to make these types of decisions.

Choosing the right caregiver (assuming you have that luxury)

In some communities in Canada, actually having your own family physician— let alone being able to shop around for "the right" family physician, obstetrician, or midwife—is the stuff of which pregnancy dreams are made. Often, it's more a case of hoping someone will be able to fit you into their caseload than being able to pick and choose who will care for you and your baby.

Until the situation improves, it's a bit of a coin toss. The doctor you end up with could have a bedside manner reminiscent of the most brisk and harried checkout clerk at your not-so-friendly neighbourhood megastore or, if it's your lucky day, the most caring caregiver imaginable. "Living in an underserviced community gave us few choices about who'd look after us during our pregnancy," recalls Jennifer, 29, mother of one. "My general practitioner doesn't do any obstetrics, so he referred me to a new local obstetrician. We couldn't have made a better choice. He was fantastic: caring, patient, kind, and gentle."

Assuming you do have the luxury of choice (which means you probably live in a larger, more urban centre), here are some of the considerations you'll want to keep in mind when you're trying to decide if a particular doctor or midwife is right for you.

> *National Birthing Initiative for Canada*
>
> The Society of Obstetricians and Gynaecologists of Canada is calling for the implementation of a National Birthing Initiative for Canada. The initiative— which has been developed in conjunction with groups representing family physicians, midwives, nurses, anesthesiologists, perinatal programs, ministers of health, schools of medicine, aboriginal groups, and other concerned parties— will provide an inclusive, integrated, and comprehensive Canadian framework for providing family-centred maternity and newborn care over the long term. To obtain an update on the status of this project, visit www.sogc.org/projects/birthing-strategy_e.asp.

- **The right level of care.** If you know from the outset that your pregnancy is likely to be high risk (for example, you have a pre-existing health condition such as diabetes or high blood pressure), an obstetrician may be your best choice. But if your pregnancy is likely to be low risk, there's no reason why a family physician or midwife shouldn't be able to provide you with equally good care during your pregnancy.

If, for some reason, you unexpectedly develop a pregnancy-related complication that causes your pregnancy to be classified as high risk, your family physician or midwife will either transfer you to an obstetrician or ask him or her to consult on your case. So you needn't fear that you won't have access to the care of a specialist if you encounter any unexpected curveballs late in the game. That option will always be available.

- **A good rapport.** If you get along famously with your family physician, you may prefer to turn to him or her for your prenatal care. If you dread spending any time with your doctor, however, you may want to find someone else to care for you and your baby. There are so many important issues to discuss during pregnancy. You want to be sure that you feel comfortable with the person who'll be providing your prenatal care and (possibly) attending your baby's birth.

- **Compatible philosophies.** Look for someone who's in sync with you when it comes to important issues like pain relief during labour, episiotomy, breastfeeding, and so on. That's not to say you'll necessarily end up with "the perfect birth," of course. No one in the baby business can offer that sort of guarantee. But you want to feel confident that your caregiver is open to discussing your plans for your baby's birth with you—as opposed to imposing his or her ideas of the one–size–fits–all labour and delivery experience on you.

- **Someone who will be there for you—literally.** Research has shown that mothers and babies benefit when they are cared for by the same caregiver (or by one of a small number of caregivers) who share the same basic philosophies about pregnancy and birth. If your caregiver works in a group, you'll want to make sure that you feel comfortable with the other members of the medical or midwifery practice. After all, there's always the possibility that one of them could end up attending your baby's birth in the place of your own doctor or midwife.

- **Someone who otherwise fits the bill.** You may want to consider some other issues when you're choosing a caregiver. If, for example, you're a survivor of sexual abuse or your religious beliefs deem it inappropriate for any male other than your husband to be present at the birth of your baby, finding a caregiver who is sensitive to these issues and who is female may be very important to you.

The checklist in the following box lists some specific questions you may want to ask when you're trying to determine whether a particular caregiver is right for you:

Caregiver Checklist: Questions to Ask

The practice

☐ How long have you been in practice? How many births have you attended? What percentage of your patients' babies do you end up delivering yourself?

☐ Do you see patients in a clinic situation or in your private practice?

☐ Do you have evening or early morning office hours?

☐ What days are you available in your office? Who sees your patients on days when you are not in the office?

☐ Do you take routine phone calls at a certain time of day?

☐ When do you take holidays? Do you attend a lot of conferences?

☐ Other than you, who might be present at the birth of my baby? Will I have the opportunity to meet some or all of these backup caregivers at some point during my pregnancy?

☐ How should I go about reaching you in the event of an emergency? Are there times when you may be unavailable to take my call? In that case, whom would I call instead?

☐ How often are you on call? Do you expect to be on call around the time that my baby is due?

☐ Do you involve residents, interns, or student midwives in your practice? If so, what role would they play in my care?

☐ What hospitals and/or birth centres are you affiliated with? (Just a handful of Canadian communities have birth centres and they tend to be based in larger urban areas. However, there is a growing movement toward integrated maternity care, where obstetricians, family physicians, midwives, and/or nurse practitioners work as a team to ease Canada's maternity-care shortage and to ensure that those providing maternity-care services are able to get some time off.)

☐ Do you attend home births? (While midwives routinely attend home births, only a handful of doctors are willing to do so.)

Pregnancy-related policies and procedures

☐ What's your standard schedule for prenatal appointments? (Most pregnant women are seen every four to six weeks during early pregnancy; every two to three weeks after 30 weeks; and every one to two weeks after 36 weeks.)

☐ Under what circumstances would you decide to see me more often than this? Note: If you've previously experienced the death of a baby through miscarriage, stillbirth, or neonatal death, you might want to ask whether the caregiver would be willing to schedule additional appointments if you required added reassurance between appointments.

☐ How much time do you set aside for each appointment? (Doctors tend to schedule about 10 minutes for prenatal appointments, while midwives typically spend 45 minutes to an hour with each client.)

☐ Do you routinely screen for symptoms of depression during pregnancy and the postpartum period?

☐ What types of tests are you likely to recommend over the course of my pregnancy (for example, ultrasound, maternal serum screening, amniocentesis, gestational diabetes, group B strep)?

☐ Under what circumstances, if any, would you need to transfer me into the care of another health-care provider? Under what circumstances would it be possible for you to coordinate shared care with a specialist?

☐ Do you see your obstetrical patients for health problems that are not pregnancy-related, such as coughs or colds?

Approaches to birth and postpartum care

☐ Do you encourage your patients to write birth plans? What advice would you offer if I decided to write one?

☐ Under what circumstances do you induce labour? What percentage of women in your practice are induced? How many days past the due date do you wait before discussing induction? What is the rate of failed induction at the hospital?

☐ How much time would you expect to be able to spend with me while I'm in labour?

☐ Do the majority of women that you care for have medicated or non-medicated births? Which methods of pharmacological and non-pharmacological pain relief do they tend to use the most often (for example, epidurals vs. labouring in water)?

☐ Do you encourage women to attempt unmedicated deliveries?

☐ Have you worked with a doula (a professional labour support person)?

☐ Do you routinely use continuous electronic fetal monitoring during labour? What percentage of women in your care receive continuous electronic fetal monitoring?

☐ What percentage of women in your care receive episiotomies?

☐ How often do the women in your care end up delivering through Caesarean section? (Note: A doctor who specializes in high-risk pregnancies may have a higher-than-average Caesarean rate just by virtue of the nature of his or her practice.) What are the most common reasons for Caesarean sections in your practice?

☐ What percentage of women attempting a vaginal birth after Caesarean (VBAC) are able to deliver vaginally?

☐ Would you expect my baby to be able to remain with me after the birth? Do you encourage skin-to-skin contact, and do you delay newborn procedures for the first hour?

☐ Do you or members of your health-care team provide breastfeeding support? What is your best advice on how I could obtain this support in our community?

☐ Under what circumstances should I contact you during the postpartum period?

While you'll want to spend some time making sure that a particular caregiver is right for you, don't wait too long to make up your mind or you could find out that his or her practice is full. Jane, a 33-year-old mother of two, encountered this frustrating situation: "When I was nine weeks pregnant with my first child, I phoned the nearest midwifery practice to inquire. I was already too late to secure the services of a midwife! The second time around, I phoned the practice as soon as I knew I was pregnant." If the caregiver you want is all booked up, consider getting on the waiting list. Some women book with more than one caregiver in order to get the type of care they want, so spots do open up.

Midwife or doula?

Confused about the difference between a midwife and a doula? Here's what you need to know. Registered midwives are health professional who provide frontline care to women and their babies during pregnancy, labour, birth, and the postpartum period. They are responsible for overseeing the care of women experiencing low-risk pregnancies and are able to conduct physical examinations, order screening and diagnostic tests, and attend normal vaginal deliveries. According to the Canadian Association of Midwives, "Midwives work in collaboration with other health professionals and consult with or refer to medical specialists as appropriate. The midwifery model of care promotes normal birth, enables women to make informed choices, and provides continuity of care and support throughout the childbearing experience. Midwives attend births in hospitals, birth centres and at home."

Doulas are trained professionals who, in the case of a birth doula, offer continuous physical, emotional, and informational support to the mother before, during, and just after birth; or who, in the case of a postpartum doula, offer emotional and practical support during the postpartum period. Research has proven that labours are shorter, women experience fewer complications, and babies are healthier and breastfeed more easily when a doula attends a birth. What's more, a postpartum doula can help ease the transition that occurs with the arrival of a new baby while reducing the risk of mood disorders.

Hospital or home birth?

Something else to keep in mind when you're shopping around for a caregiver is where you intend to give birth.

You may have strong feelings one way or another. "My biggest fears were that once I was at a hospital, I'd be lost among the other expectant mothers and treated as though I were part of a baby-making assembly line rather than a person partaking in the making of a miracle," explains Bevin, 27, who recently gave birth to her first child. If you're hoping to give birth at home, you should plan to use the services of a midwife. The Canadian Association of Midwives (www.canadianmidwives.org; 1–514–807–3668) can refer you to your provincial or territorial midwifery college or association so that you can inquire about the availability of midwives in your part of Canada.

If you're planning to give birth in a hospital, you may have the choice of using the services of either a doctor or a midwife, depending on the legislation regulating midwifery in your part of Canada. Visit the Canadian Association of Midwives website for the latest updates on the status of midwifery in every Canadian province or territory.

And as to the age-old debate about whether home birth is as safe as hospital birth, that debate continues, but the positions held by some members of the medical community have become a little less rigid in recent years.

A commentary in the February 5, 2002, issue of the *Canadian Medical Association Journal,* by Régis Blais, MD, a professor in the Department of Health Administration at the Université de Montréal, noted, "The mode of delivery, including the setting and the caregiver, is a very personal choice of expectant parents. When a health care system is able to provide various types of quality care at a reasonable cost, choices should be offered to parents. As with all therapeutic decisions, this should be a fully informed choice based on scientific evidence and personal preferences."

And the Society of Obstetricians and Gynaecologists of Canada had this comment on home birth in its March 2003 Policy Statement on Midwifery: "The SOGC recognizes and stresses the importance of choice for women and their families in the birthing process. The SOGC recognizes that women will continue to choose the setting in which they will give birth. All women should receive information about the risks and benefits of their chosen place for giving birth, and should understand any identified limitation of care at their planned birth setting. The SOGC endorses evidence-based practice and encourages ongoing research into the safe environment."

Home birth

If you decide to plan a home birth, your midwife will likely advise you to have the following types of supplies on hand. You can purchase many of these items all at once if you purchase a birth kit:

- two or more sets of clean sheets (a set for use during the delivery and a set for use after the birth)

4.2 Hospital Birth vs. Home Birth: Assessing Your Options

PROS

Hospital Birth	Home Birth
All the high-tech medical equipment is on hand in case you or your baby need it.	You're able to give birth in the privacy of your own home, surrounded by people you care about, and you won't have to share your room with strangers.
You can be prepped for an emergency Caesarean in a matter of minutes, assuming the obstetrician and the anesthesiologist are at the hospital when the emergency arises.	You don't need to head for the hospital when you're in labour.
You have more options for pain relief.	You have greater control over your birthing experience.
You can relax and enjoy your baby without worrying about the rest of the world.	You may be more relaxed, which can help reduce your need for pain medications during labour.
	There's less chance of picking up a postpartum infection or developing intrapartum fever.
	You're less likely to be subjected to unwanted medical interventions.
	The person you have worked with throughout your pregnancy is likely to be in attendance at your birth.

CONS

Hospital Birth	Home Birth
Despite an effort to create more home-like birthing environments, many hospital birthing centres still feel sterile and clinical.	If an acute emergency were to arise during labour, you would have to be transported to the hospital. While your midwife is capable of performing certain types of interventions en route to the hospital, he/she can't perform an emergency Caesarean section, if one is needed. Valuable time may be lost in transit, although the hospital staff will be busy preparing for your arrival in order to ensure they're ready for you when you arrive.
You may find it difficult to relax in the hospital environment, which can increase your need for pain-relief medications during labour.	
You may find yourself having to hop in the car and head for the hospital when you're in the heat of labour, which can be painful and upsetting.	You don't have access to the same range of pain relief options that would be available to you in a hospital.
Rigid hospital policies may interfere with your plans for the birth. What's more, your plans may have to be sacrificed if there is a shortage of beds or other resources.	

There's a greater risk of infection in a hospital setting than at home.

You may be subjected to certain interventions (e.g., electronic fetal monitoring, artificial rupture of membranes, augmentation of labour, or a Caesarean delivery) simply because the technology is available. (Some studies have shown that women giving birth in a hospital setting are sometimes subjected to these types of interventions without any specific medical reason.) There may not be time for informed consent conversations before these interventions take place, and you might even be asked to sign a "consent to treatment" form in advance of your due date.

In some situations, the lack of immediate access to the resources available in a hospital setting can result in a tragic outcome. In planning a home birth, you need to be prepared to assume this risk. Your midwife will screen you for as many potential problems as he or she can, but not all situations can be predicted ahead of time.

- waterproof pad, shower curtain or large plastic tablecloth to prevent the mattress of your bed from being damaged
- disposable absorbent pads or large diapers to absorb amniotic fluid and blood during labour and the birth
- clean towels and washcloths
- sterile gauze pads
- a dozen or more pairs of disposable gloves
- umbilical cord clamps
- a 60- or 80-millimetre (3-ounce) bulb syringe for suctioning mucus from the baby's mouth and nose
- a large bowl to catch the placenta
- receiving blankets for the baby
- sanitary napkins

Note: If you're planning a water birth, you'll also need to round up some additional supplies: a portable birthing tub (unless you intend to use your existing bathtub, Jacuzzi, or hot tub), a water thermometer (to ensure that the temperature remains around 37°C/100°F), a flashlight that works underwater (so that the caregiver can view the birth), an inflatable plastic pillow (to keep you comfortable), a fishnet (to scoop out placental fragments and other remnants from the birth), and plenty of clean towels.

So how do you go about deciding if you're a good candidate for a home birth? This is definitely one of those issues you'll want to talk over with your partner and your doctor and/or midwife, but—in general—you would be considered a good candidate for a home birth if

- you are in good medical condition and your pregnancy is considered low risk;
- you have a qualified caregiver lined up to attend the birth, and this person has all the necessary emergency medical supplies (such as oxygen, resuscitation equipment, and so on);
- you're willing to take on the added responsibility for having all the necessary birth-related supplies on hand and you understand that you might have to head to the hospital if unexpected complications arise;
- your home is reasonably close to a hospital (ask your caregiver what he/she suggests, given local climate and driving conditions);
- your partner and/or children will support you in giving birth at home and you have additional people lined up to assist you before, during, and after the birth;
- home birth feels like the right choice for you.

Bevin, 27, who recently gave birth to her first child, was immediately sold on the idea of having a home birth. It just took a bit longer for her partner, Ben, to become enthused: "I knew right away that I didn't want to give birth in a hospital—I have a fear of doctors and hospitals—but trying to convince Ben that there were other options was almost like trying to pull a semi-truck with dental floss.

"In the end, Ben listened to my arguments in favour of a home birth. I did a ton of research and presented my case to him. I also pointed out that we're just six minutes away from the closest hospital and 15 minutes from the biggest hospital, should anything go wrong. He finally agreed reluctantly, and our doctor recommended a very experienced midwife. By our second visit with her, Ben was actually convinced that having a home birth was probably better than going to the hospital!"

Marinda, 30, was similarly determined to deliver her second baby at home. She'd gone with a hospital birth the first time around, but wanted to have

home birth update

In its statement concerning home birth, the Canadian Association of Midwives states that "available scientific evidence demonstrates that home birth with midwives is a safe and viable option for healthy low-risk women." A study published in the September 2009 issue of the *Canadian Medical Association Journal* supports that conclusion. Researchers, who studied over 2,800 planned home births attended by British Columbia midwives over a four-year period, found that women giving birth at home were less likely to experience labour-related interventions and postpartum complications than women giving birth in hospital.

baby number two somewhere other than in the clinical hospital setting. "I had my second child at home in our bedroom, which was cozy and dimly lit and extremely relaxing," she recalls. "Three hours after the birth, everyone in the house was trying to sleep and the midwives were gone."

LeeAnne and her partner had planned to deliver their child at home, but ended up having to abandon those plans. "Unfortunately, because I tested positive for group B strep, we had to be at the hospital," she explains.

Home birth isn't necessarily for everyone. Some women prefer to give birth in a hospital because they feel reassured knowing that all the high-tech medical equipment—and the option of medicinal pain relief—is close at hand, should they need them. "I simply felt safer giving birth knowing that the necessary medical equipment and specialists were nearby if I needed them," recalls Marie, a mom of three. "In the end, my hospital birth felt almost as 'natural' as a home birth, but in order for me to relax and feel ready to give birth, I needed to feel safe, and, for me, that meant giving birth in a hospital setting."

Your First Prenatal Checkup

Regardless of whether you intend to give birth at home or in hospital, and to be cared for by a midwife, family physician, or obstetrician, you'll want to get in to see your caregiver as soon as possible after you find out that you're pregnant. This is particularly important if your pregnancy was unplanned and you weren't able to schedule a pre-conception checkup, because you'll want to have a chat with your caregiver about all the important issues—for example,

- any chronic health problems or conditions you may have;
- any medications you're taking (both prescription and over-the-counter);
- the state of your general health;
- your gynecological and obstetrical history;
- your family medical history;
- your general nutrition and lifestyle habits (such as whether you smoke, drink, or use drugs, and whether you exercise regularly).

During your initial prenatal checkup or pregnancy confirmation visit, your doctor or midwife will

- confirm your pregnancy by doing a urine or blood test or by conducting a physical examination to look for changes in your uterus and cervix that would indicate you're pregnant;

- estimate your due date by considering such factors as the date of your last menstrual period, the types of pregnancy symptoms you've been experiencing, physical changes to your uterus and cervix, and any information you can provide concerning the possible date of conception (you may have this information if you've been using ovulation predictor kits or charting your fertility signals);
- perform a blood test to determine your blood type and to check for anemia, hepatitis B, HIV (if you request it), syphilis, antibodies to rubella (German measles), or chicken pox (varicella), and—depending on your ethnic background and family history—certain genetic diseases;
- take a vaginal culture to check for infection (some caregivers do this routinely; others do it only if there's a specific reason);
- do a Pap smear to check for cervical cancer or precancerous cells (if you've had this test within the past year, your doctor or midwife is unlikely to repeat it. Some doctors and midwives try to avoid performing Pap smears during pregnancy because they can result in a small amount of spotting, which isn't harmful to the pregnancy, but can be quite alarming to a mom-to-be nonetheless);
- check your urine for signs of infection, blood sugar problems, and excess protein;
- weigh you to establish a baseline so that your weight gain during pregnancy can be monitored;
- take your blood pressure;
- talk to you about how you are feeling physically;
- ask you how you and your partner are feeling about the pregnancy (when a pregnancy is unplanned, there is a greater risk of prenatal depression);
- ask you if you're being abused or threatened by your partner or anyone else in your life (you can turn to your doctor/midwife for nonjudgmental support if you're a victim of intimate partner violence);
- ask you whether you have any questions or concerns (you'll want to get in the habit of bringing a list of questions to each appointment so you can get all those questions answered).

Note: Your doctor or midwife will record details about your pregnancy on your prenatal record. He or she may also provide you with a patient version of this record so that you can keep your own pregnancy records as well. If you aren't given such a record during your initial prenatal appointment, you may want to use the one at the back of this book. (See Appendix D.)

domestic violence during pregnancy

According to the Society of Obstetricians and Gynaecologists of Canada, more than one in twelve pregnant women report being abused by their partners during pregnancy. Women who are abused during pregnancy are at risk of becoming depressed or suicidal, of experiencing pregnancy complications or a fetal death, or of being murdered themselves. And children whose mothers are subjected to violence are more likely to experience developmental difficulties and to be abused themselves. Women who are in same-sex relationships, women of colour, Aboriginal women, women with disabilities, or women who are immigrants or refugees may experience different forms of intimate partner violence than other women and may find it more difficult to reach out for help. To find out about intimate partner violence resources in your community, including how to make a safety plan, visit the Canadian Network of Women's Shelters and Transition Houses at endvaw.ca/get-help.

What your due date really means

One of the most important bits of information you'll walk away with at the end of your first prenatal checkup is your doctor or midwife's best guess about when your baby will be born—your so-called "estimated date of confinement," or due date.

To calculate this all-important date, your caregiver will consult a due date chart or due date wheel and will either add 266 days or 38 weeks to the date you ovulated, or add 280 days or 40 weeks to the date of the first day of your last menstrual period (assuming, of course, that you have a textbook 28-day cycle).

Because these calculations tend to be more accurate if they're based on the timing of conception rather than the date of your last menstrual cycle, it's important to let your doctor or midwife know if you have a temperature chart or ovulation predictor kit result that could help to pinpoint the timing of ovulation. If your due date is calculated based on the date of your last menstrual period, it's important to let your caregiver know if your cycles tend to be longer or shorter than normal.

Now, before you reach for your smartphone and enter "have baby" into your calendar, remember that babies don't have a whole lot of respect for due dates. Studies have shown that just 5 per cent of babies bother to show up on schedule—although, to be fair, 85 per cent do manage to make their grand entrance within a week of their due date. And newborns don't pay much attention to the clock either. (Thought I'd give you an early heads up on that.)

4.2 Your Estimated Date of Delivery

The row of boldface numbers indicates the date of the first day of your last menstrual period. The date underneath indicates your approximate due date (assuming that you have a 28-day menstrual cycle). If your cycle is anything other than 28 days in length, your doctor or midwife will likely adjust your due date by adding or subtracting the appropriate number of days.

Please note that one month runs into the next in the second line of this chart. In other words, if your last menstrual period started on January 31st and you managed to conceive, your baby would be due on November 7th.

	1	2	3	4	5	6	7	8	9	10	11	12	13	14	15	16	17	18	19	20	21	22	23	24	25	26	27	28	29	30	31	
January	1	2	3	4	5	6	7	8	9	10	11	12	13	14	15	16	17	18	19	20	21	22	23	24	25	26	27	28	29	30	31	January
October	8	9	10	11	12	13	14	15	16	17	18	19	20	21	22	23	24	25	26	27	28	29	30	31	1	2	3	4	5	6	7	November
February	1	2	3	4	5	6	7	8	9	10	11	12	13	14	15	16	17	18	19	20	21	22	23	24	25	26	27	28				February
November	8	9	10	11	12	13	14	15	16	17	18	19	20	21	22	23	24	25	26	27	28	29	30	1	2	3	4	5				December
March	1	2	3	4	5	6	7	8	9	10	11	12	13	14	15	16	17	18	19	20	21	22	23	24	25	26	27	28	29	30	31	March
December	6	7	8	9	10	11	12	13	14	15	16	17	18	19	20	21	22	23	24	25	26	27	28	29	30	31	1	2	3	4	5	January
April	1	2	3	4	5	6	7	8	9	10	11	12	13	14	15	16	17	18	19	20	21	22	23	24	25	26	27	28	29	30		April
January	6	7	8	9	10	11	12	13	14	15	16	17	18	19	20	21	22	23	24	25	26	27	28	29	30	31	1	2	3	4		February
May	1	2	3	4	5	6	7	8	9	10	11	12	13	14	15	16	17	18	19	20	21	22	23	24	25	26	27	28	29	30	31	May
February	5	6	7	8	9	10	11	12	13	14	15	16	17	18	19	20	21	22	23	24	25	26	27	28	1	2	3	4	5	6	7	March
June	1	2	3	4	5	6	7	8	9	10	11	12	13	14	15	16	17	18	19	20	21	22	23	24	25	26	27	28	29	30		June
March	8	9	10	11	12	13	14	15	16	17	18	19	20	21	22	23	24	25	26	27	28	29	30	31	1	2	3	4	5	6		April
July	1	2	3	4	5	6	7	8	9	10	11	12	13	14	15	16	17	18	19	20	21	22	23	24	25	26	27	28	29	30	31	July
April	7	8	9	10	11	12	13	14	15	16	17	18	19	20	21	22	23	24	25	26	27	28	29	30	1	2	3	4	5	6	7	May
August	1	2	3	4	5	6	7	8	9	10	11	12	13	14	15	16	17	18	19	20	21	22	23	24	25	26	27	28	29	30	31	August
May	8	9	10	11	12	13	14	15	16	17	18	19	20	21	22	23	24	25	26	27	28	29	30	31	1	2	3	4	5	6	7	June
September	1	2	3	4	5	6	7	8	9	10	11	12	13	14	15	16	17	18	19	20	21	22	23	24	25	26	27	28	29	30		September
June	8	9	10	11	12	13	14	15	16	17	18	19	20	21	22	23	24	25	26	27	28	29	30	1	2	3	4	5	6	7		July
October	1	2	3	4	5	6	7	8	9	10	11	12	13	14	15	16	17	18	19	20	21	22	23	24	25	26	27	28	29	30	31	October
July	8	9	10	11	12	13	14	15	16	17	18	19	20	21	22	23	24	25	26	27	28	29	30	31	1	2	3	4	5	6	7	August
November	1	2	3	4	5	6	7	8	9	10	11	12	13	14	15	16	17	18	19	20	21	22	23	24	25	26	27	28	29	30		November
August	8	9	10	11	12	13	14	15	16	17	18	19	20	21	22	23	24	25	26	27	28	29	30	31	1	2	3	4	5	6		September
December	1	2	3	4	5	6	7	8	9	10	11	12	13	14	15	16	17	18	19	20	21	22	23	24	25	26	27	28	29	30	31	December
September	7	8	9	10	11	12	13	14	15	16	17	18	19	20	21	22	23	24	25	26	27	28	29	30	1	2	3	4	5	6	7	October

By the 36th week of pregnancy, the volume of your uterus is 1,000 times greater than it was before you conceived.

Multiple pregnancy

While 40 weeks tends to be the typical duration of a singleton pregnancy, women who are carrying more than one baby typically deliver a few weeks ahead of that. Twins usually make their debut at 36 weeks, triplets at 32 weeks, and quadruplets at 30 weeks. Some multiples arrive considerably earlier than that, of course, just as some singletons make an early appearance.

There are some theories as to why multiple pregnancies are likely to result in an earlier delivery:

The placentas of multiples tend to age more quickly and to function less efficiently, which is thought to directly or indirectly lead to a shorter gestation.

The uterus has its limits. Even though it's capable of expanding tremendously during pregnancy, it can only stretch so far. As Barbara Luke and Tamara Eberlein note in their book *When You're Expecting Twins, Triplets, or Quads,* "The combined weight of several babies, several placentas, and a whole lot of amniotic fluid eventually signals to the body that it's time for labor to start, no matter how much longer the calendar says pregnancy should continue. By the time she reaches 32 weeks, the uterus of a mother carrying twins is already as large as that of a singleton mom at the full 40 weeks. For the mother of triplets, the uterus is stretched to full-term size by 28 weeks. And with quadruplets on board, a woman's uterus reaches full-term size as early as 24 weeks."

Early Pregnancy Worries

If there's one thing you can say about pregnancy it's this: it's a great training ground for the worries of parenthood. And Mother Nature doesn't like to waste any time, which is why she jumps in with the worries right away—around the time the pregnancy test comes back positive. If you're not second-guessing all those crazy-making early pregnancy symptoms, wondering about what's normal and what's not; or worrying about your partner's reaction (or lack thereof) to The Big News; or freaking out about whether you're looking at a DIY delivery (since every doctor and midwife in town seems to be fully booked for the month you're due); then chances are you've moved on to one of the following early pregnancy worries.

I'm worried that I'll experience a miscarriage

If there's one concern that's pretty much universal among newly pregnant women, it's the fear of having a miscarriage. While the majority of pregnant women will

> *no pressure, mom*
>
> Think pregnant women today have a lot to worry about? A century ago our pregnant ancestors had to concern themselves not only with what they ate or drank, but also any immoral thoughts that happened to pass through their heads. The experts of the day told them in no uncertain terms that their every thought, word, and deed would have lasting effects on the developing fetus: "Low spirits, violent passions, irritability, frivolity, in the pregnant woman, leave indelible marks on the unborn child," warned B.G. Jeffris and J.L. Nichols in their best-selling 1893 family planning manual *Safe Counsel or Practical Eugenics.*

go on to have a healthy baby, a significant number of women—somewhere between 15 and 20 per cent of those whose pregnancies are confirmed by a positive pregnancy test—will have their hopes and dreams shattered.

Although it is easy to fixate on this figure, it's important to turn it on its head and look at it from the other perspective: you have an 80 to 85 per cent chance of *not* miscarrying. Yes, I know, it would be a lot more reassuring if those chances were somewhere in the neighbourhood of 100 per cent, but they're still pretty good odds nonetheless. I mean, if someone offered you a comparable crack at winning the lottery, you'd be lining up to buy a ticket in a flash.

The fact that some women experience spotting during their first trimester only adds to the worry about miscarriage. While it's only natural to panic if you have bleeding during pregnancy (even spotting that's so light it barely shows up on the toilet paper), in general, light bleeding is generally less worrisome than heavier bleeding accompanied by cramping or the passage of tissue.

Light spotting can be caused by cervical bleeding (for example, if your cervix got bumped during intercourse or started to bleed while your caregiver was performing an internal examination, because there's additional blood supply and blood flow to your cervix while you're pregnant) or by the passage of small amounts of uterine tissue (which occasionally happens in early pregnancy). It can also occur very early on in pregnancy—about seven days after conception—when the fertilized egg first attaches to the uterine wall. Note: Not all women experience this type of spotting, which is known as "implantation bleeding."

Because any amount of vaginal bleeding can be a sign of an impending miscarriage or an ectopic pregnancy (you should suspect the latter if you also experience abdominal pain, particularly abdominal pain which is worse on one side; light-headedness; and an urge to have a bowel movement), you'll want to report any spotting to your doctor or midwife as soon as possible. Your caregiver may want you to come in for a physical examination, a blood test, and/or an ultrasound to try to figure out if you are, in fact, miscarrying. Until you find out for sure what's going on, try not to hit the panic button. Many women who experience first-trimester bleeding end up giving birth to healthy babies eight or nine months down the road. (Less than half of the women who experience first-trimester bleeding actually miscarry.)

Here's something else you need to know about another worrying first-trimester symptom: it's not at all unusual to experience period-like cramping around the time that your first missed menstrual period was due. This cramping is simply your body's response to the hormonal changes of early pregnancy. As long as it isn't accompanied by any bleeding (one of the warning signs of miscarriage) or sharp pain limited to one side of your abdomen (one of the warning signs of an ectopic pregnancy), there's generally no cause for concern.

I don't feel pregnant anymore

After spending weeks coping with morning sickness, swollen breasts, and overwhelming fatigue—all the joys of early pregnancy—you wake up one morning to discover that all your pregnancy symptoms have disappeared. You can't decide whether to celebrate or to start freaking out.

While it's true that a sudden disappearance of pregnancy symptoms can indicate a missed miscarriage (in which the developing baby dies but is not immediately expelled from the mother's body), that's not the only reason your symptoms could have disappeared. They tend to spontaneously disappear around the end of the first trimester anyway.

If you're really concerned (a not-uncommon reaction if you've experienced miscarriages or other losses in the past and you're particularly anxious about this pregnancy), call your doctor or midwife to schedule an extra appointment. Your risk of experiencing a miscarriage drops significantly once your doctor or midwife is able to pick up your baby's heartbeat via ultrasound (something that can be performed transvaginally when you're just six weeks pregnant) or Doppler (a hand-held ultrasound device that can usually pick up the baby's heartbeat by the start of the second trimester). One study showed that your risk of experiencing a miscarriage drops to less than 2 per cent once your baby's heartbeat is detectable via ultrasound when you're 10 weeks pregnant.

CHAPTER 5

Operation Healthy Mother, Healthy Baby

The moment the sperm and the egg hooked up in the darkest recesses of your Fallopian tube, you signed on for a secret mission—a mission so secret, in fact, that for the first few weeks of your pregnancy, you didn't even know you'd been recruited.

Secret spy stuff aside, your mission over the next nine months is pretty straightforward: to do everything in your power to maximize your chances of enjoying a healthy pregnancy.

While doing everything by the book doesn't necessarily guarantee that you'll end up with a picture-perfect outcome, you're definitely putting the odds in your (and Baby's) favour.

The No-Worry Guide to Eating during Pregnancy

Sure, there are entire books written about the dos and don'ts of eating during pregnancy, but that doesn't mean prenatal nutrition has to be super-complicated, super-intimidating, or super-boring.

What you absolutely need to know can be summed up in one short paragraph. Eat two to three extra servings of food each day using

Canada's Food Guide to Healthy Eating as your blueprint. Increase your fluid intake by 50 per cent (from 8 glasses of water a day to 12 glasses a day). Take a multivitamin that's designed to meet the needs of pregnant women (one that has adequate iron and folic acid). Zero in on foods that are rich in iron, folic acid, calcium, vitamin D, and essential fatty acids. Gain the amount of weight that's right for you. And steer clear of foods that could make you and your baby seriously ill. (The immune system changes that go along with being pregnant leave you extra susceptible to food-borne illness right now.)

As you can see, there's no need to give your diet a major makeover (unless you know in your gut that it needs it). Nor is there any need to force down foods that you loathe or that simply have no appeal right now (the result of early pregnancy hormones affecting your senses of taste and smell) or that won't stay down anyway (if you're experiencing the nausea and vomiting of pregnancy that affects up to 80 per cent of pregnant women to varying degrees). That said, pregnancy may require a bit more nutritional planning for certain moms-to-be. Your health-care provider may recommend that you see a nutritionist or dietitian if

- you are following a specific diet as a result of allergies, food intolerances, diabetes, or digestive problems;
- you are vegetarian (you don't consume milk products or eggs, or any type of meat, fish, or poultry);
- you are pregnant with twins, triplets, or more babies;
- you are having difficulty eating due to nausea;
- you have a long-standing history of dieting and your body may be depleted of certain important nutrients;
- you are gaining weight very rapidly or you're not gaining weight at all;
- you are under 17 or over 35.

The basics

During pregnancy, you and your baby need a balanced diet that is made up of carbohydrates, proteins, fats, vitamins, minerals, and water. You can obtain these nutrients by choosing a variety of foods from each of the food groups in *Canada's Food Guide*: Vegetables and Fruit, Grain Products, Milk and Alternatives, and Meat and Alternatives.

Canada's Food Guide to Healthy Eating, which was updated in 2007, now takes into account the fact that Canadians come from many different cultural backgrounds and may want to choose a variety of different foods as a result. The new-and-improved guide can help you to make pregnancy-friendly choices while allowing you to eat in ways that feel comfortable and familiar to you. And while you're eating these comfortable foods during pregnancy, you'll be introducing your baby to these foods. Researchers believe that babies acquire culture-specific flavour preferences through amniotic fluid and later through breast milk. This helps to smooth the transition from life inside the womb to breast-feeding to solid food because Baby is already familiar with what's on the menu.

Visit www.myfoodguide.ca to find out more about *Canada's Food Guide* and to design a food guide that's right for you during pregnancy.

Dietary fibre

Your body's need for fibre jumps to 28 grams (1 ounce) per day during pregnancy—up from 20 to 25 grams (0.7 to 0.9 ounces) per day during your pre-pregnancy days. To avoid constipation (a problem for 11 per cent to 38 per cent of moms-to-be) you'll want to ensure that your diet is rich in dietary fibre (indigestible carbohydrates such as starchy vegetables, legumes, seeds, cereal grains, and whole-grain cereals). Dietary fibres help to produce bulkier and softer stools. Tip: Choose fibre-rich whole-grain products such as whole wheat bread, oatmeal, brown rice, whole-grain pasta, seeded rye, barley, quinoa, wheat berries, bulgur, millet, and kasha as opposed to instant grains and refined carbohydrates (cookies, soda pop, instant rice, and instant oatmeal) and you'll be amazed by how much better you feel. Just make sure you're matching that increased fibre intake with both fluids (12 cups, or 3 litres, of liquid per day, which can be in the form of water, milk, juice, or soups) and physical activity (unless your health-care provider advises otherwise).

Fruits and vegetables

It's time to set your inner fruit and vegetable goddess loose in the produce aisle if you haven't already. Dark and brightly coloured fruits and vegetables are your best bet, nutritionally speaking, because they are richer in vitamins and minerals. It's also a good idea to choose whole fruit rather than fruit juice so you can benefit from the added fibre, and fresh rather than canned produce, when you have the choice (many canned fruits have sugar added, and canned vegetables tend to be higher in salt).

Healthy fats

Your body needs a steady supply of healthy fats to help your baby grow. Fats play a particularly important role in the development of your baby's brain. Not all fats are good fats, however. You'll want to steer clear of trans fats (hydrogenated or partially hydrogenated fats) and to limit your consumption of saturated

salt?

In the past, sticking to a salt-free diet was a pregnancy rite of passage. Previous generations of women were told to restrict their salt intake during pregnancy in the name of minimizing edema (water retention), but we now know that doing so can actually make edema worse. While that kind of extreme regime is no longer the norm for most moms-to-be (thankfully), it's generally wise to avoid going wild with the salt shaker. Other ways to limit your salt intake during pregnancy include limiting your consumption of highly processed foods like packaged rice, soup, and pasta mixes; salty snacks; and salty seasonings.

fats (like butter, lard, whole milk dairy products, and high-fat meats such as sausage and bacon). If you don't eat fish, which is an excellent source of brain-friendly DHA (docosahexaenoic acid), try to work other sources of DHA such as walnuts, canola oil, flaxseed oil, or Omega-3 enriched eggs into your diet. See the section that follows for more about fish and essential fatty acids.

Meals and snacks that will go the distance

Including a protein source (eggs, meat, poultry, fish, tofu, beans, legumes, low-fat dairy products, nuts, peanut butter) with every meal and snack will give you the energy you need to get through your day and will help to stabilize your mood. And, speaking of meals and snacks, you should plan to have something to eat at least once every three hours throughout the day (every two hours if you're pregnant with twins). This will help to minimize nausea and keep you from getting too ravenous. Here are a few meal and snack ideas:

- pre-washed vegetables such as baby carrots, cauliflower, and broccoli with cheese cubes;
- low-fat cottage cheese teamed up with fresh vegetable sticks;
- bread sticks or crackers topped with hummus;
- pita pocket with vegetables, cheese, salsa, or hummus;
- low-fat yogourt with whole-grain cereal;
- peanut butter or soy butter spread on apple slices, a banana, or celery sticks.

Water

Water has an important role to play in keeping you healthy even when you're not pregnant. When you are pregnant, it works overtime, carrying nutrients to your body and your baby, flushing out waste products, keeping you cool, preventing constipation, and helping to control swelling. You'll know that you're consuming enough water (approximately 12 cups, or 3 litres, a day) if your urine is light in colour and you never get a chance to feel thirsty. You may find that drinking in between meals rather than during meals (or immediately before or after meals) helps to minimize nausea. If you find it tough to knock back all that water, consume some of your water in the form of low-fat milk or soup.

Don't cut down on fluids in an effort to minimize swelling. The more fluids you consume, the less fluid you're likely to retain. When you're becoming dehydrated, your body switches into conservation mode and tries to hold on to the fluids it has. The best way to wash away the problem is by consuming plenty of fluids. If that doesn't take care of the swelling, get in touch with your doctor or midwife.

Caffeinated beverages

Limit your consumption of caffeinated beverages. Caffeine is a diuretic, which means that it removes water from your body. Given that your body needs extra water when you're pregnant (12 cups or 3 litres a day as opposed to the usual 8 cups, or 2 litres), it's kind of counterproductive to be consuming caffeinated beverages—unless you don't mind pouring liquids in and flushing liquids out all day long. And then there's the fact that caffeine has a greater effect on the baby than it does on you. If caffeine leaves you feeling a little wired at times, it's having an even more powerful effect on your very tiny baby. While researchers tend to seesaw back and forth about the risks of consuming caffeine during pregnancy, the recommendations of leading health authorities tend to stay the same: limit coffee to no more than two 250-millilitre (8-ounce) cups per day. Whether coffee or tea even appeal to you is another matter. Some moms-to-be find that the mere thought of drinking their once-favourite beverage is enough to make them gag.

If you're missing your morning cup of comfort and you're looking for healthier alternatives, you might consider decaffeinated coffee (look for coffee that has been decaffeinated using a method that doesn't involve the use of chemicals), decaffeinated tea, or herbal teas that are believed to be safe for use during pregnancy (see note below). If you're craving a hot beverage that delivers more kick nutritionally, try heating up chocolate milk instead.

If you've got a serious diet pop habit, you may want to ease up on your favourite diet drink while you're pregnant. While there is no scientific evidence to prove that consuming moderate amounts of NutraSweet (aspartame), Splenda (sucralose), and other artificial sweeteners approved for use in foods in Canada is harmful to a pregnant woman or her baby, some women choose to err on the side of caution by avoiding these products during pregnancy. The only women who definitely have to steer clear of products containing aspartame are women with phenylketonuria (PKU)—a metabolic disorder. These products fill you up without providing any nutrients cautions the Dietitians of Canada. So, sure, have the occasional fix if you can't imagine nine and a half months without a glass of your beverage of choice, but don't consider your favourite diet drink to be a substitute for a more nutrient-rich beverage like a fruit-and-yogourt smoothie or a good old body-cleansing glass of water.

Talk to your doctor or midwife about the safety of various types of herbal teas before self-administering what can, in fact, be powerful medicinal products. While some studies have been conducted on the risks and benefits of certain herbal teas during pregnancy, there is still much to be learned, and caution should even be taken when consuming the following teas that are considered by Health Canada to be safe if consumed in moderation (500 to 750 millilitres, or 2 to 3 cups per day): citrus peel, ginger, lemon balm, linden flower (not recommended for anyone with a pre-existing cardiac condition), orange peel, or rose hip. If you have plant or pollen allergies, you should avoid any teas made from herbs related to plants to which you are allergic.

---

feeling irritable?

Becoming dehydrated doesn't just leave you feeling irritable. It can make your uterus irritable, too. And an irritable uterus (a uterus that is prone to non-productive contractions, which are contractions that don't result in the dilatation or effacement of your cervix) can make for an even more irritable you. If you become dehydrated and you notice that your uterus is contracting, drink two very large glasses of water. That should take care of the problem. If it doesn't, call your health-care provider. She will want to rule out the possibility of preterm labour (see Chapter 9).

The big five: The nutrients you need most during pregnancy

There are certain nutrients that tend to receive star billing during pregnancy because they have particularly key roles to play in orchestrating the mammoth changes that are going on inside your body. I'm talking about folic acid, iron, calcium, vitamin D, and essential fatty acids.

It can be difficult to meet your body's demands for all these nutrients through food sources alone. That's why Health Canada recommends that all women of child-bearing age take a folic acid supplement (containing at least 0.4 milligrams of folic acid) and that women who are pregnant or planning to become pregnant take a multivitamin containing at least 16 to 20 milligrams of iron as well.

Now let's zero in on each of these nutrients so that you can get a sense of what each one has to offer you and your baby, and how you can find ways to work them into your meals and snacks without turning your eating habits upside down.

Folic Acid

Function: Folic acid is needed for cell production and repair. It is needed to make DNA and RNA, the building blocks of cells. Folic acid also supports your expanding blood volume.

RDA during pregnancy: The recommended dietary allowance (RDA) for folic acid during pregnancy is 400 micrograms or higher, depending on your risk factors as assessed by your health-care provider.

Benefits: Folic acid reduces the risk of open neural tube defects, which occur if the neural tube fails to close properly during the 21st to 28th days following conception. The risk is reduced when you start taking a daily multivitamin containing folic acid three months before you conceive and continue to do so during at least the first month of pregnancy. Note: It's important to eat folate-rich foods in addition to consuming a folic acid supplement.

A number of studies show that taking multivitamins with folic acid also reduces the risk of other types of birth defects (cardiovascular and limb defects, cleft palate, oral cleft, congenital hydrocephalus, and urinary tract anomalies) and possibly even the risk of developing pre-eclampsia.

Taking folic acid in late pregnancy may also help to reduce the risk of preterm delivery and low birth weight.

Where to find it: You'll have to make a conscious effort to add folic acid to your diet. According to the Motherisk Clinic at the Hospital for Sick Children in Toronto, a typical woman of child-bearing age obtains just 0.2 milligrams per day from her diet.

Excellent sources, containing more than 0.055 milligrams of folic acid per serving, are cooked fava, kidney, pinto, roman, soy, and white beans, chickpeas, lentils, cooked spinach, asparagus, romaine lettuce, orange juice, canned pineapple juice, and sunflower seeds. Good sources (more than 0.033 milligrams per serving) are cooked lima beans, corn, bean sprouts, cooked broccoli, green peas, Brussels sprouts, beets, oranges, honeydew melons, raspberries, blackberries, avocados, roasted peanuts, and wheat germ. Other foods containing folic acid (0.011 milligrams or more) include cooked carrots, beet greens, sweet potatoes, snow peas, summer or winter squash, rutabaga, cabbage, cooked green beans, cashews, roasted peanuts, walnuts, eggs, strawberries, bananas, grapefruit, cantaloupe, whole wheat or white bread, pork kidney, breakfast cereals, and milk.

Notes/Tips: To increase the amount of folate (folic acid) in your diet, choose more servings of whole-grain and enriched grain products and dark green vegetables and legumes, and continue to take your prenatal vitamin or folic acid supplement (whichever your health-care provider recommends).

peanuts

Peanuts and peanut products are a good source of both protein and folic acid. They can also be a source of allergy concern for approximately 1 per cent of the population. If you or your partner has a strong family history of food allergies or other major allergies such as asthma, atopic dermatitis, or allergic rhinitis, talk to your health-care provider about whether peanuts or peanut products are a good choice for you during pregnancy. Some research has indicated that babies with an increased risk of allergies may be adversely affected by prenatal exposure to peanuts or peanut products.

Iron

Function: Iron is an essential item in proteins such as enzymes and hemoglobin. Almost two-thirds of the iron in the body is taken up by the hemoglobin used to circulate red blood cells. Hemoglobin transports oxygen to tissues and cells.

RDA during pregnancy: Your iron needs increase as your pregnancy progresses. You will need more iron during the second and third trimesters than you did during the first trimester.

The RDA for iron during pregnancy is 27 milligrams per day. The RDA is set at a level that allows women to start storing iron early on in pregnancy. That way, they can build up a reserve of the iron they'll need to take them through their third trimester.

Eating according to *Canada's Food Guide* and taking a daily multivitamin that has 16 to 20 milligrams of iron will meet the iron needs of most pregnant women, but some women may need more iron than others. Talk to your health-care provider to find out how much iron is right for you.

Benefits: Consuming adequate iron during pregnancy helps to ward off fatigue, prevent cardiovascular stress, and maintain your resistance to infection. It also prevents your baby from becoming anemic. Fetal anemia can lead to premature birth and low birth weight. It can also result in a baby being born with serious, even life-threatening complications.

Where to find it: We are able to obtain iron from two types of food sources: animal sources (so-called "heme iron") and plant sources ("non-heme iron"). Most of the iron we eat is in the non-heme form. About 60 per cent of the iron found in meat, poultry, and fish is in the non-heme form, with the other 40 per cent being in the heme form. The iron found in eggs and plant-based foods, such as legumes, vegetables, fruit, grains, nuts, and iron-fortified grain products, is only in the non-heme form. Heme iron can provide up to one-third of the total dietary iron that the body absorbs.

Excellent non-heme sources of iron (3.5 milligrams per serving or more) are cooked beans, white beans, soybeans, lentils, and chickpeas; clams and oysters; pumpkin, sesame, and squash seeds; and iron-enriched breakfast cereals. Good heme sources of iron (2.1 milligrams per serving or more) are ground beef or steak and blood pudding, and good non-heme sources are canned lima beans, red kidney beans, split peas, enriched cooked egg noodles, and dried apricots.

Other foods containing heme iron (0.7 milligrams per serving or more) include chicken, ham, lamb, pork, veal, halibut, haddock, perch, salmon, shrimp, canned sardines, tuna, and eggs. Other non-heme sources are peanuts, pecans, walnuts, pistachios, roasted almonds, roasted cashews, sunflower seeds, cooked egg noodles, bread, pumpernickel bagels, bran muffins, cooked oatmeal, wheat germ, canned beans (drained), canned pumpkin, raisins, peaches, prunes, and apricots.

Notes/Tips: Your iron needs double when you're pregnant. Your blood volume has increased, you are supporting your baby as well as the placenta, and your body is stockpiling iron in anticipation of blood loss that occurs at the time of birth.

During the third trimester, your baby starts to draw upon your iron stores so he can stockpile enough iron to carry him through the first six months of life. At that point, he'll be ready to start making the transition to solid foods.

You'll maximize absorption of your iron supplement by taking it on an empty stomach (or with a glass of orange juice), but you may find that it's too hard to handle that way when you're pregnant. If that's the case, take it with foods that are known to enhance the absorption of iron rather than to inhibit it. (See below.)

To boost your iron intake, choose more servings of meats and alternatives, as well as whole-grain and enriched grain products. As noted above, iron from animal sources is more readily absorbed than non-heme iron from plant-based foods.

To maximize non-heme iron absorption from foods, combine foods that are rich in non-heme iron with foods that are rich in vitamin C, which enhances iron absorption. The effect is strongest when foods containing vitamin C are eaten with foods containing high levels of non-heme iron inhibitors. For instance, a glass of orange juice can help minimize the effect of phytate in breakfast cereal and calcium in milk.

Polyphenols from tea and coffee; phytate from legumes and certain vegetables, unrefined rice, and grains; certain proteins found in soybeans; and calcium at levels greater than 300 milligrams interfere with the absorption of non-heme iron. Calcium inhibits the absorption of both types of iron (heme and non-heme). Furthermore, non-heme iron competes with other metals (zinc, copper) for transfer across the gut.

Don't take a calcium supplement or calcium-containing antacids with meals. Too much calcium can interfere with iron absorption. If the supplement is taken one to two hours after a meal, you won't experience the same problem.

Meat, fish, and poultry can also improve non-heme absorption. Even modest amounts of these foods can improve the absorption of non-heme iron in a meal.

Drink tea or coffee one to two hours between meals rather than with meals as these drinks can interfere with iron absorption.

---

iron deficiency

Iron deficiency is quite common during pregnancy. You're more likely to be low on this important nutrient if

- you're carrying more than one baby;
- you're pregnant for the third or subsequent time (particularly if those pregnancies were spaced closely together);
- your diet is low in meat, fish, poultry, or vitamin C;
- you're in the habit of drinking tea or coffee close to mealtime—something that can interfere with the absorption of iron;
- you take acetylsalicylic acid (ASA) or other non-steroidal anti-inflammatory drugs on a regular basis;
- you have a history of heavy menstrual bleeding or your iron stores were depleted prior to pregnancy for other reasons;
- you're involved in endurance sports (which contribute to iron loss through sweat) or marathon running (which contributes to iron loss through the breaking down of blood cells);
- you give blood three or more times each year.

Calcium

Function: Calcium aids with muscle contractions, blood vessel expansion and contraction, the secretion of hormones and enzymes, and the transmission of impulses throughout the nervous system. It also maintains your bones and provides for the development of your baby's skeletal system.

RDA during pregnancy: The RDA for calcium ranges from 700 milligrams to 1,300 milligrams per day. Pregnant and nursing women really don't need more calcium than their non-pregnant and non-lactating counterparts because their bodies are much more efficient at absorbing and making use of calcium.

Benefits: Taking calcium helps to reduce the risk of pre-eclampsia and fetal lead poisoning (because calcium reduces the amount of lead circulating in the mother). It helps to bring down blood pressure in both the mother and the baby.

Where to find it: Excellent sources (275 milligrams per serving or more) are milk, Swiss cheese, tofu set with calcium sulphate, plain yogourt, whole sesame seeds, and fortified plant-based beverages. Good sources (165 milligrams per serving or more) are cheeses such as mozzarella, cheddar, edam, brick, parmesan, gouda, feta, processed cheese slices, and processed cheese spread; flavoured yogourt; canned sardines; and canned salmon (including bones). Other foods containing calcium (55 milligrams per serving or more) include creamed cottage cheese, ricotta cheese, cooked or canned legumes (such as beans), cooked bok choy, kale, turnip greens, mustard greens, broccoli, oranges, cooked scallops, cooked oysters, almonds, and dried sunflower seeds.

Notes/Tips: Calcium absorption increases when you are consuming adequate amounts of vitamin D. But, the more calcium you consume at one time, the less efficiently it is absorbed.

To boost your calcium intake, choose more servings from the milk products food group or try adding milk powder to recipes (7 tbsp, or 100 grams, of powdered milk contains as much calcium as 1 cup, or 235 millilitres of fluid milk) or use milk when you're making soup. You can also obtain calcium by consuming fortified orange juice, eating sardines, or taking a calcium supplement.

Weight-bearing activities like walking can help your body to store more calcium, provided that such activities are performed at least three times per week. Smoking, leading a sedentary lifestyle, and consuming too much protein, salt, or caffeine interfere with the body's ability to store calcium.

Vitamin D

Function: Vitamin D helps to improve calcium and phosphorus absorption. It also plays a role in cell metabolism, the regulation of cell growth, and immunity. Vitamin D deficiency has been linked to reduced fetal weight gain; osteoporosis; asthma; autoimmune diseases such as rheumatoid arthritis, multiple sclerosis, and inflammatory bowel diseases; diabetes; impaired muscle function; reduced resistance to tuberculosis; and an increased risk of developing specific types of cancer.

RDA during pregnancy: For most people, the RDA for vitamin D is 600 IU per day.

Benefits: Your supply of vitamin D during pregnancy is important for the long-term health of your baby. Reduced bone density in 9-year-old children, the severity of asthma in 3-year-old children, and susceptibility to type 1 diabetes have been linked to low vitamin D status during fetal life. Studies also suggest that infants of mothers who were vitamin D or calcium deficient during pregnancy may be at risk for enamel defects in primary and permanent teeth in spite of adequate supplementation later.

---

lactose

If you're following a lactose-free diet because you have difficulty digesting the sugar in milk, you may find that you're able to digest small servings of dairy products while you're pregnant. Some studies have shown that pregnancy improves a woman's ability to digest lactose.

If, however, you continue to have difficulty digesting lactose, you'll need to focus on obtaining calcium from as many non-milk food sources as possible: tofu, calcium-fortified bread or juice, dark green leafy vegetables, sardines, salmon, and so on.

Here are some other ways to cope with lactose intolerance during pregnancy:

- Look for lactose-free dairy products and tablets or drops that can help you to process the lactose in milk.
- Try eating yogourt that contains acidophilus (active cultures that can actually aid in the digestion of lactose).
- Try drinking milk at mealtime rather than on its own—something that can help to eliminate some people's lactose-intolerance problems.
- Stick to very small servings of dairy products that are naturally low in lactose, like aged cheese (not fresh, processed, or cottage cheese) or yogourt. You might even try drinking a small serving of milk. The smaller the serving, the less likely you are to run into problems.
- Take a lactose-free calcium supplement. They're an inexpensive source of calcium that can be easily digested by lactose-intolerant people looking to boost their calcium intake.

Where to find it: Excellent sources of vitamin D are evaporated milk, fortified soy beverages, margarine, and fatty fish such as salmon. Good sources include egg yolks.

Notes/Tips: Vitamin D is obtained from food and produced by the skin when the skin is exposed to sunlight of sufficient intensity. Obtaining 30 to 40 minutes of sunlight exposure to the face and arms is the best way of obtaining your recommended daily amount of vitamin D. (The usual advice about timing your exposure to avoid the risk of sunburn and excessive exposure to harmful UV rays, and using sunscreen even though its effect on vitamin D absorption is not yet known, still applies.) Because getting your vitamin D from the sun is not possible for much of the year in Canada, or practical if you're juggling work and family responsibilities, there's a nutritional Plan B: supplementing with 600 IU of vitamin D.

---

milk and vitamin D

Women who restrict their milk intake during pregnancy in an effort to avoid gaining too much weight or to prevent their babies from developing allergies (only an issue for 1 per cent of mothers) significantly reduce their intake of a key pregnancy nutrient—vitamin D—and tend to give birth to lighter babies. This was the key finding of a McGill University study reported in the *Canadian Medical Association Journal* in April 2006. If a woman is restricting her milk intake, it's important that she increase her intake of vitamin D from other sources, the researchers emphasized.

Essential Fatty Acids

Function: Omega-6 and Omega-3 fatty acids play a key role in brain development and visual function.

RDA during pregnancy: Not established.

Benefits: Women who consume adequate amounts of DHA (one of the most important Omega-3 fatty acids found in fish oil) during pregnancy are less likely to experience a preterm delivery or give birth to a low birth weight baby. And mothers with a history of postpartum depression may be able to minimize symptoms of depression following subsequent births by taking DHA supplements during subsequent pregnancies.

Where to find it: Include sources of essential fatty oils such as soybean, canola, grapeseed, and flaxseed oils; non-hydrogenated margarines; soy-based

---

fish

Fish is an excellent source of high-quality protein, it's low in saturated fat, and it provides significant amounts of Omega-3 fats and other essential nutrients, such as vitamin D, zinc, and iron. Some studies have demonstrated that pregnancy lasts longer (giving a baby more time to develop and grow) and child neurodevelopment scores are higher when mothers eat fish during pregnancy. On the other hand, eating fish can result in the baby being exposed to harmful toxins like methyl mercury or PCBs. So what's a pregnant woman to do?

fish (continued)

- Consume fish in moderation, according to the International Institutes of Medicine, which concluded in a 2007 review that the benefits of eating fish are greater than the benefits of not eating fish, provided that women choose the recommended types and amounts. Here's a summary of those recommendations, as adapted by Health Canada:
  - Continue eating at least 150 grams (5.5 ounces) of cooked fish each week during pregnancy, as recommended in *Canada's Food Guide*.
  - Choose types of fish that generally have low levels of contaminants, such as salmon, trout, herring, haddock, canned light tuna, pollock (Boston bluefish), sole, flounder, anchovy, char, hake, mullet, smelt, Atlantic mackerel, and lake white fish.
  - Choose fish such as char, herring, mackerel, salmon, sardines, and trout which are high in Omega-3 fatty acids.
  - Limit your intake of tuna (fresh and frozen), shark, swordfish, marlin, orange roughy, and escolar to no more than 150 grams (5.5 ounces) per month, and your intake of canned (white) albacore tuna to no more than 300 grams (10.5 ounces) per week. Note: This advice does not apply to canned light tuna. Canned light tuna contains other species of tuna such as skipjack, yellowfin, and tongol, which are low in mercury. Pregnant women do not have to limit the amount they eat of these types of canned tuna.
  - Fish obtained through recreational activities are not covered by federal food safety regulations, and PCBs can be a concern in addition to mercury if you eat fish like trout, salmon, or bass that are caught through sport fishing. Some studies have indicated that prenatal exposure to high levels of PCBs can result in low birth weight, decreased IQ, and learning difficulties. Many provinces monitor wild foods, particularly sports fish and wild game, for signs of chemical contamination and issue bulletins advising the public about their findings. Contact your provincial or territorial ministries of health and natural resources to inquire about the availability of such information in your jurisdiction.
  - If you never eat fish and you are wondering what else you can do to work DHA into your diet during pregnancy, think eggs rather than fish supplements. According to Health Canada, fish oil supplements should not be considered equivalent to eating fish. Chickens are quite efficient at converting ALA (alpha-linolenic acid) to DHA and therefore Omega-3 eggs can contribute significant amounts of DHA to the diet. If you do decide to take a fish oil supplement, look for a Natural Product Number (NPN) on the product label. This proves that the fish oil supplement has been government approved for safety, efficacy (potential therapeutic benefit), and quality. Note: Don't take cod liver oil during pregnancy, particularly if you are already taking a multivitamin supplement. You could end up consuming too much vitamin A, something that increases the risk of birth defects.

products (tofu or veggie burgers, for example); and salad dressings made from non-hydrogenated oils such as canola or soybean oils in your diet. Limit your intake of fried foods, higher fat commercial bakery products, and snack foods. Essential fatty oils such as DHA are found in fatty fish such as salmon, mackerel, and sardines.

Notes/Tips: Western diets are relatively rich in Omega-6 fatty acids, but low in Omega-3. Marine foods such as fish are a good source of Omega-3 fatty acids. (Omega-3 fatty acids from fish inhibit prostaglandins and related compounds that are involved in cervical ripening and the subsequent triggering of labour.)

The supporting cast: other key nutrients

Here's the lowdown on some other important nutrients—both vitamins and minerals—that also play a key role during pregnancy.

Note: Don't exceed the recommended daily allowance of vitamins and minerals per day. Large doses of certain types of vitamins—particularly vitamin A—can be harmful to the developing baby. This is one of those situations in which more is definitely not better.

Vitamin A

Function: Vitamin A is necessary for immune function, vision, the reproductive system, and genes.

RDA during pregnancy: 770 micrograms per day.

Benefits: Vitamin A plays a role in determining infant size and the length of pregnancy. It also supports the development of the embryo.

Where to find it: Sources are vegetables, fruit, and liver.

Notes/Tips: Too little vitamin A can result in decreased birth weight or congenital abnormalities. Too much can result in birth defects such as cleft lip or cleft palate, and abnormalities of the central nervous system, heart, and thymus.

---

liver

Liver is another one of those nutrient-rich foods that needs to be consumed in small quantities. It's full of iron and folic acid, and it is the single largest food source of vitamin A. That's why there's cause for concern: a 85-gram (3-ounce) serving of beef liver contains 12 times the recommended daily allowance of vitamin A. A 1995 study found that women who consumed four times the recommended daily dose during the first two months of pregnancy were twice as likely to give birth to a baby with birth defects.

Vitamin B12

Function: Vitamin B12 aids in red blood cell formation and in brain and nervous system function.

RDA during pregnancy: 2.6 micrograms per day.

Benefits: The B12 you ingest crosses your placenta to help in the development of your baby's brain and spinal cord.

Where to find it: Vitamin B12 is naturally found in animal products—meat, poultry, fish, eggs, milk, and milk products—and is added to fortified breakfast cereals.

Notes/Tips: A vitamin B12 deficiency increases the risk of abnormalities in the baby, including neural tube defects.

Vitamin C

Function: Vitamin C enhances iron absorption, recycles vitamin E, and performs other important body maintenance functions.

RDA during pregnancy: 85 micrograms per day.

Benefits: An adequate consumption of vitamins C and E is linked with a reduced risk of pre-eclampsia in at-risk women. Vitamin C deficiency is associated with an increased risk of premature rupture of membranes (PROM) and infection.

Where to find it: Vegetables like baked potatoes, tomatoes, peppers, and broccoli, and citrus fruits, strawberries, and kiwis.

Notes/Tips: Women who smoke or who are under a lot of stress may benefit from additional vitamin C.

Choline

Function: Choline promotes brain development and memory function during the early years of life.

RDA during pregnancy: 450 milligrams per day.

Benefits: Sufficient choline in your diet may reduce the risk of neural tube defects.

Where to find it: A single egg provides roughly half of the recommended daily intake of choline during pregnancy. Other places to turn for this brainy nutrient include beef and chicken liver.

Notes/Tips: Choline deficiency is related to pre-eclampsia, premature birth, and low birth weight.

Iodine

Function: Iodine is a component of the thyroid hormone, which regulates your body's metabolic rate.

RDA during pregnancy: 220 micrograms per day.

Benefits: Your intake of iodine is necessary for the healthy development of your baby's brain, as well as her thyroid function after she's born.

Where to find it: Sources of iodine are seafood, seaweed, and iodized salt.

Notes/Tips: An iodine deficiency affects maternal and fetal thyroid function. Severe deficiencies can lead to low birth weight, preterm birth, congenital abnormalities, miscarriage, stillbirth, and perinatal and infant death.

Magnesium

Function: Magnesium strengthens your bones and your immune system, allows your nerves and muscles to function normally, allows your bowels to function regularly, and regulates your heart rhythm.

RDA during pregnancy: 350 milligrams per day for women 30 years of age and under; 360 milligrams per day for women over 30 years of age.

Benefits: Magnesium plays a role in developing your baby's bones, cartilage, teeth, and ears.

Where to find it: Dark leafy greens and roasted nuts are excellent sources of magnesium. Whole grains and legumes are also good sources.

Notes/Tips: A magnesium deficit can lead to pregnancy-induced hypertension (PIH), preterm labour triggered by uterine hyper-irritability, and fetal growth abnormalities.

Zinc

Function: Zinc helps the body with immune function, protein synthesis, wound healing, DNA synthesis, and cell division.

RDA during pregnancy: 11 micrograms per day.

Benefits: Zinc supports healthy growth and development. Zinc deficiency is associated with an increased risk of congenital anomalies (including neural tube defects) as well as other pregnancy and birth complications.

Where to find it: Zinc is naturally present in some foods (oysters, red meat, poultry, beans, nuts, crab, lobster, whole grains, and dairy products), added to others, and available as a dietary supplement.

Notes/Tips: The body doesn't have any way of storing zinc, so you need a steady intake of this mineral.

Iron may affect zinc absorption, although iron-fortified foods don't have a significant impact on zinc absorption. Also, taking iron supplements between meals helps decrease iron's effect on zinc absorption.

High zinc intake can inhibit copper absorption, sometimes producing copper deficiency and associated anemia.

Vegetarian and vegan diets

Vegetarian eating has become so popular—and you may be feeling so healthy—that you may not even recognize the fact that you need to consider some special issues if you're following a vegetarian (semi-vegetarian, pollo-vegetarian, pesco-vegetarian, lacto-ovo-vegetarian, or ovo-vegetarian) or vegan diet during pregnancy. Here are the key points to keep in mind.

Your body requires extra protein when you're pregnant—enough to support your baby's rapid growth and development. This can be as simple as adding nuts and seeds to salads, cooking with lentils, or working additional tofu into meals.

If you don't eat meat, you may need to make a special effort to ensure you're obtaining adequate quantities of vitamins B12, B2, and D, calcium, iron, and zinc. Your iron needs nearly double when you are pregnant. Combine iron-rich foods with foods that are rich in vitamin C. (See earlier section on iron for more specific advice.) You may also want to ask your health-care provider to recommend a vitamin B12 supplement and to check your hemoglobin regularly to ensure you aren't becoming anemic. Note: If you consume a lot of foods that inhibit iron absorption (tea, coffee, and calcium) and if you avoid all foods of animal origin, you may find it helpful to consult with a dietitian.

Ensure that you're getting enough calcium, which is important for your health and for the creation of healthy bones and teeth in your developing baby. If you don't drink milk, try soy, rice, and almond beverages that are fortified with vitamins A, D, B12, riboflavin, as well as calcium and zinc; or orange juice with added calcium.

a question of timing

It's important to eat well throughout pregnancy. You want your baby to receive a steady flow of nutrients during all the key stages of development. If nutritional deficiencies occur early in pregnancy, brain growth and development may be compromised; if they occur later in pregnancy, lung growth may be affected. Whenever nutritional deficiencies reach a critical point, oxygen and nutrients are directed to the baby's brain at the expense of other organ and body systems.

Continue to take a folic acid supplement in addition to eating a diet that's rich in folate (spinach, legumes, and orange juice).

Not wanted at the dinner table: Avoiding food-borne illness

Your immune system has to make some accommodations in order to allow your body to play host to your baby and your baby's various support systems during the nine months of pregnancy. In the overall scheme of things, this is good. Miraculous, actually. But it does have its downsides at times, one of them being that these immune system changes leave you more susceptible to food-borne illness (a.k.a. food poisoning). It's not a huge deal, once you're aware of this fact and know which foods to avoid. That's what this next section is about.

The two main offenders

Food-borne illness is a concern to everyone these days, but two particular types of food-borne illnesses pose a specific threat during pregnancy: listeriosis (caused by the bacterium *Listeria monocytogenes*), which can be found in certain types of soft cheeses, ready-to-eat meats, and unpasteurized milk, and which is capable of surviving in cold temperatures; and toxoplasmosis (caused by the parasite *Toxoplasma gondii*), which can occur if raw or undercooked meat is eaten or other contaminated raw foods are eaten, or if the parasite is contracted through the handling of contaminated soil or kitty litter (see tips below). The symptoms of both listeriosis and toxoplasmosis are similar: nausea, vomiting, stomach cramps, diarrhea, and fever. If you have listeriosis and it spreads to your nervous system, you may also develop a headache, a stiff neck, confusion, a loss of balance, or convulsions.

Listeriosis. According to the Centers for Disease Control and Prevention, listeriosis occurs 20 times as often in pregnant women as in other healthy adults. You don't have to be exhibiting signs of listeriosis for your baby to be affected: sometimes the illness is transmitted to the baby via the placenta without the mother exhibiting any symptoms of illness at all. When the illness is diagnosed (via a blood test), antibiotics are given to the mother (during or after pregnancy) or the newborn or both. If left untreated, listeriosis can lead to premature birth, miscarriage, or stillbirth, or it can cause pneumonia, septicemia (a bacterial blood infection), or meningitis in a newborn baby. Note: If you've previously experienced a miscarriage or other loss because of exposure to listeriosis during pregnancy, this is unlikely to occur in a subsequent pregnancy. Researchers believe that past exposure to listeriosis provides some measure of immunity against the disease.

To reduce your risk of contracting listeriosis, avoid

- soft cheeses such as Feta, brie, Camembert, Roquefort, blue-veined, queso blanco, queso fresco, or queso panela unless the package specifically states that the cheese was made with pasteurized milk;
- refrigerated pâté or meat spreads (as opposed to canned pâtés, which are designed for a longer shelf life);
- refrigerated smoked seafood, unless it has been thoroughly cooked (and consume it promptly because *Listeria* thrives at refrigerator temperature);
- hot dogs and deli meats (including ham, turkey, and salami), unless they have been reheated until they are steaming hot;
- raw (unpasteurized) milk or foods containing raw milk.

Toxoplasmosis. If you develop toxoplasmosis during pregnancy, you have a 50 per cent chance of passing it on to your baby. While antibiotic treatment can reduce the severity of symptoms in the newborn, toxoplasmosis can have a devastating impact on the developing baby. Many babies who are born with toxoplasmosis develop eye infections, enlarged livers and spleens, jaundice (yellowing of the skin and eyes), and pneumonia. Some experience seizures, severe vision loss, cerebral palsy, developmental problems, and other difficulties.

To reduce your risk of contracting toxoplasmosis, keep the following things in mind:

- Don't eat raw or undercooked meat, and wash your hands with soap and water right after handling raw meat.
- Aside from eating undercooked meat, the other key source of toxoplasmosis is cat feces—an important point to bear in mind if you have a cat (ask someone else to change the kitty litter) or if you enjoy gardening (wear gloves). To reduce the risk of kitty bringing unwanted parasites into your home, avoid feeding your cat raw or undercooked meat.

Other foods to avoid

Listeriosis and toxoplasmosis aren't the only bacteria that can get a mom-to-be into trouble. They're just the two main offenders. Here's a quick run-through of the other types of foods you should plan to avoid during pregnancy, along with the lowdown on their bacterial accomplices:

Foods that are made from raw or undercooked eggs. One in 20 eggs contains salmonella (a bacterium that can lead to the food-borne illness known as salmonellosis), so cook your eggs thoroughly and avoid eating foods that are made with raw or undercooked eggs, like eggnog, Caesar salad, and hollandaise sauce, until after Baby arrives.

Sushi and other raw fish (especially shellfish such as oysters and clams).
Shellfish may be contaminated with raw sewage, which can lead to severe gastrointestinal illness. Cook fish thoroughly, so that you can kill off any disease-causing bacteria or parasites.

Raw sprouts and unpasteurized juices. Raw vegetable sprouts (including alfalfa sprouts and radishes) and unpasteurized fruit and vegetables juices may be super-healthy, but they can also be loaded with bacteria (including salmonella and E. coli), which could cause you to become seriously ill. If you were to pass the bacterial infection on to your developing baby, you could end up with a very sick newborn—a baby suffering from diarrhea, a fever, and possibly even meningitis.

Improperly canned or preserved food. These may lead to botulism, a muscle-paralyzing disease caused by a toxin made by the bacterium *Clostridium botulinum*. Canned foods need to be heated long enough and to high enough temperatures to kill spores that can otherwise grow and produce the toxin. If something goes wrong during the canning or food preservation process (home or commercial), bacteria can grow inside the containers. If you open up a can of food from the store (or a jar of pickles from Aunt Jen) and the contents look more toxic than tasty, odds are that's what's happened.

Raw or undercooked meat or poultry. These can cause a plethora of food-borne illnesses, including listeriosis, toxoplasmosis, E. coli, campylobacter infections, and salmonella. To reduce the risk of food contamination and food-borne illness, follow these guidelines.

- Keep it clean—your hands and your cooking area. That means washing your hands thoroughly with soap and water before, during, and after handling food, and thoroughly disinfecting all food preparation surfaces before and after you work with food. All food surfaces should be disinfected using household bleach.
- Wash all raw fruits and vegetables thoroughly before serving.
- Keep raw and cooked foods separate, to avoid cross-contamination. (Just one drop of juice from raw chicken meat can lead to campylobacteriosis,

a nasty form of food-borne illness that is characterized by cramping, fever, nausea, vomiting, and bloody diarrhea.)

- Know how to cook and store various types of foods (and at what temperature).
- Refrigerate or freeze foods promptly after eating.
- Check the temperature of your refrigerator. It should be below 4°C (39°F).
- Keep your refrigerator clean. The warmer and dirtier your fridge gets, the more readily bacteria will thrive.
- Pay attention to the best-before dates on foods. Go through your fridge on a regular basis so that you can use up foods while they are still at their best (as opposed to pitching them out when they are past their prime).
- If in doubt, throw it out. Take advantage of your heightened sense of smell during pregnancy. If a food smells like it may have gone bad, err on the side of caution. Don't play food-poisoning roulette.

Your Pregnancy Gain Plan

Everyone knows that weight gain is part of the pregnancy package, along with the possibility of stretch marks. But what you might not realize is just how much weight gain you should be shooting for and why. That's because there's no such thing as a one-size-fits-all pregnancy "gain" plan—nor should there be. After all, if you glance around the waiting room at your midwife's clinic or doctor's office, you'll see that there's no such thing as a one-size-fits-all pregnant woman.

Weight gain during Pregnancy

There are so many messages out there warning us about the horrors of gaining weight that it can take a bit of time to do the mental mind switch required to embrace the physical changes of pregnancy—a time in your life when gaining a healthy amount of weight is a good thing.

The recommendations for weight gain during pregnancy for Canadian women changed in 2009, when Health Canada decided to adopt the brand new guidelines that had just been introduced by the U.S.-based Institutes of Medicine. The new guidelines specify target ranges for weight gain, based on pre-pregnancy body mass index (BMI), and a recommended rate of weight gain per week during the second and third trimesters. It is assumed that all women, regardless of pre-pregnancy BMI, will gain 1.1 to 4.4 pounds (0.5 to 2.0 kilograms) during the first trimester The guidelines also specify target ranges for weight gain for some, but not all, mothers who are expecting multiples.

Of course, not every pregnant woman manages to gain weight in this prescribed fashion. You may end up losing rather than gaining weight during the first trimester if you're experiencing a particularly nasty bout of morning sickness. And, as your pregnancy progresses into the second and third trimesters, you may find there are some weeks when you gain 2 or 3 pounds (1 to 1.5 kilograms) and others when you don't manage to gain any weight at all. What matters is the overall pattern of your weight gain—that you're slowly but surely gaining weight as your belly begins to blossom.

How much food you need during pregnancy will be determined by your activity level and your pre-pregnancy weight. Plan healthy meals and snacks based on *Canada's Food Guide to Healthy Eating* and pay attention to your body's hunger and fullness signals, as opposed to following any rigid pregnancy eating plan that may or may not meet your body's need for food.

5.1 Weight Gain during Pregnancy		
Pre-pregnancy BMI Category	**Recommended rate of weight gain (per week) during the 2nd and 3rd trimesters**	**Recommended total range of weight gain during pregnancy**
Underweight BMI <18.5	1.0 lb/week 0.5 kg/week	28–40 lbs 12.5–18 kg
Normal weight BMI 18.5–24.9	1.0 lb/week 0.4 kg/week	25–35 lbs 11.5–16 kg
Overweight BMI 25.0–29.9	0.6 lb/week 0.3 kg/week	15–25 lbs 7–11.5 kg
Obese BMI ≧30	0.5 lb/week 0.2 kg/week	At least 15 lbs 7 kg

Notes:

- Calculations assume a total of 1.1–4.4 lbs (0.5–2.0 kg) of weight gain in the first trimester.
- A narrower range of weight gain may be advised for women with a pre-pregnancy BMI of 35 or greater. Consult with your health-care provider if you fall into this category.
- Health Canada offers the following weight gain advice to women who are expecting twins: "The 2009 Institute of Medicine (IOM) report titled *Weight Gain During Pregnancy: Reexamining the Guidelines* provides provisional guidelines for women carrying twins: normal-weight women should gain between 37–54 lbs (17 and 25 kg), overweight women, between 31–50 lbs (14 and 23 kg) and obese women, between 25–42 lbs (11 and 19 kg) . . . Based on the IOM review of evidence, there is insufficient information available to develop guidelines for underweight women carrying twins and for women carrying more than two fetuses." The Society of Obstetricians and Gynecologists of Canada (SOGC) recommends a weight gain of 35 to 45 lbs (16 to 20.5 kg) with a twin pregnancy.
- You can calculate your BMI using this formula (BMI = weight(kg)/height(m)^2) or use the BMI calculator available on the Health Canada website: www.hc-sc.gc.ca/fn-an/nutrition/prenatal/bmi/index-eng.php

Source: Canadian Gestational Weight Gain Recommendations, Health Canada, 2009.

Healthy eating during pregnancy doesn't have to be a nine-month exercise in deprivation. Sure, this is one time in your life when you might want to kick your doughnut-for-breakfast habit. And it goes without saying that you shouldn't be trying to live on decaf coffee and doughnuts alone. Each of these foods can be enjoyed in moderation, provided you're also consuming ample quantities of healthier foods. What you want to do is find the sensible middle ground between deprivation and overindulgence. (The deprivation mindset can put you on the fast track to Binge Avenue, while overindulgence can quickly snowball into unhealthy weight gain.) Learning to guesstimate portion sizes (and relating those portion sizes back to *Canada's Food Guide*) is a valuable first step.

It takes approximately 80,000 extra calories to grow a baby. To ensure that your body is getting enough food to meet your baby's needs, you should plan to increase your intake by 100 calories per day during the first trimester and 300 calories per day during the second and third trimesters. If you're planning to breastfeed, you'll need even more food after your baby arrives: an extra 450 calories per day.

Of course, if you're particularly active or your metabolism is very high, this still may not be enough food for you and your baby. And if you're quite overweight and you're trying to keep your weight gain at the low end of the recommended range for your pre-pregnancy BMI (see Table 2.1 on page 25), you may not need this many extra calories per day. You may have to experiment a little until you figure out how much food your body requires to gain weight at a slow but steady pace.

5.2 Where the Weight Goes

Here's what your body does with a 35-pound (15-kilogram) pregnancy weight gain (which is typical for a normal-weight woman):

Baby	7.7 lb (3.5 kg)*
Breasts	1.1 lb (0.5 kg)
Maternal stores of fat, protein, and other nutrients	9.1 lb (4.2 kg)
Placenta	1.6 lb (0.7 kg)
Uterus	2.4 lb (1.1 kg)
Amniotic fluid	2.0 lb (0.9 kg)
Blood	5.0 lb (2.3 kg)
Body fluids	6.1 lb (2.8 kg)

* This figure is based on the weights of male Canadian newborns born between 38 and 42 weeks of pregnancy. Female babies tend to weigh slightly less.

Too much of a good thing

It's possible to get a little too enthusiastic about the weight gain during pregnancy thing (to forget that you're eating for someone who will, at term, weigh 8 pounds (3.5 kilograms) or so—not another full-sized adult).

Health-care experts have always known that gaining too much weight during pregnancy could be a problem, but, in recent years, they've gone from considering it a temporary problem that a post-baby pep talk from your health-care provider could take care of ("Here are your postpartum exercise guidelines and your postpartum nutrition guidelines. Now go enjoy that new baby!") to realizing that excess weight gain during pregnancy is a serious problem that can have long-lasting health implications for both mother and baby.

Before I run through the risk factors related to excess weight gain during pregnancy, I want you to keep some important points in mind: a risk factor is not the same thing as a diagnosis. Being 10 pounds (5 kilograms) overweight is not the same thing as being 110 pounds (50 kilograms) overweight, and weight isn't the single, defining measure of a person's health. Oh yeah, one more thing: Being motivated to make healthy choices for the well-being of yourself and your baby is a good thing. Being freaked for the rest of your pregnancy because you've gained too much weight (or you're not at your ideal weight) is not.

Okay, then. Here's the list of risk factors related to gaining excessive weight during pregnancy (in relation to the guidelines set by health authorities such as Health Canada). Once again, we're not talking guaranteed doomsday forecasts here, but rather information you should have so that you can make the most informed choices possible related to nutrition, weight gain, and so on.

Gaining excess weight during pregnancy increases the likelihood that you will experience such pregnancy-related complications as high blood pressure, pre-eclampsia, and gestational diabetes, particularly if you're already starting out pregnancy overweight or obese.

It increases the odds that you'll give birth to a baby who is large for gestational age. This, in turn, increases the risk that you may require a Caesarean delivery or experience prolonged labour and, rarely, birth trauma or worse.

It means you're less likely to lose your pregnancy weight, which could make it more difficult to conceive (if you're planning to get pregnant again). It also increases the odds that you will experience pregnancy- and birth-related complications during subsequent pregnancies, if you embark on those pregnancies overweight or obese. (See above.) You also face an increased risk of experiencing other health-related problems, simply by virtue of being overweight or obese.

eating for more than two

It's just as important for a mom-to-be who is pregnant with twins, triplets, or more to focus on eating a variety of nutrient-rich foods as it is to focus on gaining a particular amount of weight. Here are the key things to remember.

- Eat mini-meals rather than big meals. As your pregnancy progresses and your babies take up more and more real estate in your abdomen, you'll likely find that it's impossible to eat an entire meal all at once.
- Realize that your weight-gain pattern will be individual. The rate of gain and the total weight gain are both important figures, but it's unlikely your weight gain will be on target every week. Some weeks you may overshoot and some weeks you may not gain anything at all. What you're looking for is a general pattern indicating that your weight gain is roughly on target.

It means that your children are more likely to become overweight. The body system responsible for regulating appetite after birth starts tuning in to nutrition-related signals prior to birth. These signals can permanently alter the set point of appetite regulation in humans. Researchers at the Children's Hospital of Philadelphia and the University of Pennsylvania School of Medicine found that children born to mothers who gained more than the recommended amount of weight during pregnancy were 48 per cent more likely to be over-weight at age 7 than children whose mothers stayed within the recommended range for weight gain.

The best-laid plans

So you've already gained two trimesters' worth of weight—and you're only at the end of the first trimester? Now what? Don't panic, for starters. (Or, worse, decide it's a lost cause anyway and decide to deal with your frustration about the extra weight by noshing whatever food keeps calling your name.)

Talk to your health-care provider about the early weight gain (to ensure that there isn't a medical reason for that sudden jump on the scale). Then try to get back on track as best you can. Balanced and healthy nutrition is your best bet for achieving the slow, steady weight gain based on your pre-pregnancy BMI (see Table 2.1 on page 25).

While you might be tempted to diet during pregnancy in order to avoid having to deal with extra pounds later on, it's simply not worth the risk. Dieting during pregnancy puts a stress on the metabolism, which can be detrimental to fetal development, maternal health, and breastfeeding capability.

A study conducted at Johns Hopkins Bloomberg School of Public Health found that women who are fatigued, stressed, and anxious tend to consume more calories, and they have a particular fondness for carbohydrates. But what they gain in carbs they tend to sacrifice on the nutrient front. They miss out on folate (folic acid) and vitamin C. If you feel like you're doing a lot of stress-related eating, you may want to talk to your health-care provider about how you're feeling and experiment with non-food-related ways of managing stress. (See the section on coping with stress, later in this chapter.)

Gaining too little

You don't want to go overboard in the weight-gain department, but gaining too little can be a problem, too.

Mothers who gain less than the recommended amount of weight during pregnancy are more likely to give birth prematurely or to give birth to a low birth weight baby (a baby who weighs less than 5.5 pounds or 2.5 kilograms). Low birth weight babies face an increased risk of coronary disease, stroke, type 2 diabetes, high blood pressure (hypertension), and osteoporosis.

And researchers working in the newly emerging field of developmental science have discovered that a mother's diet before and during pregnancy may have a greater impact on the life-long health of her baby than previously believed. Not gaining enough weight may program your baby's body to store food in a way that can lead to obesity later in life. Researchers have found that fetuses that sense famine-like conditions as a result of their mothers' low calorie intakes may program their bodies to store fat more efficiently. After birth, these babies are less sensitive to sensations of fullness. They tend to grow more quickly and to store more fat.

Slow growth in the uterus leads to biological differences between small babies and their larger counterparts. Such differences include reduced kidney function, fewer cells in the heart and blood vessels, elevated cholesterol ratios, and higher blood pressure.

So what can you do if you're gaining too little weight? If you can't eat a lot in one sitting normally, it's going to get even worse when your stomach is crowded by your baby, so get used to eating frequent small meals. Plan ahead and have enough food at work and on the go so you can snack every couple of hours. Save your salad for after the main course to make sure you have room for that higher-calorie entree. Eating high-calorie foods is one way to gain more weight, but do it wisely: skip the French fries and stick to nutritious foods like nuts and avocados. Speak to a dietitian if you're really having trouble gaining weight.

When no food is appealing

Nausea and vomiting of pregnancy (a.k.a. morning sickness) can put you off eating or make it difficult to make what you've eaten stay down. In most cases, babies continue to thrive even if their moms are feeling downright miserable. This is because the baby is extremely small during the early weeks of pregnancy and doesn't require a lot of calories and nutrients. (Your body ensures that your baby's needs are met at this point by taking nutrients from whatever foods you're able to consume and drawing upon your nutritional stores.) Here are some nutrition tips that may make it easier for you to find something that appeals, or, at least, is a little less unappealing. (See Chapter 7 for more about nausea and vomiting of pregnancy and a particularly severe form of morning sickness known as *hyperemesis gravidarum*.)

Ensure that you are consuming adequate amounts of vitamin B (a water-soluble vitamin found in chickpeas, beef liver, tuna, salmon, and other food sources). Nausea and vomiting in pregnancy may be a result of long-term B6 deficiency. The solution? Supplement with 50 mg of vitamin B6 twice daily.

Eat mini-meals every two to three hours rather than larger meals three times per day. Not only are smaller meals easier to digest, more frequent meals will prevent your blood sugar from dropping too low, which can actually trigger nausea and send your moods cascading in all directions.

Choose carbohydrate-rich foods like fruit, fruit juices, breads, whole-grain cereals, rice, and pasta. Team a complex carbohydrate up with a serving of protein for lasting energy and fewer blood sugar dips.

Avoid greasy or fried foods and foods with overpowering odours. If you find that cooking odours in general make you queasy, stick to foods that can be eaten raw (sandwiches and salads) or open a window while you're preparing your food.

Eat soups and drink liquids between meals so that you won't fill up on these foods at mealtime. Otherwise, you may not eat enough other food to keep your blood sugar from diving before the next meal or snack.

Remain in an upright, seated position after eating. If you lie down, it's more difficult for your body to digest your food and you may start feeling queasy.

If you're surviving on soda crackers and flat ginger ale, you're probably concerned that you're depriving your baby of crucial nutrients. This is one worry you can scratch off the list fairly easily. In most cases, morning sickness is far harder on the mother than the baby. If your baby had to rely on what you were able to keep down on a meal-to-meal basis, there might be cause for concern. Fortunately, Mother Nature in her infinite wisdom has prepared for just such an

---

eating disorders

If you are currently struggling with an eating disorder or you've struggled with body image concerns or an eating disorder in the past, let your health-care provider know. You may want some extra support during and after your pregnancy. Research has shown that women who experience an eating disorder during pregnancy tend to gain less weight during pregnancy, are at increased risk of developing severe nausea and vomiting of pregnancy (*hyperemesis gravidarum*), are more likely to give birth to low birth weight babies, and are three times as likely to develop postpartum depression as other new moms. If you haven't struggled with your eating disorder for some time, there's plenty of reasons for optimism. Women whose eating disorders are in remission can expect to enjoy similar pregnancy outcomes to other women who have not experienced eating disorders. You can find out more from the National Eating Disorder Information Centre. Reach them by phone at 1–866–NEDIC–20 (633–4220) or visit their website at www.nedic.ca.

---

emergency by stockpiling nutrients in your body. So even if it's been a couple of weeks since you were able to stomach anything more exciting than soda crackers, your baby is still dining away on nutrients from all the multi-course meals you enjoyed during your pre-morning sickness days.

Morning sickness poses a threat to the developing baby only if it happens to be particularly severe and unrelenting. In 1 out of every 300 pregnancies a woman will develop a more serious form of morning sickness known as *hyperemesis gravidarum* (Latin for excessive vomiting in pregnancy). The symptoms of *hyperemesis gravidarum* include heavy vomiting (such as the inability to keep any food or drink down for more than 24 hours); reduced frequency of urination; dehydration; dryness of the mouth, skin, and eyes; extreme fatigue, weakness, or faintness; and confusion. The condition is generally treated with a combination of IV fluids and anti-nausea medications, but it's far better to nip the problem in the bud than to try to treat it after the fact. Be sure to let your doctor or midwife know if you're having a rough time with morning sickness.

You can find out more about both *hyperemesis gravidarum* and garden-variety morning sickness (a.k.a. nausea and vomiting of pregnancy) in Chapter 7.

Work it, Baby: Prenatal Fitness

While there's nothing you can really do to "train" for labour, studies have shown that your labour is likely to be shorter and less complicated if you're in good physical condition when those first contractions hit. That's why pregnant women are encouraged to make exercise part of their regular routine unless their health-care providers advise otherwise. The goal, however, is to maintain your current level of physical conditioning during pregnancy—not to embark on a boot-camp style training program.

Your doctor or midwife is likely to recommend that you refrain from exercising during pregnancy if

- you're carrying triplets or other higher-order multiples;
- you've been diagnosed with pregnancy-induced hypertension (high blood pressure) or pre-eclampsia;
- your membranes (amniotic sac) have ruptured prematurely;
- you're currently experiencing premature labour;
- you've had problems with premature labour during a previous pregnancy;
- you've been diagnosed with a condition known as incompetent cervix, in which the cervix dilates prematurely;
- you've been having persistent problems with vaginal bleeding throughout your second or third trimester or both—something that could indicate a possible placental problem;
- you have been diagnosed with placenta previa (after the 28th week) or other types of placental problems;
- you're experiencing significant pubic or lower back pain;
- your baby isn't growing as quickly as expected for a baby of that gestational age (a condition known as intrauterine growth restriction);
- you have uncontrolled type 1 diabetes or a cardiovascular or respiratory disorder that is not currently under control.

Your health-care provider *may or may not* recommend exercise during pregnancy, depending on your specific situation, if

- you have a history of miscarriage or preterm birth;
- you have a cardiovascular or respiratory disorder that is currently under control;
- you are anemic;
- you are significantly malnourished or struggling with an eating disorder;
- you are carrying twins and in your third trimester;
- you have other significant medical conditions.

Assuming you get the go-ahead from your caregiver to exercise (what most moms-to-be can expect), you've got plenty of great reasons to be physically active during pregnancy. Being active during pregnancy

- helps you to maintain your pre-pregnancy fitness level or to get in the habit of being physically active (a great habit to have in place as you make the journey to parenthood).
- makes it easier for you to keep your weight gain within the target range. Studies have shown that women who work out regularly during pregnancy are less likely to find themselves stuck with a huge amount of weight to lose after giving birth.
- increases the likelihood that your baby will be a healthy weight at birth. (Newborns tend to be healthiest when they weigh in at 7.7 to 8.8 pounds, or 3.5 to 4 kilograms.) Moderate exercise during early pregnancy encourages growth of the placenta—the organ responsible for supplying oxygen and nutrients to the baby.
- improves your mood and boosts your energy level, makes it easier to sleep, reduces fatigue, stress, and anxiety, eases symptoms of depression, improves body image, and enhances overall feelings of wellness. Since pregnancy is a time when many women report experiencing intense mood swings, this is welcome news indeed!
- helps to keep your blood glucose levels stable, which can reduce your likelihood of developing gestational diabetes.
- reduces the risk that you will develop pre-eclampsia—perhaps by as much as 43 per cent.
- lowers your blood pressure, which can reduce your risk of developing pregnancy-induced hypertension (a condition that affects 12 per cent of pregnant women).
- helps to ward off a number of pregnancy-related complaints. You're less likely to be troubled by insomnia, backache, ankle swelling, fatigue, venous thrombosis, varicose veins, hip soreness, leg cramps, abdominal muscle disturbances, pregnancy-related urinary incontinence, and constipation if you're exercising regularly.
- gives your immune system a boost. One study reported a decreased incidence of colds, flu symptoms, sinusitis, and bronchitis in women who exercise during pregnancy.
- helps to prevent heart disease, diabetes, osteoporosis (bone loss), and may even help to minimize your risk of cancer.
- prepares your body for labour. Studies have shown that women who are physically fit prior to labour experience faster labours and require fewer inductions, fewer episiotomies, fewer forceps deliveries, and fewer Caesarean deliveries than their less fit counterparts. They're also

less likely to require pain relief to manage maternal exhaustion and to require artificial rupturing of the membranes to speed labour along. Their babies benefit as a result: there are fewer abnormal fetal heart rate readings produced during labour from the babies of mothers who exercised during pregnancy as compared to mothers who didn't.

- reduces the amount of time it takes your body to recover from the delivery. That means you'll be in the best possible shape for the next marathon you'll face: becoming a mother.

As beneficial as prenatal exercise can be to a pregnant woman and her baby, it's still necessary to give some thought to your workout. Here are some important points to keep in mind when you're planning your fitness program.

Make physical activity part of your daily routine. The Public Health Agency of Canada recommends at least 2.5 hours of physical activity each week. The recommendation also applies when you are pregnant and postpartum, unless your health-care provider advises otherwise. If you have difficulty finding large blocks of time for exercise, enjoy being active in 15-minute blocks of time instead. That's just as effective.

Choose your fitness activity with care. Certain forms of exercise are not recommended for pregnant women. These types of manoeuvres can result in injury because a hormone called relaxin relaxes all your joints and ligaments to make it easier for your body to give birth. You can reduce the risk of injury by incorporating a warm-up and a cool-down into your workout. And make a point of zeroing in on pregnancy-friendly exercises that will help prepare your body for giving birth (see Table 5.3)

Avoid activities that could result in abdominal trauma or other types of injuries. Remember: your increased weight, the shift in your centre of gravity, and the fact that your joints and ligaments are more relaxed all affect your coordination and balance. This can make it easier for you to fall or injure yourself. Some pregnancy-friendly fitness activities include walking, swimming, stationary cycling, cross-country skiing, low-impact and pregnancy aerobics, and stretching and strengthening activities such as yoga and pilates that have been modified to meet the needs of pregnant women. Activities that aren't recommended during pregnancy include contact sports and fast-paced team sports such as football, basketball, and volleyball; adventure sports such as parachuting, mountain climbing, and scuba diving; sports with a high risk of trauma, such as downhill skiing, horseback riding, water-skiing, surfing, and ice skating; and high-impact, weight-bearing sports such as running or jogging. You'll also want to avoid exercising at high altitudes (over 6,000 feet, or about 1,800 metres) because there is reduced oxygen available to you and your baby, and to avoid scuba diving. (Scuba diving is associated with an increased risk of miscarriage, birth defects, poor fetal growth, and preterm labour.)

> **get active!**
>
> Looking for more detailed information on exercising during pregnancy? The Canadian Society for Exercise Physiology (CSEP) has published a manual entitled *Active Living During Pregnancy: Physical Activity Guidelines for Mother and Baby*. You can order a copy by calling the CSEP at 1–877–651–3755 or by visiting the CSEP website at www.csep.ca.

To reduce the risk of injury, wear appropriate footwear.

Stick with your weight-training regime. Women who continue to perform weight-bearing exercise at 50 per cent or more of their pre-pregnancy levels tend to gain less weight, deposit less fat, retain less fat, feel better about their bodies, have shorter and less complicated labours, and recover more rapidly than women who stop exercising. Weight training is considered safe as long as the resistance level is kept light to moderate. While doing your weight train-ing, you'll want to keep your breathing controlled and modify exercises that are normally performed while you are lying on your back (in the so-called supine position) or in a semi-reclined (tilted supine) position—a position that can result in decreased oxygen available to the fetus.

Exercise smart. Rather than attempting floor exercises that might leave you susceptible to injury—deep knee bends, full sit-ups, double-leg raises, and straight-leg raises are all no-nos during pregnancy— zero in on exercises that will help prepare your body for giving birth. (See Table 5.3.)

If back pain starts to become a problem for you, work on your abdominal muscles. The weaker your abdominal muscles are, the harder your back has to work to keep your body upright.

Check for abdominal muscle separation. If you feel a ridge running from your pubic bone to your belly button that is more than two finger-widths wide, you will need to modify your exercise routine to prevent further muscle separation. (See Chapter 7 for more on this topic.)

It's not a good idea to launch a new fitness program or increase the intensity or duration of your existing program prior to the 15th week of pregnancy. Besides, you may not feel like hitting the gym at this stage of the game: "I had started exercising about a month prior to conception, but I gave it up in early pregnancy," confesses Jennifer, a 32-year-old mother of one. "I was experiencing exhaustion beyond anything I had ever felt before. It was a major accomplishment to get out of bed and get dressed. The thought of lacing up sneakers and going to the gym reduced me to tears."

Your blood volume, cardiac output, heart rate, and blood pressure increase while you're working out. To get a complete picture of how hard your body is working when you're exercising, you may want to get in the habit of using the perceived exertion scale, which asks you to monitor your rate of breathing, how sore your muscles are, and your fatigue level, in addition to your heart rate (as opposed to monitoring your heart rate alone). You can find out more about the perceived exertion scale by visiting the Canadian Society for Exercise Physiology website (www.csep.ca).

Always warm up and cool down. Ease in to your workout gradually and then wind down until your heart is beating at its regular resting rate.

Don't allow your body to become overheated. An overly high body temperature (39°C/102°F) can cause certain brain and spinal defects in babies, particularly if the overheating occurs during the first trimester of pregnancy. Decrease the duration and intensity of your workout, wear lightweight clothing, avoid exercising during the hottest times of the day or on hot, humid days, steer clear of hot tubs, saunas, and Jacuzzis, and skip your workout if you have a fever.

Consume enough liquids to keep yourself well hydrated before, during, and after exercise, and ensure that you're eating enough. If you're particularly active, the extra 300 calories a day recommended to most women during the second and third trimesters of pregnancy might not be enough for you. You may have to bump your caloric intake up further to avoid weakness, dizziness, and inadequate weight gain.

Pay attention to your body. Stop exercising immediately if you experience any or all of the following symptoms while exercising and get in touch with your health-care provider immediately: persistent uterine contractions; back pain or pubic pain that gets worse when you exercise; bloody discharge or a sudden gush of fluid from the vagina; unexplained abdominal pain; swelling of the ankles, hands, or face; headaches or vision disturbances; dizziness or faintness; extreme fatigue; heart palpitations, chest pain, or shortness of breath; and/or changes to the amount of fetal movement.

Realize that your pregnant body needs more oxygen than your pre-pregnant body (15 times as much when you're exercising, in fact)—which explains why you may find yourself huffing and puffing as you work out, even if you're in great shape. As your uterus gets bigger, it starts to crowd your diaphragm (the large muscle that separates your chest from your abdomen)—something that only increases that out-of-breath feeling.

Wear a bra that provides the support you need when you're active. Your breasts are bigger and heavier than they were before you became pregnant, and the ligaments that support breast tissue can be permanently damaged if they become overstretched. This can lead to a saggy bosom and a lot of discomfort while you're exercising.

You'll need to alter your exercise position starting in the mid-second trimester. When you lay flat on your back after the 16th week of pregnancy, your uterus rests on the vena cava—the vein responsible for returning blood from your lower body to the heart. This severely reduces the blood flow back to your heart, along with the flow of blood back to your baby. Your heart will start beating more slowly and you will feel dizzy—like you're about to pass out.

Start thinking ahead about what you will do to stay fit after the baby arrives. Ask friends with babies to share their best advice.

And now the most important piece of advice: have fun. Sign up for a prenatal fitness class so that you can get to know other pregnant women in your community. Hop on your stationary bike while you're reading your favourite pregnancy magazine. And make an after-dinner stroll with your partner part of your daily routine. Pregnancy is a time to enjoy and celebrate your body and the miracle that's taking place inside. It's the perfect time to be physically active.

5.3 The Best Pregnancy Floor Exercises	
Type of Exercise	**What It Does for You**
Squatting	Stretches your legs and opens your pelvis. Great preparation for birth if you intend to do some of your labouring and birthing in a squatting position.
Pelvic tilting or rocking	Strengthens your abdominal and back muscles. Can improve your overall posture and help to prevent or relieve backache.
Bridge (back bend with shoulders resting on the ground)	Stretches out your back muscles while also giving your pelvic floor muscles a gentle workout.
Side-lying clamshell (left side, knees bent, raise your right knee to open up the clamshell)	Exercises your abdominal muscles and your hip muscles.
Pelvic floor	Strengthens the muscles in your pelvic diaphragm (the muscles that support your uterus and bladder), helps to prevent pregnancy incontinence after childbirth (a symptom that may not show up until many years later), and can make birth easier. To practice your Kegels, locate the correct group of muscles by stopping and starting the flow of urine while urinating. (Note: Don't do this on a regular basis. You're only doing this to locate the correct group of muscles.) To perform your Kegel exercises, tighten and relax the muscles several times in a row. Work up to holding your muscles for 10 seconds before releasing them. **Caution:** Doing Kegels incorrectly can take its toll on your pelvic floor muscles. This is why a growing number of moms-to-be are opting for a prenatal consultation with a physiotherapist who specializes in women's health. Such a consultation includes training in how to do a proper Kegel—one that will leave your body stronger, not weaker. And a pelvic floor assessment can provide you with valuable information about strengthening your core muscles, preparing for birth, and postpartum recovery.

Feel the Heat

Being pregnant is like having a block heater implanted into your belly for nine and a half months. It's a welcome bonus on the coldest winter day (you can count on a heating boost of about 0.5°C to 1.0°C (0.9°F to 1.8°F), thanks to your baby's metabolism, although some of this heat is lost as a result of increased blood flow to the skin), but it's not so great to have your heater permanently switched to "on" on the hottest day in July. It's uncomfortable to exercise under such conditions, especially to the point where you're drenched in sweat. Some animal studies have indicated that becoming overheated in early pregnancy may prevent the neural tube from closing. Sure, they're animal studies rather than human studies, but why take a chance? There will be plenty of other days to sweat at the gym next July.

high-intensity workouts	The bodies of pregnant athletes are better able to respond to the demands of high-intensity workouts during pregnancy than the bodies of women who have previously been inactive or exercising at a lower level of intensity. An athlete's body is in top condition and will ensure that the baby receives adequate oxygen and energy, even when the mother is engaged in high-intensity exercise. If a less fit mother tries to exercise at high intensity, her body will respond by redirecting blood flow from the uterus to the muscles, depriving the baby of oxygen and nutrients and releasing stress hormones that can trigger preterm labour.

Quitting Time: Smoking, Drinking, and Drugs

Back in Chapter 2, I ran through a whole laundry list of reasons for not smoking, drinking, or using illegal drugs while you were trying to conceive. If you have yet to kick those habits, you have even more reasons to do so now. Here's a roundup of the latest research on this front.

Smoking

There are so many reasons to go smoke-free during pregnancy. The benefits of quitting are immediate:

- The amount of oxygen your baby receives increases after just one day of being smoke-free.
- You'll be less likely to experience pregnancy-related complications. When you smoke during pregnancy, your heart rate and blood pressure increase, your immune system is less able to fight off infection, you face an increased risk of miscarriage, ectopic pregnancy, placental abruption, placenta previa, early/late pregnancy bleeding, premature rupture of membranes, preterm labour, preterm birth, and fetal growth restriction (babies born to women who smoke during pregnancy weigh an average of 200 grams (7 ounces) less at birth than is typical), and perinatal mortality. Furthermore, you are twice as likely to experience complications during labour or birth.
- You'll be more likely to eat nutritious foods while you're pregnant.

Smoking affects your sense of taste. Smokers are less likely to eat fruit, vegetables, whole grains, and lower fat milk than non-smokers. And, to make things worse, smoking interferes with the absorption of certain nutrients.

- You'll sleep better at night. Women who smoke report increased sleep disturbances during pregnancy. They have difficulty getting to sleep, they sleep for just a short period of time, they snore loudly, they experience discomfort when they breathe, they wake up feeling less rested, and they have difficulties with early-morning awakening and excessive daytime sleepiness. Women who are exposed to second-hand smoke experience all of these symptoms except for excessive daytime sleepiness and early morning awakening.

- You'll increase the odds that your baby will be born at a healthy weight. Smoking during pregnancy increases the risk that a baby will be born prematurely, at low birth weight, small for gestational age, and with congenital health problems. Smoking is the leading cause of low birth weight, with birth weight typically dropping by 14 grams (0.5 ounces) times the number of cigarettes smoked per day. Nicotine restricts the circulation between uterus and placenta by narrowing the blood vessels. Your baby gets less oxygen and fewer nutrients, something that can limit your baby's growth and lead to health problems.

- You'll reduce the odds of your baby becoming obese or developing certain types of diseases and birth defects. Infants born to mothers who smoked during pregnancy are more likely to be lighter at birth, but, as early as age 3 to 5 years, they tend to be heavier than their peers. Research has demonstrated that the effect of maternal smoking on childhood obesity is as great as the link between frequent TV viewing or playing video games on childhood obesity. If a mother smokes more than 10 cigarettes a day while she is pregnant, the risk of her child going on to develop diabetes quadruples as compared to other babies. And women who smoke during pregnancy are nearly 2.5 times more likely to give birth to babies with oral clefts.

- Your baby will be less likely to experience behavioural issues and developmental delays that have been linked to prenatal smoking. A study by researchers at Vanderbilt University and the University of Kentucky (published in the April 2007 edition of *Environmental Health Perspectives*) linked prenatal exposure to tobacco smoke to reduced speech-processing ability in otherwise healthy newborns. Other studies have linked prenatal smoking to colicky behaviour and sleeping and feeding problems in infants; speech, hearing, and behavioural difficulties in toddlers; lowered general cognitive functioning in preschoolers; lags in language development, reduced verbal IQ, significant problems with the aspects of reading that rely on auditory skills; and attention deficit hyperactivity disorder, oppositional and aggressive behaviour, anti-social behaviour, and conduct disorders in older children.

How to quit

- Change one or two of your daily smoking routines. For example, having a cigarette when you drink coffee or when you're in your car. If you can break the association you've built up between a particular activity (driving or drinking coffee) and smoking, you'll reduce your dependency on cigarettes and find it easier to quit.
- Keep a diary of where and how much you smoke.
- Replace your old way of coping with stress (reaching for a cigarette) with new, body-nurturing ways. (See the section on stress later in this chapter for some suggestions.)
- Use the four Ds: drink water with crushed ice, breathe deeply (take a deep breath, hold for two seconds, then let it out), delay smoking for a few minutes when you get the urge, and do something else (try a different activity).
- The first three to four days are the toughest. It gets a lot easier after that. In fact, by the 10th day, your withdrawal symptoms will be gone.
- If you can't quit altogether, reducing the amount you smoke will help to improve your baby's birth weight.
- Your health-care provider can help you to come up with a personalized game plan for quitting smoking. You'll also find other helpful strategies at www.quit4life.com and www.smokershelpline.ca.
- Make your home and car smoke-free environments.
- Get support from family members, friends, professionals, and your local public health department.

Drinking

The facts about alcohol consumption during pregnancy are just as compelling. There is no known safe amount of alcohol that you can consume during pregnancy, there is no safe type of alcohol you can consume during pregnancy, and there is no safe time to consume alcohol during pregnancy.

Your baby is roughly twice as affected by any alcohol you consume during pregnancy as you are. (His metabolism is still immature. He can't burn off alcohol as efficiently as you can.) The extent to which a baby is affected by alcohol exposure during pregnancy depends on

- how much alcohol was consumed;
- how many other exposures (to alcohol and other harmful substances) have occurred during pregnancy;
- whether the baby has been exposed to viruses and other sources of infection during pregnancy;
- how efficiently the mother burns off alcohol;
- the mother's overall health;
- the baby's genetic susceptibility to alcohol;
- the timing of the exposure. First trimester exposures are most likely to result in birth defects because this is the period of critical development for organs and body systems. (See Chapter 6.) Exposures at other points in pregnancy are more likely to damage the baby's central nervous system or to affect the baby's overall growth.

Not every baby who is exposed to alcohol during pregnancy will be affected, but the damage, when it occurs, can be far-reaching.

Drinking alcohol during pregnancy increases the risk of miscarriage, stillbirth, intrauterine growth restriction, premature delivery, and giving birth to a low birth weight baby. It also increases the risk that a baby will exhibit some or all of the conditions common to fetal alcohol disorder.

A study at San Diego State University concluded that binge drinking may damage the developing baby's circadian rhythm: the internal clock that regulates sleep/wake patterns. A disrupted circadian rhythm has been linked to behavioural problems such as attention deficit hyperactivity disorder and mental disorders.

A study at University of Washington at Seattle found that children whose mothers consumed one to two drinks per day during pregnancy were more likely to exhibit learning problems, particularly with regard to mathematics and memory tasks, and behavioural difficulties, including attention problems. Other studies have noted links between alcohol exposure during pregnancy and hyperactivity, impulsivity, poor social and communication skills, and alcohol and drug use.

Researchers at Emory University in Atlanta discovered that there is an increased risk of infection in the newborn if at least seven drinks per week were consumed during pregnancy or during the three months prior to conception.

	The term fetal alcohol spectrum disorder is used to describe a cluster of conditions that frequently occur in children who were exposed to alcohol prior to birth. These include specific facial features, poor brain development, poor vision and hearing, difficulty learning, developmental problems, and neuro-behavioural problems. The term fetal alcohol spectrum disorder is starting to replace the terms "fetal alcohol syndrome" and "fetal alcohol effects" which have traditionally been used to describe the effects of varying degrees of alcohol exposure during pregnancy.
Fetal Alcohol Spectrum Disorder	

Ready to put your drinking habit on ice?

The most important thing to know is that it's never too late. Giving up alcohol at any point in pregnancy will benefit your baby. If you are having difficulty making changes to your drinking habits, get support from an encouraging, non-judgmental person. If you don't know who to talk to, try calling the Motherisk Alcohol and Substance in Pregnancy Helpline: 1–877–327–4636. Or visit the Motherisk Clinic's website at www.motherisk.org.

Get your partner on board. Moms-to-be with partners who drink are more likely to drink during pregnancy. Let your partner know that you'd appreciate it if he or she would support your decision not to drink during pregnancy by easing off on the drinking, too.

Drugs

Drugs are bad news during pregnancy. What complicates things is that drugs may be just one piece of the puzzle: a woman who is using drugs during pregnancy may be dealing with other issues as well (poor nutrition, smoking, drinking, STDs, domestic violence).

The good news is that problems caused by illicit drug use during pregnancy are completely preventable. Your best bet is to stop using them before you become pregnant or to hold off on becoming pregnant until you can avoid drugs completely during pregnancy. If you are pregnant and using drugs *other than heroin*, you are encouraged to stop using drugs right away. If you are pregnant *and using heroin* you should consult your health-care provider or a drug treatment centre about methadone treatment. If you don't know who to talk to, try calling the Motherisk Alcohol and Substance in Pregnancy Helpline: 1–877–327–4636. Or you can visit the Motherisk Clinic's website at www .motherisk.org.

Sleeping for Two

Here's proof that Mother Nature has a rather wicked sense of humour: at the time in your life when you are most in need of sleep, sleep can be frustratingly elusive. Either you find it hard to settle down to sleep in the first place or you end up tossing and turning all night. So what's an exhausted mother-to-be to do?

Well, for starters, you might want to take solace in the fact that you aren't the only pregnant woman in your prenatal class who is unwillingly burning the candle at both ends. Sleep deprivation is a pregnancy rite of passage for most moms-to-be. So what's causing the expectant mothers of the nation to toss and turn at night when they should be somewhere in Dreamland? A variety of pregnancy-related aches and pains, that's what.

The fun starts in the first trimester. By the time you're 10 to 12 weeks pregnant, rising levels of estrogen, prolactin, and progesterone can interfere with your ability to get a solid night's sleep. You may find it hard to get to sleep in the first place, thanks to your oh-so-tender breasts, and even if you do settle into a deep sleep, you're likely to find yourself trekking to the bathroom at least once in the middle of the night. You can blame your midnight strolls on both the pressure of the growing baby on your bladder and the hormonal effects of progesterone. Progesterone acts on the smooth muscle of your urinary tract, causing you to need to urinate more frequently than usual. And, of course, if you're bothered by the nausea and vomiting of pregnancy, then you may find that the queasiness you're experiencing can get in the way of a good night's sleep, too.

Fortunately, you get a bit of a reprieve in the second trimester—at least insofar as those middle-of-the-night treks to the bathroom are concerned. As the baby continues to grow, her position changes: because she's not camped out on your bladder any longer (well, at least for now), you don't have to urinate with quite the same frequency. The only bad news on the sleep front during the second trimester is that you may start snoring. Approximately 30 per cent of pregnant women start snoring during the second trimester—many for the first time in their lives. The culprit? Swelling in the nasal passages caused by rising estrogen levels.

The third trimester is, by far, the worst trimester when it comes to sleep. Studies have shown that 97 per cent of women in their third trimester report waking up at least once during the night and 92 per cent report sleeping restlessly. Heartburn, an increased need to urinate, sinus congestion, leg cramps, your baby's movements (which are most noticeable when you finally slow down at the end of the day), and difficulty finding a comfortable position all conspire against you in your quest for rest. The best way to manage sleep disturbances in late pregnancy is to practise good sleep hygiene. That means sticking to a regular sleep schedule, avoiding (or minimizing the length of) daytime naps, exercising regularly, avoiding caffeine within six hours of bedtime (assuming, of course, that you haven't kicked your caffeine habit altogether), and getting out in the daylight early in the day in order to keep your body's internal clock functioning properly. And if those never-ending middle-of-the-night bathroom visits are wearing you out, you'll want to decrease your intake of fluids right before bedtime.

When it comes to getting comfortable (no small feat at this stage of the game), the most comfortable sleep position also happens to be the one that maximizes blood flow to your baby: lying on your left side. If you have a tendency to roll forward, you could find yourself left with a nasty backache in the morning, so it's a good idea to get in the habit of tucking a pillow in-between your knees. That should help to ease some of your physical discomfort for at least an hour or two (at least in theory). Some women find that, by late pregnancy, no position is comfortable, not even floating on a sea of body pillows.

The bigger challenge, of course, is to get your mind to wind down so that you can get the sleep you need. After all, there's plenty to think about as you approach

---

sleeping comfortably

Forget about location. Position is everything, especially when it comes to finding a comfortable sleeping position in late pregnancy.

Discomfort caused by tender breasts in early pregnancy may make sleeping on your stomach impossible. This could be as good a time as any to get used to sleeping on your side. Sleeping on your left side maximizes the flow of blood and nutrients to your baby and your uterus while helping your kidneys get rid of waste and fluids.

If you're being bothered by lower back pain, take the pressure off your lower back by sleeping on your side. Make sure you sleep with your knees and your hips bent and that you place a pillow between your knees, under your abdomen, and behind your back. If you own a body pillow, you may be able to achieve a similar result by tossing your leg over the body pillow (which kind of acts like a surrogate bedmate). Your real-life bedmate may be happy to have someone else playing the role of body double at this point, particularly when you insist on changing position every hour or two all night long.

If you're having problems with heartburn, try sleeping in a semi-seated position, with your head elevated on pillows. (You may have to experiment with the number of pillows until you get just the right combo.) You'll also want to avoid spicy, acidic, and fried foods; and consume smaller, more frequent meals. (For more tips on managing heartburn and other pregnancy-related discomforts, see Chapter 7.)

the end of pregnancy. You may find yourself feeling excited about meeting your baby, nervous about the challenges that you may face while giving birth, and worried about the changes that motherhood may bring to your life. The best way to cope with this late-night parade of thoughts is to ensure that your sleep environment is sleep enhancing (dark, quiet, and slightly cool, and computer- and television-free) and that you're tired when bedtime rolls around (being physically active earlier in the day will help to take care of this). Next, come up with an evening wind-down routine that works for you. Have a relaxing bath, listen to soothing music, and read something that will help you to drift off to sleep. (And, of course, you'll want to turn your alarm clock away from you so that you won't start keeping track of how long it's taking you to fall asleep.)

dreams and nightmares

"I keep having awful nightmares about my baby. Is this mother's intuition telling me there's something wrong?"

As you've discovered, pregnancy isn't always what you'd dreamed it would be. A study conducted at the Sleep Research Centre at the Hôpital du Sacré-Coeur de Montréal found that 59 per cent of pregnant women experienced dreams in which their baby was in danger.

Other studies have revealed that pregnant women tend to experience vivid dreams that can be both intense and disturbing. Sleep researchers pin part of the blame on that wacky cocktail of pregnancy hormones responsible for so many other pregnancy-related complaints.

During pregnancy (especially during the last trimester) you spend a greater percentage of your sleep time in REM (the stage of sleep when you're most likely to dream and to wake up easily). And because you tend to wake up more often in the night when you're pregnant—either because you have to make a trip to the bathroom or because your hips are sore from sleeping on your side—you tend to remember more about your dreams, including the parts you'd rather not.

Hormones aren't solely responsible for these often disturbing dreams, however, as studies have shown that fathers-to-be also experience their fair share of pregnancy-related nightmares. Clearly there's so much mental work to be done during the nine months of pregnancy that parents' brains end up putting in a fair bit of overtime!

Try not to let your dreams worry you. The fact that you've had a baby-related nightmare does not in any way mean that you're destined to experience it in real life. So if you wake up feeling panicked in the middle of the night, go heat up a glass of warm milk in the microwave and focus on how well your pregnancy is going in the real world.

Sleep and health

Be sure to let your health-care provider know if you're missing out on sleep on a regular basis. If you're not sleeping well, you may find yourself dealing with some of the fallout of sleep deprivation during the day: difficulty concentrating, difficulty making decisions or solving problems, forgetfulness, irritability, and depression. You may also find yourself experiencing some physical symptoms: gastrointestinal complaints, food cravings (which can be accompanied by increased weight gain), and daytime sleepiness.

Too many nights of poor-quality sleep can start to affect how well you are functioning and feeling. Sleeping for less than six hours a night during the last three to four weeks of pregnancy can increase the length of labour and increase your likelihood of requiring a Caesarean section.

Sleep disorders during pregnancy

Snoring may be annoying (particularly to your partner). But sleep disorders like sleep-disordered breathing and obstructive sleep apnea can be downright worrisome and necessitate a check-in with your health-care provider.

Sleep-disordered breathing (gasping, choking, and having difficulty breathing while you sleep) affects 15 per cent of women in late pregnancy and is more likely to occur in women who had high pre-pregnancy BMIs and who experience a lot of weight gain around the neck during pregnancy. It is linked to an increase in daytime sleepiness.

Some women develop obstructive sleep apnea (OSA) (a more severe form of sleep-disordered breathing) during pregnancy. OSA occurs when the tissue in the back of the throat collapses and blocks the airway. The muscles inside the throat relax as you sleep. Gravity then causes the tongue to fall back and it ends up blocking the airway. This prevents air from getting into the lungs. When you notice that you're not breathing, you wake up. This cycle can occur a couple of times each night or many hundreds of times per night. Sleep apnea must be treated as quickly as possible in order to prevent the developing baby from experiencing growth restriction as a result of the reduced flow of oxygen. Continuous positive airway pressure (CPAP) is the recommended treatment method. Women who develop sleep apnea during pregnancy need to be followed after pregnancy to ensure that the condition resolves once they lose the extra weight they gained during pregnancy. A follow-up sleep study is generally ordered for two to three months after the birth. In the meantime, treatment may be required to prevent the new mother from experiencing severe sleep deprivation.

restless leg syndrome

Ask anyone who has ever experienced restless leg syndrome to describe their experience with this particular pregnancy complaint and they'll probably start twitching as they recall it. Restless leg syndrome (RLS) is a condition in which leg twitches occur every 20 to 40 seconds. They often occur just as you are trying to fall asleep, and they can be severe enough to wake you and your bedmate from the deepest, most refreshing sleep.

Note: RLS has been linked to being deficient in iron or folic acid at the time of conception. If you are experiencing RLS, you may want to find out if you are currently deficient in one or both minerals and, if you are, whether your health-care provider recommends any changes to your nutrient intake.

(Don't Get Too) Stressed about Stress

Stress is never a good thing. It can sap your energy, make it difficult for you to sleep, cause headaches and backaches, lead to unhealthy eating (either eating too much or too little), and generally take the joy out of life.

When you're pregnant, it can go from being a drag to being a health hazard, if stress gets bad enough. When stress is sudden and massive or chronic and unrelenting, the risks of such pregnancy-related complications as premature birth, low birth weight, birth-related complications, and poor fetal growth and development increase. Prolonged exposure to maternal stress may also increase the baby's risk of developing such adult-onset disorders as type 2 diabetes, hypertension (high blood pressure), coronary artery disease, end-stage renal disease, and depression.

Now, just to be clear, the kind of stress that comes from juggling deadlines at work or dealing with a very annoying relative isn't typically the type of stress that is going to cause you any grief. You're more likely to experience stress-related pregnancy complications if you are subjected to what psychologists describe as a negative life event (the death of someone close to you, a devastating relationship breakup, a serious illness, losing your job, a catastrophic event). And your odds of that event having an impact on your baby are greater if that event occurs early on in your pregnancy. Chronic stress can lead to complications if that stress is severe (you're living in poverty or you're involved in an abusive relationship).

Of course, it's best to avoid any stress during pregnancy—and in a perfect world, you'd be able to do that. But until someone figures out how we can arrange to be pregnant in a perfect world, we'll have to continue to settle for being pregnant on this decidedly imperfect planet and learning to manage the stress that goes along with that. Here are some tips.

Don't get stressed about stress. Rather than obsessing about all the things that could happen to you if you were subjected to chronic and unrelenting stress or sudden and massive stress, focus on strategies for becoming the least stressed pregnant person you know (or a reasonable facsimile of that). Fake it until you make it, in other words.

Shine some light on your darkest worries. If there are any worries lingering in the darkest recesses of your pregnant mind, shine some light on them so that others can help you deal. Set up an appointment with your health-care provider to go through all the concerns that are causing your stress levels to soar. It's the first step to putting an action plan in place. And don't worry if some of those worries aren't 100 per cent pregnancy-related. If they're on your mind and they are affecting your health during pregnancy, your health-care provider will want to help you find a solution. That solution may mean making a referral to another professional: a credit counsellor, a couples' therapist, or whoever else may be best able to meet your needs at this time.

Set realistic expectations for yourself. Sometimes pregnancy stress is caused by a desire to measure up to extremely high standards—and the frustration that results if you have to wave the white flag because morning sickness, fatigue, or other early-pregnancy symptoms have sapped you of your usual energy. Where is it written that pregnant women have to be superhuman beings for all 40 weeks of pregnancy? In no credible book or study I've ever read.

Don't work too hard. You're not indispensable at work, no matter what you do. And they're going to have to get used to making do without you soon anyway.

Go with the pregnancy flow. That way, when you feel like crashing on the couch after dinner rather than tackling the items on your to-do list, you won't have to feel stressed out or guilty. You can congratulate yourself for listening to your body and nurturing yourself and your growing baby.

Make peace with your hormones. Understand that the hormonal changes of pregnancy make it more difficult to manage stress. (You've no doubt heard about the legendary mood swings of pregnancy. Well, they're legendary for a reason.) Recognize that mood swings are a common part of pregnancy and may serve a function: they alter our perception and help us see things in a more baby-centred way.

Take the best possible care of your physical health. Leading a healthy life-style makes it easier to manage stress. That means eating well, getting enough sleep, and being physically active (which relieves stress and helps to eliminate discomforts that can themselves be a source of stress).

When you're feeling low, ask for what you need. Even if it's just quiet time or a cuddle. But also make sure to spend time with your partner when you're not tired and stressed.

Remember what the Beatles said. We get by with a little help from our friends. We humans are social creatures. Simply becoming isolated (perhaps as a result of early pregnancy fatigue) can be stressful. We start to feel like we're stranded on Pregnancy Island, with no way to get off. The solution is obvious, once someone points it out: send a text message to your nearest and dearest, inviting them to visit you (and pamper you) on your Island until you start feeling better. (Which you will, very soon. That's what the second tri-mester is for.) Don't rely on your partner exclusively. Have a friend look out for you, someone who will get you out, and laugh and cry with you.

Master a variety of different relaxation techniques. Some of the techniques other moms-to-be have found helpful include progressive muscle relaxation, deep breathing, guided mental imagery, mindfulness meditation, biofeed-back, and yoga.

Practise your relaxation breathing. Practise relaxation breathing on a reg-ular basis. Not only will it serve you well on labour day, it can also help to keep your stress level down while you're still pregnant. Put one hand on your abdomen and practise breathing all the way into your abdomen so that your hand rises and falls while you breathe. Once you've mastered that, try breathing deeply and pausing slightly before you exhale. Then, as you exhale, slowly count to four. After five to ten minutes, you'll find that your breath-ing gradually slows down, your body starts to relax, and your mind begins to feel calmer.

Try meditation. Studies have shown that meditation can help to reduce stress, relieve pain, lower both your blood pressure and your heart rate, and improve the quality of your sleep. When you're ready to meditate, simply find a comfortable, distraction-free place to sit, set a timer for five minutes (you'll gradually want to work up to 20 minutes), place your hands on your belly, close your eyes, and focus on the sound of your breathing until the timer goes off.

Go for a massage. Having a massage helps to relieve backaches, leg cramps, headaches, and other pregnancy-related aches and pains. Plus, it soothes and relaxes the nervous system by releasing endorphins into your body. So if you've ever needed a reason to book a massage or hand that bottle of massage oil to your partner, you've now got the perfect excuse: motherhood! Note: You can find out more about pregnancy massage and other relaxing spa treatments in Chapter 8.

Work that stress out of your system using hand weights or resistance bands. The activity will give you something to focus on other than how stressed you're feeling. Pick up a book or an instructional video so that you can be sure that you're performing the routines safely, and heed any advice your health-care provider has given you about exercising during pregnancy.

Make a cup of tea. Tea has an amino acid in it called theanine, which can have a calming effect on the body that can last two to three hours.

Turn off information overload every once in a while. Stop reading those pregnancy books, turn off the news, and don't answer the phone.

Sign up for childbirth classes. Fear of the unknown can be a major source of stress, so obtaining answers to as many pregnancy, birth, and baby-related questions as possible may help to ease your anxiety level considerably. Tip: If you can, try to find childbirth classes that feature a few early bird classes scheduled for early pregnancy on top of the usual late-pregnancy childbirth preparation classes. These classes are terrific because they give you a sneak preview of the physical and emotional changes of pregnancy. Then, a month or two before the birth, your class will reconvene to prepare for labour, birth, and early parenthood.

Line up a pregnancy mentor. Much of the stress of pregnancy comes from being unsure about what's normal and what's not during this strange yet wonderful time in your life. In addition to turning to your doctor or midwife for support and information, you might want to take the advice of Jennifer Louden, author of *The Pregnant Woman's Comfort Book* (HarperCollins), and line up a pregnancy mentor—a woman who is either pregnant herself (ideally a few months ahead of you) or who has recently given birth. Having someone to turn to for this from-the-trenches advice can help to alleviate a lot of your anxiety.

Start putting together your own pregnancy and parenting support network. I'm not talking about anything formal with meetings and minutes and official T-shirts (although the T-shirt part would be fun). I'm talking about hand-picking your own pregnancy and baby advice and help team. Now bear in mind that you want to recruit the right kinds of supporters: people who are there to lend a helping hand and to share that invaluable gem of wisdom at the perfect moment, but who won't bombard you with unwanted advice or question your judgment every step of the way. Your support network will be unique. It may be made up of family and friends, with behind-the-scenes support from your health-care provider, your childbirth educator, your prenatal fitness instructor, your doula, and so on. Some team members may come and go (you have to say your goodbyes to your midwife at some point, as much as you'd love to stay in monthly or weekly contact forever); some may still be part of your team when your baby is heading off to college. Putting this kind of support in place isn't just good for your stress level, by the way. It's good for the health of you and your baby. You'll reduce your risk of becoming depressed before and after the birth and increase the odds that your baby will be born at a healthy weight.

Depression During Pregnancy

It wasn't that long ago that people had difficulty even grasping the concept of prenatal depression. ("What does she have to be depressed about? She's having a baby!") Now it's common knowledge that as many as one in eight pregnant women experience depression at some point during pregnancy. And people know that biology, genetics, and environment can all play a role in perinatal mood disorders, as they do in other types of mood disorders.

A study published in the January 2010 issue of the *American Journal of Obstetrics and Gynecology* added to what is known about depression during pregnancy by identifying some key risk factors for depression during pregnancy: maternal anxiety, life stress, a history of depression, a lack of social support, an unplanned pregnancy, domestic violence, living on a lower income, having less education, smoking, being single, and being involved in a poor-quality relationship. Fertility treatments and high-risk pregnancies can also be risk factors because of the anxiety they create.

Because a woman's life circumstances can change at any time, moms-to-be are increasingly being monitored for symptoms of depression and other perinatal mood disorders on an ongoing basis—and for good reason. Between 10 and 20 per cent of women develop a mood disorder during the perinatal period (which consists of pregnancy plus the year following the birth). Women with perinatal mood disorders experience feelings of anxiety, sadness, depression, panic, frustration, and confusion. Other symptoms may include feeling overwhelmed, trouble sleeping or sleeping too much, changes in appetite, feeling hopeless, crying uncontrollably, feeling guilty or worthless, lack of interest in family and friends, lack of concentration, anxiety or irritability. In very rare cases (less than 0.2 per cent), symptoms may include thoughts of harming the baby or oneself. Many women with depression experience acute anxiety before delivery.

If you think you might be struggling with a perinatal mood disorder, it is important to talk to your health-care provider. Perinatal mood disorders can be treated, and there are a variety of treatment options available: everything from talk therapy to support groups (which have proven to be very successful in the management of prenatal depression) to bright light therapy to medication. The sooner you talk to your health-care provider, the better: wait lists for perinatal psychiatrists can be long, and the sooner treatment begins, the more positive the outcome for both mother and baby. (Complications associated with depression during pregnancy include inadequate pregnancy weight gain, not obtaining adequate prenatal care, increased substance use, and premature birth. And complications associated with stress, depression, and anxiety include lower birth weight, decreased Apgar scores—a score that assesses the baby's well-being at birth—smaller head circumference, and small-for-gestational-age babies.)

Friends and family members have an important role to play when a woman is dealing with depression during pregnancy. They can

- listen, support, and encourage her and remind her that it's not her fault that she is struggling with a perinatal mood disorder;
- offer help with tasks that may be difficult for her to manage while she's feeling overwhelmed (such as making nutritious meals, keeping track of prenatal appointments, troubleshooting other sources of stress in her life);
- encourage her to take care of her physical health (obtaining adequate sleep, going for walks) because these activities will give her a psychological boost as well;
- continue to reach out to her, even if she doesn't return phone calls or e-mails (she needs to know that people care, even if she doesn't have the energy or focus to maintain her side of the relationship right now);
- remind her that she won't feel this way forever. Many women have lived through this and are now leading happy lives once again. She can, too.

Note: If medication is recommended, your health-care provider will weigh the benefits of treatment against the risks of prescribing a particular medication during pregnancy. When making your decision about medication use during pregnancy, remember that *not* treating depression can pose a risk to the health of both mother and baby.

Staying Healthy during Pregnancy

Your body has enough to deal with in pregnancy, so the last thing you'll want is a nasty cold or the flu. At worst, most illnesses will only be another inconvenience to deal with on top of the leg cramps, heartburn, and sleeplessness—reason enough to avoid them. However, some illnesses that your body fought easily before you were pregnant, such as high fevers, urinary tract infections, and food poisoning, could be dangerous to your baby now, so it's especially important that you take precautions to stay healthy. It's also important that you keep your health-care provider informed about what's going on with your health.

Take steps to avoid illness

The very same immune system changes that make it possible for your body to play host to your baby for the nine months of pregnancy leave you more susceptible to infection and illness. While you are pregnant, your immune system has to learn how to differentiate between the baby (which it doesn't want to attack) and foreign invaders, such as diseases, which it still wants to fight off, in order to keep you and your baby healthy. The immune system responds more vigorously to bacterial infections than it does to viral infections. As a result, viral infections and illnesses that your body can usually fight off without too much difficulty can pose a threat to the well-being of your baby.

Given your compromised immune system, taking the usual measures to avoid illness is even more important: wash your hands, eat well, exercise, avoid stress, and somehow get as much rest as you can. When winter rolls around, talk to your health-care practitioner about getting a flu shot. Be picky when you choose something to eat out of the fridge: if it's past the expiry date, toss it out. As well, make sure you prepare and store food properly to avoid food-borne illnesses. And you'll want to steer clear of sick co-workers and family members, not to mention that fellow bus passenger who's coughing up a lung.

5.4   When to Call Your Health-Care Provider

You should get in touch with your health-care provider right away if you experience any of the following symptoms or warning signals:

• Cramps or stomach pains that are painful and persistent

• Contractions that don't appear to follow the pattern of Braxton Hicks contractions

• Fever, chills, dizziness, vomiting, or a bad headache

• Blurry vision or spots before your eyes

• Sudden or severe swelling of the feet, hands, or face

• Bleeding or the passage of fluid from the vagina (a trickle or a gush)

• An increase in the amount of vaginal discharge

• Pain or pressure in your lower back

• A feeling like the baby is pushing down

• A sense that something just isn't quite right, and you feel the need to ask questions about what's going on with your body and your baby

---

flu vaccine

The influenza vaccine (a.k.a. the flu shot) is recommended for all pregnant women who will be in their second or third trimester during flu season. Possible risks of contracting the flu during pregnancy include pneumonia, reduced fetal growth, preterm labour, and maternal and fetal mortality. The vaccine doesn't provide total protection against the flu. When the vaccine and the viruses in circulation during a particular flu season are similar, the vaccine can prevent the flu among 70 to 90 per cent of healthy adults under 65. Even if you do get the flu, the vaccine can still protect you against flu-related complications by minimizing the severity of the illness. That's good news if you're having a baby and your immune system is in pregnancy mode.

Effects of infectious diseases and viruses on pregnancy

Most women breeze through pregnancy, feeling healthier than they've ever felt. But it is possible to contract a potentially serious illness. Here's what you need to know:

Varicella (chicken pox) and shingles. Exposure to chicken pox can lead to serious complications during pregnancy. Pneumonia is the most common maternal complication, something that is likely to become more severe if the mother is a smoker, has pre-existing lung disease or is already experiencing immune system problems, or has an extensive rash; or if the onset of chicken pox occurs during the third trimester of pregnancy. Hospitalization may be required if chest symptoms, neurological symptoms other than a headache, a hemorrhagic rash, bleeding, significant mucus membrane involvement, or other serious symptoms occur. Maternal death is a risk if the symptoms become extremely severe. Possible effects for your baby include prematurity, skin lesions, neurological abnormalities, eye anomalies, skeletal abnormalities, gastrointestinal and genitourinary anomalies, limb deformities, low birth weight, meningoencephalitis, miscarriage, and stillbirth. The most common birth defect associated with the chicken pox is limb abnormalities. (The incidence is 1 per cent if the mother contracts the chicken pox before 20 weeks of pregnancy.) Microcephaly, cataracts, and vocal cord paralysis are other possible effects. The good news is that 85 to 90 per cent of pregnant women are immune to chicken pox and shingles.

At your first prenatal visit, tell your health-care provider if you have never had chicken pox—a simple blood test can tell whether you're immune or not. If you suspect that you have been exposed to it during your pregnancy (either face-to-face contact for at least five minutes or indoor contact for more than an hour with someone who is contagious) and you don't know whether or not you're immune (for example, you haven't had chicken pox and you haven't lived in the same house with someone who has had chicken pox or shingles), call your health-care provider right away. Your doctor can administer a special type of immune globulin (VZIG) to prevent you from getting a severe infection. Chicken pox is most dangerous to the baby if you contract it shortly before or after giving birth.

Cytomegalovirus (CMV). CMV is commonly contracted in childhood, so you're probably immune to it, although it can be reactivated later in life. If you do contract it, the symptoms are usually mild, and include a sore throat, fatigue, fever, and swollen glands. If you are infected during pregnancy, the risks to your baby are low, but they could include miscarriage, intellectual disabilities, psychomotor retardation, developmental abnormalities, progressive hearing impairment, respiratory illness, jaundice, intrauterine growth restriction, failure to thrive, and eye infections. CMV is most likely to cause a problem if you contract it for the first time when you're pregnant.

Measles. Most women have been immunized against this disease, so it's very rare for a pregnant woman to contract it. If you do contract it, the symptoms will occur in two stages: first, a runny nose, cough, fever, and sensitivity to light; second, small white spots inside the mouth, then a red rash that starts on the face and moves down the body. Measles in a pregnant woman can result in fetal loss and prematurity.

Mumps. Mumps is another disease that has been virtually eliminated in North America due to immunization. Symptoms include swelling in the cheeks and jaw, muscle aches, fever, and fatigue. In the unlikely event that you do contract it while pregnant, it can cause miscarriage and preterm labour, and will increase your baby's risk of developing adult-onset diabetes.

Human parvovirus B19 (fifth disease or slapped cheek disease). Parvovirus B19 is a virus that is responsible for erythema infectiosum, a common childhood illness that is most commonly spread through respiratory secretions or via hand-to-mouth contact. The transmission rate of maternal parvovirus B19 from mother to baby is 17 to 33 per cent. Most babies infected recover on their own with no harmful effects. When there are harmful effects, however, they may include miscarriage (before 20 weeks, the rate is 14.8 per cent; after 20 weeks, the rate is 2.3 per cent), congenital anomalies (central nervous system, craniofacial, and eye anomalies), and fetal hydrops (fluid accumulation in fetal tissue) due to fetal anemia and heart failure. Most children born to mothers who were exposed to parvovirus B19 during pregnancy do not experience any long-term consequences.

If you suspect that you have been exposed to parvovirus B19 infection, you should arrange to be assessed to find out if you're immune to this particular illness or if you have a current infection. If, like 50 to 65 per cent of women of reproductive age, you have immunity, you can relax because you won't develop an infection and the virus won't have any impact on your pregnancy. If you have had a recent parvovirus B19 infection, you will be referred to an obstetrician or a maternal-fetal specialist who can talk to you about how your baby might be affected by exposure and arrange to conduct ultrasounds for 8 to 12 weeks after exposure to monitor for the development of fetal hydrops. If fetal hydrops develops, an intravascular transfusion may be recommended.

Rubella (German measles). You've likely been immunized against rubella—the Centers for Disease Control and Prevention consider it eradicated in the United States. It is a mild disease with symptoms of a fever, red rash, achy joints, and swollen lymph glands. Rubella can have very serious effects on the developing baby if a woman contracts the virus during pregnancy: miscarriage, fetal infection, stillbirth, fetal growth restriction, neuromotor deficits, pneumonitis, diabetes mellitus, thyroid dysfunctions, progressive panencephalitis, deafness (60 to 75 per cent), cardiac defects (10 to 20 per cent), eye problems (10 to 25 per cent), central nervous system disorders (10 to 25 per cent), and behavioural problems. The types of effects are determined by the gestational age at which maternal infection occurs, and the likelihood of infection also varies with the timing of exposure. During the first trimester, infection rates are nearly 80 per cent. This rate of infection drops to 25 per cent in the late second trimester, increases to 35 per cent at 27 to 30 weeks' gestation, to then become almost 100 per cent from 36 weeks of gestation on. The risk of birth defects is 90 per cent before 11 weeks, 33 per cent at 11 to 12 weeks, 24 per cent at 13 to 15 weeks and 0 per cent after 16 weeks. Fetal growth restriction only becomes a concern in cases of third-trimester infection.

The rubella vaccine is not recommended for use during pregnancy. The vaccine has the potential to cross the placenta and infect the fetus. The Society of Obstetricians and Gynaecologists of Canada (SOGC) recommends that you hold off on becoming pregnant for a period of 28 days following immunization. The vaccine can, however, be administered during pregnancy and to the children of pregnant women, with certain exceptions. The vaccine should not be administered to anyone with a history of febrile illness, immunodeficiency, or a history of an anaphylactic reaction to neomycin.

If you do happen to become pregnant after receiving your rubella immunization, try not to panic. According to the SOGC, there have been no reports of congenital rubella syndrome in babies born to women who were inadvertently vaccinated during early pregnancy.

Note: Inactive vaccines, such as the pneumococcal, influenza, diptheria, tetanus, and hepatitis B vaccines, are considered safe for use during pregnancy.

Sexually transmitted infections. These can be transmitted to the developing baby during pregnancy or at the time of birth. Chlamydia, syphilis, and herpes are linked to higher-than-average rates of stillbirth, premature labour, and other complications.

Urinary tract infections (UTIs). Urinary tract infections are relatively common (they are experienced by 2 to 13 per cent of pregnant women, but just 1 to 2 per cent of pregnant women experience symptoms). When symptoms occur, they include frequent urges to urinate, pain when urinating, and foul-smelling, cloudy urine. UTIs are caused by the anatomical changes of pregnancy, which lead to a pooling of the urine. Untreated UTIs can lead to more severe infections (pyelonephritis) in 20 to 40 per cent of cases, which can, in turn, lead to premature birth, low birth weight, and, occasionally, stillbirth. Prompt treatment with antibiotics is important, as is ongoing screening for symptomless infections. These antibiotics are safe during pregnancy.

Vulvovaginitis. Vulvovaginitis is the term used to describe fungal infections that occur in the vaginal mucous membranes. Vulvovaginitis is particularly common during pregnancy (the incidence rate is 30 per cent for pregnant women versus 15 to 20 per cent for non-pregnant women) for a few reasons: there is extra glucose in the cells in the vagina, estrogen levels are elevated, allowing candida (yeast) to thrive, and the immune system isn't working as well as it does when the body is in a non-pregnant state, making it easier for infection to set in. The infection can be passed to your baby during birth, causing thrush.

HIV. The Society of Obstetricians and Gynaecologists of Canada recommends that all pregnant women be screened for HIV during pregnancy. A mother who is HIV-positive has a 25 per cent risk of transmitting the virus to her newborn if no treatment is administered. It is possible to reduce this transmission rate by 90 per cent through treatment, according to the SOGC.

vaginal discharges

There's no need to be alarmed if you experience an increase in the amount of leukorrhea (the odourless white mucus discharge produced by the vagina) while you're pregnant. The hormonal changes of pregnancy cause your vaginal secretions to become wetter and more abundant.

There is, however, cause for concern if your vaginal discharge becomes greenish-yellow, foul smelling, or watery. These types of discharges may indicate that you've developed an infection that requires treatment, or that your membranes have ruptured prematurely. In either case you'll need to seek medical attention, since certain types of vaginal infections can increase your risk of experiencing various pregnancy-related complications. For example, bacterial vaginosis (an infection characterized by a thin, milky discharge with a fishy odour) is associated with an increased risk of premature labour, premature rupture of the membranes (PROM), and preterm delivery. Fortunately, bacterial vaginosis and other similar types of infections can usually be treated quickly and easily with oral antibiotics. Tip: You may want to talk to your health-care provider about the advisability of taking acidophilus to try to pre-empt a yeast infection triggered by antibiotics.

If you test positive for HIV, you should be treated with antiretroviral therapy between 15 and 19 weeks of pregnancy. A Caesarean section is only recommended as a method of delivery for those pregnant women who haven't received optimal antiviral therapy. If you haven't been treated during pregnancy, you should be offered a preventative dose of HIV prophylaxis during labour, and a preventative dose of HIV prophylaxis should be given to the baby postpartum. This reduces the risk of transmission by 12 to 13 per cent.

Other steps to staying healthy

Here are some other important points to keep in mind when it comes to staying healthy during pregnancy.

Schedule a rendezvous with your dentist

The hormonal changes of pregnancy increase your odds of developing periodontal disease (gum and bone problems in the mouth). So if you haven't spent any quality time with your dentist for as long as you can remember, schedule a rendezvous as soon as you can.

Book a checkup during your first trimester so you can have your teeth cleaned and your oral health assessed. If your dentist suggests medication as part of your dental treatment, make sure she knows that you're pregnant so that she can double-check that the medication is considered safe for use during pregnancy. If you require dental work, the best time to schedule it is during the second trimester. X-rays of your mouth should only be taken in an emergency, according to the Canadian Dental Association. Note: Abdominal X-rays, CAT scans, and diagnostic procedures involving radioactive dyes should also be avoided during pregnancy.

Brush and floss. I know. You're tired of hearing that boring dental health message, but it's extra important when you're pregnant. You're likely to find that your gums become more sensitive during the second and third trimesters and that they may even start bleeding when you brush your teeth. (What you're experiencing is pregnancy gingivitis, a common condition that typically disappears after you give birth.) The solution, in the meantime, is to brush your teeth at least twice a day, using a soft toothbrush and a fluoride toothpaste, and to continue to floss. (Your gums are more sensitive to bacteria along the gum line, so you want to get rid of as much of that bothersome bacteria as possible.) If you can't brush and floss after enjoying a snack on the go, eat some cheese, rinse your mouth with water, or chew a piece of sugarless gum.

Earlier studies pointing out a possible link between periodontal disease and preterm birth were refuted by a study of 823 pregnant women published in the

November 2, 2006, issue of the *New England Journal of Medicine*. The researchers concluded that periodontal treatment during pregnancy is safe, and having your teeth cleaned during pregnancy rather than after pregnancy doesn't appear to affect the likelihood that you will have a preterm birth.

Eat well

Ensure that your body is receiving the nutrients it needs to maintain your oral health and to help your baby to build strong teeth and bones. The key nutrients from an oral-health perspective are calcium, vitamins A, C, and D, as well as adequate protein and phosphorus.

Discuss complementary and alternative medicine with your health-care provider

Be sure to let your health-care provider know about your use of complementary and alternative medicine (CAM) so that she'll have a full picture of what types of health care you are receiving. That way, the two of you can discuss the safety of various CAM therapies during pregnancy.

Some CAM therapies, such as meditation, acupuncture, chiropractic treatment, deep breathing, massage therapy, and yoga, have many demonstrated benefits and have become so integrated with North American medicine that they are hardly considered alternative at all. Other CAM therapies may be well established, but may not yet have accumulated the body of research required to demonstrate their safety and effectiveness.

Here are some questions you may want to think about when you are considering a new CAM therapy or a new CAM practitioner:

- What scientific studies have been conducted to assess the safety and effectiveness of this therapy? Is this treatment considered to be safe and effective for pregnant women and their babies?
- What potential side effects (or interactions with other medications or herbal products) have been reported?
- What is the training, experience, and skill level of the CAM practitioner? What licences or certifications does this person have? Are they from accredited institutions?
- Do you feel comfortable with the practitioner? Was the practitioner able to answer your questions to your satisfaction?
- How much will the treatments cost? How many treatments will be required? Does the treatment plan seem reasonable and acceptable to you?

Hold off on getting that body art

Because of the increased risk of infection at the piercing site, body piercings and tattoos should be avoided during pregnancy. If infection were to occur, it could spread to your bloodstream and be carried to your baby. If non-sterile equipment is used during the piercing procedure, infections such as hepatitis B or C or HIV may also be transmitted.

There are a few additional issues to consider on the tattoo front as well. First, the jury's still out when it comes to the effects of tattoo inks and dyes on the developing baby. Second, not all health-care providers feel comfortable inserting an epidural through the site of a recent tattoo, so you'll want to inquire about hospital policy if both a pregnancy tattoo and a childbirth epidural are in your plans for the upcoming months.

Skip the hot stuff

Hold on. I'm not talking about that kind of hot stuff. We'll be having that conversation in Chapter 8. What I'm talking about is your body getting overheated from really vigorous exercise or a too-high fever. Whatever it is, it's bad for your baby, particularly if it occurs during early pregnancy. (A maternal fever of 38.9°C (102°F) lasting more than 24 hours during the first month of pregnancy increases the odds of a baby being born with a neural tube defect by 10 times. Cleft lip and cleft palate are associated with a high maternal fever, and cardiovascular disorders are associated with a high maternal fever plus influenza. That's why health-care experts advise pregnant women to avoid any activity that might result in overheating (a temperature of over 38.3°C/101°F). That includes exercising vigorously on a hot day, soaking in a hot tub, or hitting the sauna. It's also important to treat a fever, either by using an appropriate fever-relief medication or by using other methods of bringing down your temperature—stripping off layers of clothing, soaking in a lukewarm bathtub, and so on.)

Don't douche

Not only does douching increase your chances of experiencing an ectopic pregnancy and of developing pelvic inflammatory disease, some commercial douching preparations contain substances that could be harmful to the developing baby. Since I've been harping about not douching since the beginning of this book, this time around, for variety's sake, I'm going to hand the microphone over to Natalie Angiers, author of one of my all-time favourite books, *Woman: An Intimate Geography.* Here's what she has to say on the whole subject of douching: "Don't douche, ever, period, end of squirt bottle."

Staying Safe at Home

Home is where we go to relax and unwind, where we let ourselves be who we are. Because we're so comfortable in our own skin on our own turf we sometimes overlook the hazards in our own backyard or in our own bathroom. Here's a quick guide to staying safe and healthy in your home during pregnancy.

Medications

Old habits die hard. It's easy to stumble into the bathroom in the middle of the night on auto-pilot, open the medicine cabinet, and pop an old, familiar cold remedy into your mouth only to realize in horror, seconds later, that the rules that govern all your daily decisions recently changed: you're pregnant!

To avoid such a scenario, you may want to consider moving all of the medications that are temporarily off-limits to a lockbox. (That's where you'll want to store your medications once baby arrives on the scene anyway.)

Here are some other tips on medication use during pregnancy.

- Don't assume that it's business as usual when it comes to any prescription or over-the-counter medications you've been taking for a long time. If your pregnancy was unplanned and you are taking one or more medications, get in touch with your health-care provider right away to find out if it is still safe for you to take these medications during pregnancy. Some of the ingredients in common over-the-counter drug products can be harmful—even toxic—to the developing baby.

- Don't stop taking medications that have been prescribed to you without checking with your health-care provider first. Your caregiver may need to gradually reduce your dose of a particular medication or switch you to a different medication. Or she may weigh the risks of having you remain on the medication against the risks of going off it and decide that it's in the best interests of you and your baby for you to remain on the medication throughout the rest of your pregnancy. Your health-care provider will also consider

  - whether there is a single-action, short-acting medication available (as opposed to a long-acting medication) that will achieve the same therapeutic result;

  - whether there is a topical or inhaled version of the medication (as opposed to a systemic version) that will achieve the same therapeutic result;

  - whether a particular medication has a proven history of use during pregnancy without any adverse reactions as compared to a newer medication (for which there may not be the same amount of history available);

- – what the lowest effective dose of the safest available medication would be, given what is known about the various medications available at this time.
- • Make sure that anyone who is in a position to recommend or prescribe medications to you at any point during your pregnancy is aware that you are pregnant. And be sure to let them know just how far along you are. It's particularly important to minimize exposure to medications during the first trimester (when body systems are being established and organs are developing), if at all possible.

Herbal products

Herbal products may be derived from natural products, but that doesn't mean that they're necessarily safe to use during pregnancy. Because most herbal products are classified as dietary supplements, they are not regulated in the same way that pharmaceutical products are even though they can have powerful medicinal effects.

Very few controlled studies have been conducted to date on herbal products—and even fewer have studied the safety of these products during pregnancy. That's why it's generally best to avoid using an herbal product during pregnancy unless your health-care provider is able to reassure you that it won't pose any risk to you or your baby.

You may also want to consult the following sources to find out what is known about the effects of a particular herbal product on a pregnant woman and her baby:

The Motherisk Clinic: The Motherisk Clinic maintains a database summarizing what is known about the safety of various herbal products during pregnancy. You can contact the clinic—which is based at Toronto's Hospital for Sick Children—by calling 1–416–813–6780.

The Licensed Natural Health Products Database (LNHPD): The LNHPD contains product-specific information on those natural health products that have been issued a product licence by Health Canada, indicating that the product has been assessed by Health Canada and has been found to be safe, effective, and of high quality when used as recommended. The database includes information on licensed natural health products, such as vitamin and mineral supplements, herb and plant-based remedies, traditional medicines (such as traditional Chinese medicines or Ayurvedic medicines), Omega-3 and essential fatty acids, probiotics and homeopathic medicines as well as many everyday consumer products, such as certain toothpastes, antiperspirants, shampoos, facial products, and mouthwashes. You can find out more about the LNHPD by visiting the Health Canada website.

Toxins

It's easy to overlook the number of toxic substances we come into contact with in our homes and in our neighbourhoods: paints, solvents, lawn-care products, and other powerful chemicals in the environment. These are synthetic substances that our bodies—and our babies—simply don't know how to handle.

While scientists used to believe that the placenta acted as a filter, preventing harmful substances from reaching the baby, we now know that the baby is affected by environmental exposures during pregnancy and that those exposures can have far-reaching effects.

Research is still emerging in this area, but so far we know that prenatal exposure to environmental toxins can change the immune system, heighten sensitivity to allergens, and may result in low birth weight, premature birth, and reproductive abnormalities including infertility.

Not every baby exposed to a toxin will experience health problems. Genetic susceptibility, the timing of the exposure, the combined effects of various substances to which the developing baby has been exposed, and other unknown factors all come into play in determining how and to what extent a baby will be affected.

To minimize your exposure to chemicals in your home, take the following steps:

- Place mats inside and outside each door in your house so that you can knock as much dirt off your shoes when you enter your home. Then switch to indoor shoes or slippers (or go barefoot) when you're indoors so that you won't track in pesticides and other toxins from outdoors.
- If you live in an older home, let the water run for a minute before you take any water for drinking or for cooking. Stick to cold water. Hot water will remove higher levels of lead from the pipes.
- Have your soil tested for the presence of lead and other toxins before you plant any vegetables or fruit trees.
- If your house needs to be painted, use non-toxic paints, wear a face mask and protective clothing, and work in a well-ventilated area. If you have lead-based paint in your home, have it removed by a professional.

Ditto for dealing with any toxic mould problems in your home. And arrange to stay elsewhere while the work is being done to avoid exposing yourself and your baby to dangerous toxins.

- Minimize your use of consumer products containing lead: for example, lead-wicked candles, certain cosmetics, inexpensive jewellery, and other household items. Pay attention to consumer product alerts and recalls so that you can take back any products you own that have been found to contain lead.

- Choose alternatives to soft vinyl products so that you can minimize the amount of PVC and phthalates found in your home. Phthalates are used to soften plastic. Research has indicated that these chemicals have a tendency to take on hormone-like qualities in the human body.

- Use glass containers rather than plastic containers for reheating food. Microwave-safe plastic containers shouldn't leach chemicals to the same degree as other plastic containers, but the best way to reduce chemical leaching from plastic exposures is to avoid reheating food in plastic containers, period. And never reheat food in a plastic container (or using plastic wrap or a plastic bag) that isn't designed for use in a microwave oven. You could end up leaching phthalates from the plastics into your food.

- Use non-toxic cleaners, solvents, and paints wherever possible. If you need to use a toxic product, purchase the minimum quantity required for the job and follow the product instructions carefully to minimize the risk to your health.

- Don't use pesticides or herbicides, even if they're still permitted in your community. They contain deadly toxins that have been associated with learning, behavioural, and developmental disabilities; immune system problems; and reproductive disorders.

- Be aware of the hazardous substances associated with your hobbies, such as painting or photography. Use non-toxic alternatives, if available, or use toxic products in well-ventilated areas. Note: Depending on the risks associated with some of the chemicals involved (call the Motherisk Clinic at 1–416–813–6780 or visit www.motherisk.org), you may want to put some of your hobbies on hold until after you have your baby.

- Wash fruit and vegetables (and peel, if appropriate) to remove any pesticide residue. Note: Organically grown produce doesn't have to be peeled.

- Stick to Health Canada's guidelines concerning fish consumption during pregnancy. (See the section on essential fatty acids earlier in this chapter.) Fish is an important source of essential fatty acids, so you don't want to eliminate it from your diet entirely, but it's important to avoid consuming excess quantities and to steer clear of certain types of fish that are known to be particularly high in mercury.

- Avoid pesticide-based head lice treatments. Ask your pharmacist to recommend a pesticide-free alternative instead.
- Ask your dentist to use alternatives to mercury-based fillings in your teeth.
- Err on the side of caution when it comes to threats to your health or your baby's health at home and at work. (See the discussion about hazards in the workplace later in this chapter.)
- Join forces with others who share your concern about the environment and its effect on the health of pregnant women and their babies to press governments for stricter pre-market testing of products containing synthetic chemicals. As Mohawk midwife Katsi Cook once noted, "Women are the first environment."

To find out more about the risks posed by various types of environmental toxins on human health, you may want to visit the websites of the Canadian Association of Physicians for the Environment: www.cape.ca and Science and Environmental Health Network: www.sehn.org.

Diseases carried by pets and other animals

The litter box. Both cat feces and raw meat may contain a parasite called

---

prenatal lead exposure

Prenatal lead exposure is harmful to the developing baby—one of the reasons why lead was removed from gas and paints in the late 1970s. Each 10 microgram per decilitre increase in blood lead levels leads to an average five-point decrease in IQ levels. Lead exposure during pregnancy is also associated with miscarriage, preterm birth, low birth weight, and neurobehavioural-cognitive deficits. It can also have an impact on male fertility, leading to decreased sperm counts and motility, and impotence and lack of libido in adult males.

Any new lead exposures that occur during pregnancy are shared with the baby. Any toxins that are stored in a pregnant woman's bones—the result of a lifetime of environmental exposures—can be mobilized and shared with her baby as her body draws upon her calcium stores to meet the needs of her developing baby. Ensuring an adequate calcium intake through food sources can help to minimize this effect. See the section on nutrition during pregnancy, earlier in this chapter, for advice on maximizing your calcium intake during pregnancy.

toxoplasmosis, which can be very harmful to the developing baby. (See the section on food-borne illnesses earlier in this chapter.) It's best to avoid changing kitty litter at all while you're pregnant, but if you absolutely have to do it because no one can take over this task for you, wear gloves and then wash your hands thoroughly.

Contaminated garden soil. The same rule applies to gardening, by the way: wear gloves. Some friendly neighbourhood cat may have chosen your garden for a litter box. Wear gloves when you're gardening and be sure to thoroughly wash the soil off any vegetables you harvest from your garden, just in case the soil has been contaminated with cat or other animal feces.

Rodent problems. If you have a mouse or rat infestation problem at your house, deal with it right away. A pet rodent, such as a hamster, might need to find a temporary new home. Rodents can spread diseases that can be harmful to the developing baby. One such disease is caused by the lymphocytic choriomeningitis virus (LCMV). LCMV infection can result in hydrocephalus (excess fluid in the head), developmental problems, blindness, and even death. Hire a pest-control company to deal with the problem or ask another family member to set traps (as opposed to using chemicals that can be dangerous to a pregnant woman and her baby).

Accidents and falls

While it's best to avoid any sort of abdominal trauma while you're pregnant, you may find it reassuring to know that your baby is well protected from day-to-day tumbles. This is because your body is designed to protect your developing baby. Your uterus is made up of a thick wall of muscle that helps to keep your baby safe. What's more, within the uterus, your baby is cushioned by the amniotic fluid that he or she floats around in. And during the early weeks of pregnancy, your baby has some added protection: the uterus is hidden away behind the thick pelvic bone. When you stop to consider all the things that can be harmful to the developing fetus, you may be tempted to hide under the covers for the next nine months. It's easy to become paranoid, but it's important to keep things in perspective: the odds of ending up with a healthy baby in your arms nine months down the road are decidedly in your favour.

Domestic violence

No woman wants to consider the possibility that she could be abused by her partner during pregnancy, but abuse is a fact of life for pregnant women across

> About 6 to 7 per cent of women who are pregnant are involved in a car crash during their pregnancy. A study reported in the April 2008 issue of the *American Journal of Obstetrics and Gynecology* concluded that the proper use of seatbelts by all pregnant women (the seatbelt buckled under the abdomen) would prevent approximately 84 per cent of serious adverse injuries to the fetus and fetal deaths due to car accidents.

Canada every single day. Maybe it's happened to a friend of yours. Maybe it's happening to you.

According to Health Canada, 21 per cent of women who have been abused were abused during pregnancy. Forty per cent of these women reported that the violence first started during pregnancy. A study of pregnant women in Toronto found that 6.6 per cent were being abused during their current pregnancy and 11 per cent had been abused prior to this pregnancy. A similar study of pregnant women in Saskatoon found that 5.7 per cent were being abused during their current pregnancy and 8.5 per cent had been abused during the year prior to pregnancy.

In many cases, domestic violence begins during pregnancy, with the frequency and severity of episodes often increasing while a woman is pregnant. The abuse may be triggered by the physical and emotional changes of pregnancy. The abuser may resent these changes or having to share the woman's attention with the baby, may fear losing control over the woman, particularly as the woman's health-care provider and others encourage her to make the healthiest choices for herself and her baby, and may be stressed by the financial changes associated with pregnancy.

Physical attacks during pregnancy may target the areas associated with pregnancy (the pregnant woman's breasts, abdomen, and genitalia) as a way to channel pregnancy-related anger and to hide the injuries associated with the assault.

Effects of domestic violence during pregnancy

According to the Society of Obstetricians and Gynaecologists of Canada, domestic violence (a.k.a. intimate partner violence) during pregnancy cause the following:

- a delay in the pregnant mother seeking prenatal care
- insufficient pregnancy weight gain
- infections during pregnancy (vaginal, cervical, kidney, uterine)
- worsening of chronic illnesses
- maternal stress and depression
- an increased risk of the pregnant mother being suicidal

- abdominal trauma
- first- and second-trimester bleeding
- miscarriage
- hemorrhage
- premature rupture of membranes (PROM)
- intrauterine growth restriction
- premature labour and birth
- placental abruption
- complications during labour
- low birth weight—the birth of a baby weighing less than 5.5 pounds (2.5 kilograms)
- injury to or death of the developing baby

Other effects of domestic violence during pregnancy

Not surprisingly, moms-to-be who live with the threat of violence are more likely to experience depression and thoughts of suicide, to eat poorly, and to turn to alcohol, cigarettes, and illicit drugs as a means of coping with their stress.

For women with a history of sexual abuse, giving birth may be extremely traumatic. The pain associated with the contractions, the sense of loss of control, and the pelvic/genital exams by multiple health-care providers may trigger painful memories, causing women to disassociate or react with fear, panic, or other extremes of emotion.

What every woman needs to know about domestic violence

Domestic violence doesn't have to be physical to be abusive. Domestic violence can involve other types of behaviours that are designed to threaten, intimidate, or control you. Domestic violence is all about power and control. An abusive partner might . . .

- attack you verbally by calling you names and humiliating you in front of others.
- belittle your accomplishments and whittle away at your self-esteem.
- keep tabs on where you are and what you are doing every minute of the day.
- isolate you from family and friends.
- prevent you from accessing health care (doctor, midwife, dentist).
- stalk or harass you.
- threaten to hurt people you love or to harm your pets.

- threaten you with a weapon or other objects.
- destroy your property.
- refuse to have sex with you or force you to engage in sex.
- force you to become pregnant or to have an abortion.
- limit your financial independence or use your credit cards without permission.

Abuse is never justified. It can't be excused because someone simply lost their cool because they got too angry, they're under too much stress, or they were drunk. Abuse is wrong and it's a crime.

Nothing you said or did justifies the abuse. No one deserves to be hit, humiliated, or stolen from—and especially not by someone who claims to love them. And accepting an apology in order to buy yourself some peace is a painful price to have to keep paying over and over again.

You can't fix someone else. An abusive individual is the only one who can deal with the underlying issues that trigger the abuse. The individual has to want to deal with the problem. To make the kinds of changes involved in tackling a problem like this requires guts and hard work—and dealing with all the muck that gets dredged up during therapy. You can't want that change for someone else. They have to want it for themselves. Change truly must come from within.

- Don't settle for apologies and promises in lieu of action. You deserve so much more.
- You have to put the safety of yourself and your baby ahead of any other concerns. The effects of abuse during pregnancy are far reaching. Abuse affects your baby and it affects you. Abuse always causes harm.
- The abuse is likely to continue after your baby is born. Sixty-four per cent of women who were abused during pregnancy reported that the violence escalated during pregnancy, and 95 per cent of women who were abused during the first trimester reported that the violence escalated after the baby was born. Sixty-two per cent of the women involved in this particular study required medical care for injuries during the postpartum period.
- Children whose mothers experience intimate partner violence face a greater risk of developmental difficulties and of being abused themselves.
- Every woman who is being abused needs a safety plan. In addition to

thinking about who you would call for help and where you would go if things got out of control, you need to have access to certain important items (you may want to leave them in the care of a friend, family member, or your lawyer just in case): birth certificates, health cards, passports, immigration papers and other key identification for you and your children (originals or photocopies); school and immunization records; bank, tax, and key financial records (lease or rental agreement, house deed, mortgage payment book, insurance papers); credit cards; cash, keys for house, car, safety deposit box; photograph of partner; address book; prescriptions/medications; clothing for you and your children; and children's items.

Support is available for women who are thinking about leaving an abusive relationship. Consult your phone book for local services. Inspired by the Best Start pamphlet *Abuse in Pregnancy: Information and Strategies for the Prenatal Educator.*

Staying Healthy at Work

Gone are the days when a woman was expected to resign from her job the moment she found herself "in the family way." Pregnant women are as much a part of the modern workplace as smartphones.

According to the SOGC, most women experiencing low-risk pregnancies can safely continue to work outside the home. If, however, your job is physically demanding (for example, it requires repeated stooping and bending, repeated climbing of ladders, poles, or stairs, or heavy lifting), exposes you to radiation, toxins, or other harmful substances (see Table 5.6), or involves shift work or prolonged standing, you might want to consider switching jobs or requesting a job modification for all or part of your pregnancy. Jobs such as these can modestly increase your chances of miscarrying, going into labour prematurely, or having a low birth weight baby.

Even if your job doesn't present any obvious threat, you'll still need to make an effort to take care of yourself while you're on the job. Here are a few tips:

Realize that you may have to spill the beans sooner than you had intended. If you are routinely exposed to cigarette smoke, infectious diseases, heavy metals, toxic chemicals, oil-based paints, radiation, anaesthetic gases, or other harmful substances at work; your job is highly stressful, strenuous, or physically demanding; you have to stand for more than three hours per day at work or you have to do a lot of bending, stooping, stair or ladder climbing, or heavy lifting; you work in an extremely hot, cold, or noisy environment; or you work long hours (more than 40 hours a week) or rotating shifts, you should plan to meet with your employer to discuss job modifications as soon as possible. You may be worried about how your employer or coworkers will react. Don't let that stop you from taking proper care of yourself and your baby. (Table 5.5 will help you to assess how pregnancy-friendly your employer is right now—and where there may be room for improvement.)

Get up and move around as often as you can—at least once every couple of hours. Sitting down for more than three hours at a stretch can lead to fluid retention in your legs and feet, reduced blood flow to your baby, muscle strain (particularly in your lower back), and tension in your back and shoulder areas.

Find a position that's comfortable for you while you're working at your desk. Place a pillow behind the small of your back, prop your feet up on a

---

5.5   How Pregnancy-Friendly Is Your Workplace?

Does your employer . . .

- demonstrate a positive attitude toward workers who are pregnant?
- offer emergency first-aid training and CPR training to all employees so that they know how to deal with health-related emergencies at work?
- have an emergency response plan that spells out what to do if an employee is in need of emergency medical care?
- protect workers from reproductive hazards, including tobacco smoke, and encourage workers to check Workplace Hazardous Materials Information System (WHMIS) sheets so that they can be informed about the hazards posed by all materials used in the workplace? (Visit the Health Canada website or the website of your provincial or territorial ministry of occupational safety and health to find out more about WHMIS.)
- provide suitable protective gear to all workers, including pregnant women?
- ensure that the workplace is properly ventilated and that the temperature and noise levels do not exceed recommended levels?
- suggest job modifications so pregnant workers can avoid heavy lifting, prolonged standing, working excessive hours, and exposure to reproductive hazards?
- schedule short breaks at least once every two hours and make it possible for pregnant workers to rest during those breaks?
- offer family-friendly policies such as part-time and flex-time work options, job sharing options, and employee and family assistance programs so that pregnant workers can find creative ways to balance their working lives with their need to attend prenatal appointments, adjust to the physiological changes of pregnancy, and take the best possible care of themselves and their babies?

5.6 Hazards in the Workplace

Here are a few of the more common workplace hazards that pose a risk to the pregnant worker or her baby.

Type of Risk	Potential Effect on Pregnant Worker	Potential Effect on Developing Baby
Anaesthetics		Miscarriage
Carbon monoxide		Miscarriage, premature birth, congenital malformation
Solvents such as benzene, trichloroethylene, carbon tetrachloride, vinyl chloride, chloroprene, epichlorohydrin, carbon disulfide	Increased susceptibility to poisoning (liver, kidney, blood, central nervous system problems)	Miscarriage, premature birth, congenital malformation, visual impairment, learning and behaviour problems
Toxic metals, lead, mercury, cadmium	Increased susceptibility to poisoning (liver, kidney, blood, central nervous system problems)	Miscarriage, stillbirth, premature birth, low birth weight, congenital abnormalities, learning and behaviour problems
Physical Hazards		
Biological hazards (e.g., exposure to German measles, measles, mumps, bacteria in a hospital or laboratory setting)		Miscarriage, congenital malformation
Extreme heat and humidity	Increased susceptibility to respiratory, gynecological, and urinary tract infection	Miscarriage, premature birth, neural tube defects
Ionizing radiation (e.g., radiology department at a hospital)		Central nervous system abnormalities, intellectual disabilities

Sources: Organization of Teratology Information Specialists (www.otispregnancy.org), Illinois Teratogen Information Service (www.fetal-exposure.org), March of Dimes (www.marchofdimes.com), and Motherisk (www.motherisk.org).

footstool or an open desk drawer (to relieve pressure on your lower back), and make sure you take regular breaks.

Take steps to avoid carpal tunnel syndrome. If you spend a lot of time at a computer or doing other repetitive motions, make sure that your workstation is designed to reduce the risk of carpal tunnel syndrome (a condition in which the nerves in the wrist become compressed by fluids retained by the surrounding tissues). If you find yourself experiencing any of the telltale symptoms, such as numbness and tingling in your hand, pain in your wrist or arm, weakness in your hand and thumb, and more intense symptoms when using your hands and at night, deal with the problem immediately by resting and elevating your hand. Your health-care provider may suggest that you wear a splint to avoid further damage. Sure, the condition is likely to resolve itself once you've had your baby and your fluid balance returns to normal (provided you haven't done any lasting damage to the nerves in your wrist by then). But that's many months from now.

Dress for comfort, not style. You've got the rest of your life to try to squeeze into high heels and power suits. For now, focus on comfort. Wear low-heeled, comfortable shoes and loose-fitting clothing (ideally natural fibres, which tend to be more comfortable when you get overheated, as most pregnant women do). If you dress in layers you can remove a layer or two to adjust your temperature up and down.

Eat, drink, and be merry. Make a point of stopping for snacks and meals at regular intervals, no matter how crazy things may be at the office. Keep a refillable bottle of water on your desk so that you can remember to keep yourself well hydrated. And try to keep your stress level to a minimum. (That may be easier said than done.)

---

travelling for work

If your job is likely to require some out-of-town travel during your pregnancy, make sure you bring along a copy of your prenatal record. That way, if you run into unexpected pregnancy complications, the doctor on call at the emergency ward at the nearest hospital will have the information he or she needs to provide you and your baby with the best possible prenatal care.

Most airlines have policies prohibiting women from flying during the last two months of pregnancy unless they have a doctor's certificate—something you'll definitely need to keep in mind when you're scheduling business trips.

You'll also want to consider your own comfort before you agree to attend that conference halfway around the world when you're six and a half months along. Don't forget to consider what happens when you travel in the real world—as opposed to what your itinerary outlines. Missed connections, an impromptu overnight camp-out in the airport, and all the other joys of travel—with a baby bouncing on your bladder all the while.

Master the art of the power nap. If you're feeling drop-dead exhausted (a not uncommon condition during the first and third trimesters, by the way), then try to squeeze in a nap during your lunch hour or afternoon break. If that's not possible, make flopping down on the couch for half an hour a sacred part of your daily arriving-home-from-work ritual.

Get your Zs. You can't expect to function well on the job if you're sleep-deprived, so be sure to hit the hay early enough to get a good night's sleep. Your sleep needs increase while you're pregnant. Instead of getting away with seven or eight hours a night—what a typical woman of child-bearing age requires—you may find that you need nine or ten hours.

Until now, I've been focusing on health and safety: yours and Baby's. In the next few chapters, I'm going to broaden that focus a little by bringing life-style into the picture. We'll still be talking about what's going on with your baby and your body (starting with your baby's development, week by week, and the A-to-Z roundup of pregnancy symptoms). First stop: your incredible growing baby.

CHAPTER 6

Your Incredible Growing Baby

"When my baby started moving inside me—the best feeling in the world, by the way—I'd worry if it was less active or didn't move for a while. One day I was so upset that the baby hadn't moved much that I put on my *Mozart for Mothers-to-Be* CD: one set of headphones for me and another on my tummy. The baby started kicking immediately. I was so relieved."

—JENNIFER, 27, CURRENTLY PREGNANT
WITH HER FIRST CHILD

Ever wish you had a window in your belly so you could look inside and see what is going on with your baby? This chapter offers the next best thing: detailed information about how your baby changes and grows as your pregnancy progresses. This week-by-week and month-by-month guide also highlights the ways your body anticipates and prepares to meet your baby's needs for pregnancy, birth, and breastfeeding, while continuing to meet your own needs at the same time.

You can track these exciting changes starting with the first day of your last menstrual period (LMP) or in terms of your baby's gestational (or fetal) age. Gestational age is measured from the first day of conception (if known) or calculated based on menstrual cycle length or ultrasound results. Fetal development is commonly tracked in relation to gestational age—the age of the developing embryo (weeks four to eight) or fetus (weeks nine to thirty-eight). (Weeks one to three are generally referred to as the fertilization period or pre-embryonic period.)

Your health-care provider, however, will likely refer to the number of weeks since your last period, so I've used LMP dates here. If at any point you want to know the gestational age, just subtract two weeks from the LMP date.

The First Trimester: The Beginnings of Life, and the Start of a Whole New Way of Life

Before ovulation

Week 1

Your pregnancy journey begins on the first day of the last menstrual period you'll have for a while, whether you know it yet or not. There's no fetal age yet, since you haven't even conceived, but this is the time when your baby is the proverbial twinkle in your eye. Your due date will be calculated by adding 280 days (40 weeks) to the first day of your last period. Note: Your health-care provider may adjust your due date, based on the length of your menstrual cycle or the results of an ultrasound or other test.

Week 2

This is prime time when it comes to conception. If you're actively trying to conceive, you may be having sex every day or every other day this week. To maximize your odds of conceiving, you'll want to have an abundance of healthy sperm on hand when ovulation occurs. (See Chapter 3 for more about getting pregnant.) Intercourse lasts for four minutes, on average, and during the big event, blood volume in the penis typically increases by 50 per cent.

Before pregnancy, your uterus (which will be measured by your caregiver in centimetres) measures 7.5 × 5 × 2.5 centimetres and is capable of holding approximately 2 teaspoons (10 millilitres). By the end of your pregnancy it will measure 20 × 25 × 22.5 centimetres and be capable of holding an incredible 21 cups (5 litres) or more.

Pre-embryonic stage: The first three weeks of development

Week 3

Your baby's fetal age is calculated from this point onward (assuming, of course, you conceive). Your pregnancy (as calculated from the first day of your last menstrual period) is typically two weeks farther along than your baby's fetal age. Ovulation occurs and, if this is your cycle to conceive, conception will occur.

The total quantity of semen ejaculated is approximately half a teaspoon to one and a quarter teaspoons (2 to 6 millilitres), and each quarter teaspoon (about

1 millilitre) of semen holds an average of 100 million sperm. Sperm gain their ability to swim (at a speed of 2 to 3 millimetres (0.08 to 0.12 inches) per minute) once they hit the female reproductive tract, hitching a ride via cervical mucus, which tends to be super-stretchy around the time of ovulation. Cervical mucus is designed to protect, nourish, and transport sperm; it may even help to filter abnormal sperm. Sperm is packaged in semen, which is rich in fructose, providing the sperm with a source of energy and added protection against the acidic vaginal environment. Some sperm survive up to 80 hours, but most don't survive more than 48 hours.

Only 1 per cent of sperm reach the egg right away. Other sperm find their way to the egg during the next few days, guided by an attractant found in the follicular fluid of the egg follicle. Several hundred helper sperm are needed to assist the successful sperm in making it through the outer membrane of the ovum. At that point, physiochemical changes occur, making the membrane impenetrable by additional sperm.

Your baby's first home is made nice and cushy in the next stage of the process. The corpus luteum, or yellow body (which is the portion of the dominant egg follicle that is left behind in the ovary), begins to secrete large quantities of progesterone. This blast of hormones causes the uterine lining (or endometrium) to thicken in preparation for implantation and uterine secretions to increase. The endometrium needs to be thick so that it can supply nutrition and oxygen to the ball of cells (or blastocyst) until the placenta is ready to take over this function.

The single-celled zygote (which consists of 46 chromosomes: 23 from the female and 23 from the male) starts making its way down the Fallopian tube toward the uterus. While it travels, it begins a process of cell division known as mitosis. Within a day of fertilization, the zygote divides itself into two cells. Then it divides into four cells, then eight cells, and so on. If all goes well, the single-celled zygote will eventually develop into a 6-million-celled mature fetus, and your body will be fully prepared for labour, birth, and breastfeeding. Within five to seven days, the zygote is a much more complex being with distinct layers of cells—an outer layer and an inner layer—as well as the beginnings of an amniotic cavity and what will become an amniotic membrane. It is now known as a blastocyst.

Some pregnancies result in the conception of more than one baby. Sometimes two or more eggs are released and fertilized, resulting in the conception of fraternal (non-identical) twins, triplets, or other multiples. Or a single egg is released and fertilized, but then that egg splits in half, resulting in the conception of two identical twins. Or a combination of these events occurs, resulting in the conception of a large number of babies, some of whom are identical and some of whom are fraternal.

Your body starts preparing for a possible pregnancy during the luteal (post-ovulatory) phase of your menstrual cycle. Every month your body assumes you're going to conceive unless it receives evidence to the contrary in the form of the arrival of your menstrual period. Those incredibly inconvenient premenstrual symptoms you may experience—bloating, abdominal cramps, constipation, swelling or tenderness in the breasts, cyclic acne, headaches, increased emotional sensitivity, irritability, and tension—are associated with your rising progesterone levels.

> **progesterone**
>
> Progesterone is the hormone responsible for your pre-dinner and post-dinner pregnancy naps and the nighttime battle of the blankets (the one in which you become overheated and start removing blankets, regardless of the season). It's also responsible for your frequent treks to the bathroom. Progesterone relaxes the smooth muscle tissue throughout your body, including the muscles that control the flow of urine.

Week 4

Your baby measures a whole 0.2 millimetres (0.008 inches) from head to rump, which is the way a baby's length is measured before birth. Not that you'd be able to tell which end is the head and which is the rump. At this point your baby is just a tiny ball of cells.

A week after ovulation, progesterone causes tiny hair-like protrusions from the cells of the endometrium to group together to form smooth, flower-like protrusions called pinopodes. Their job is to create an implantation-friendly environment. They absorb liquid and make it less likely that the fertilized egg will be bumped away by the hair-like protrusions. These pinopodes only last for two days before their job is done.

The ball of fertilized cells (or blastocyst) reaches the uterus about five days after ovulation, and spends the next day just floating around. During this time, it obtains its nutrition from secretions from uterine glands. Some of the cells begin to separate into a thick inner mass and a thin outer shell. Approximately six to nine days after fertilization, the blastocyst begins to embed in the endometrium (the uterine lining), ideally on either the front or back wall of the uterus. Some women notice a small amount of light bleeding or spotting (implantation bleeding) approximately 10 days after conception.

For the next week or so, the blastocyst obtains its nourishment and oxygen from the cells that line the wall of the uterus. The blastocyst also starts to produce a hormone called hCG (human chorionic gonadotropin)—the hormone that your pregnancy test will detect. The hCG maintains the uterine lining and the corpus luteum. By the end of week four of your pregnancy, your precious little blastocyst's implantation is complete.

Your uterus begins to grow as soon as implantation occurs (even if implantation occurs outside of the uterus). As your pregnancy progresses, your uterus changes from its non-pregnant pear shape to a spherical shape, and then to a cylindrical shape. It ends up tilting and rotating to take advantage of whatever space it can find in increasingly cramped quarters.

Week 5

The ball of cells that will become your baby is growing by leaps and bounds, and will measure between 2 and 3 millimetres (0.08 and 0.12 inches) long this week. At the start of this week, it is oval or round, but within three days it becomes long and pear-shaped. By the end of the week, it will be longer and slipper-shaped (think ballet slipper, not bunny slipper).

Blood vessels begin to appear and create the beginnings of the cardiovascular system. After about seven days, a tube-shaped heart is formed and begins to beat. Three separate layers of cells, which are the building blocks of the various types of body tissue, are laid down: the ectoderm layer, used to create skin, hair, nails, and the nervous system; the mesoderm layer, used to create the major structural tissues in the body; and the endoderm layer, used to create the cells that line the organs. Gaps appear between layers of the mesoderm, leaving room for the heart, lungs, and organs in the abdomen.

Embryonic stage: Your baby begins to develop human characteristics

Week 6

Your baby (called an embryo at this stage) is now 4 to 6 millimetres (0.16 to 0.24 inches) long and is shaped like a tiny *c*, since rapid growth of the brain and spinal cord have caused the body to curl. Some people think the embryo resembles a tiny seahorse. You may not, but at any rate you can now distinguish the head from the rest of the body. Many other amazing developments happen this week:

- The brain develops into five areas. The forebrain is prominent and cranial nerves are visible.
- The neural tube starts to fuse. It ultimately becomes the spinal cord.
- The preliminary structures of the baby's eyes and ears begin to form.

- Upper limb buds (which will become the arms) appear, followed by lower limb buds (the future legs).
- The heart is beating.
- Tiny buds that will ultimately develop into the lungs, stomach, liver, and pancreas are present.
- The basic structures of all the organ systems have been put in place, including the placenta.
- A large tail is present. (It gradually disappears as the baby continues to develop.)

The corpus luteum supports the pregnancy for the first six to seven weeks, until the placenta is fully functional.

Your cervix undergoes some noteworthy changes during pregnancy. It becomes thicker and wider; it becomes softer (as a result of increased blood flow to the region); and it takes on a lilac tint. A greater quantity of cervical mucus is produced during pregnancy, and a mucus plug is produced to make it more difficult for infections to pass from the vagina to the uterus. Months from now, prior to or during labour, this plug will be released as part of your show. (The discharge you release before delivery, that is. Don't worry; no one is selling tickets.)

Week 7

Baby will be 7 to 9 millimetres (0.28 to 0.35 inches) long this week. The brain is developing rapidly and the head is growing at a rapid rate, too. The result? A baby that appears to be mostly head. The facial features on that giant head will become more prominent this week.

Upper limb buds (the future hands) take on paddle-like features, and lower limb buds (the future feet) take on flipper-like features. The baby's third, permanent set of kidneys are starting to form (after having already gone through two other sets), and the umbilical cord becomes clearly visible.

By week seven, the placenta is capable of producing enough progesterone to maintain the pregnancy. There is a slight dip in progesterone levels as the corpus luteum ceases to function, but then progesterone levels continue to rise once again as the placenta fully takes over.

Week 8

Your baby, who is 11 to 14 millimetres (0.43 to 0.55 inches) long, will become a boy or girl this week, as the sex organs start to take on either male or female characteristics. There is rapid growth in the hindbrain, and the external ear canal and the outer ear are formed, although they initially appear as swellings. Eye pigment has been formed, making the eye much more visible.

The upper limbs also experience a lot of growth this week: the elbow and wrist regions can be seen, as can little buds that will ultimately become fingers. Within a few days, the lower limbs will mirror this growth. Your baby's intestines are also growing rapidly—so much so that they bulge out of the tiny abdominal cavity into the umbilical cord due to space constraints.

Week 9

The bones of your 16- to 18-millimetre-long (0.63- to 0.71-inch-long) baby are beginning to harden, and the fingers are starting to separate from one another, although they are still very short and webbed. The liver becomes very prominent this week. Your baby's tail is still present, but it's getting shorter.

Week 10

Baby weighs 4 grams (0.14 ounces) now—a bit less than a sugar cube—and is 27 to 31 millimetres (1.06 to 1.22 inches) long. Half of that is head, but it's a head that is starting to look a little more recognizable:

- The face and neck are well formed by now.
- The eyelids are formed.
- The ears may be low-set on the head, but they are actually starting to look like real ears.

The fingers are separated, but still webbed. However, the toes are no longer fully joined together. Bone tissue begins to develop in lower limbs, and deliberate

fetal heart rate

Heart rate patterns have long been considered to be an important indicator of fetal well-being. Now heart rate patterns before birth are being used to suggest the rate at which children will develop through their toddler years. Scientists at Johns Hopkins Bloomberg School of Public Health, the National Institutes of Health, and Johns Hopkins Medical Institutions discovered that, after about 28 weeks of gestation, greater variation in fetal heart rate predicted better performance on a standardized developmental exam administered when the children were 2 years old, and superior language abilities when the children were 2 and a half years old. They published the results of their research in the November/December 2007 issue of the journal *Child Development.*

limb movements begin to appear. Your baby's stubby tail will (thankfully) disappear this week.

Your baby's heart is working hard. The fetal heart rate (FHR) can range anywhere from 110 to 160 beats per minute. It's probably in the 130 to 160 beats per minute range (as compared to 90 to 140 bpm for toddlers, 80 to 110 bpm for preschoolers, and 75 to 100 bpm for children). The heart rate will gradually decrease as pregnancy progresses.

External genitalia are visible now, but don't get too excited: it's too soon to tell whether your baby is a boy or a girl.

Fetal stage: Your baby's body systems mature

Weeks 11 to 14

Your baby, who will weigh 10 to 45 grams (0.35 to 1.59 ounces) and measure 5 to 8 centimetres (2 to 3 inches) during this month, is now known as a fetus and is about to enter a growth spurt—growth in body length and limbs speeds up for the next two weeks. Baby's face is beautiful to you, of course, but it hasn't taken on the characteristics of a newborn yet. The face is broad and the eyes are still quite far apart. Over the next three weeks, the eyes will move closer together and the ears will assume their standard position as well.

During this period, bone tissue develops in the skull and in the longest bones of the skeleton, the intestines return to the abdominal cavity, and the production of red blood cells by the liver decreases and starts up in the spleen. The fetus starts to produce urine and begins to transfer waste products to you via the placenta. By the end of the first trimester, approximately 12 to 13 weeks, the placenta is fully functioning.

Your baby is beginning to make sucking motions and is starting to swallow amniotic fluid. Amniotic fluid is made up of amniotic cells, maternal blood, and fetal urine. At 12 weeks, there is approximately 30 millilitres (1 ounce) of amniotic fluid, and this will increase to approximately 1.5 litres (51 ounces) by term.

The top of your uterus (the fundus) changes from a spherical shape to a dome shape between 12 and 16 weeks of pregnancy. Your uterus has a natural tendency to want to contract, particularly once the uterus starts shifting position and practice contractions (a.k.a. Braxton Hicks contractions) begin to occur. Braxton Hicks contractions—contractions that don't result in the onset of labour—can be measured from the first trimester of pregnancy onward. They help to ensure the movement of blood to the placenta. They differ from bona fide labour contractions in that they are irregular, weak, and unsynchronized, and they occur in multiple locations at the same time. Contraction activity will increase during pregnancy by 5 per cent per week. Luckily, hormones such as progesterone, relaxin, prostacyclin, and nitric oxide (and possibly hCG, too) play a role in inhibiting contractions.

The Second Trimester: Goodbye Nausea, Hello Maternity Jeans

On the grow

Weeks 15 to 18

Baby weighs 60 to 200 grams (2 to 7 ounces) and measures 9 to 14 centimetres (3.5 to 5.5 inches) from head to rump this month. Place your bets now, if you haven't already: it's possible to tell if you're carrying a boy or a girl. The eyes and ears now resemble those of a newborn, so you'll definitely be able to recognize that you're carrying a baby and not, say, a seahorse. Slow eye movements will begin during this period.

Baby's arms are longer and more developed than the legs, and the bones are continuing to grow harder. Limb movements are becoming more coordinated, so your gymnast baby is moving around in your uterus, reaching hands up to the face and down to the toes.

Baby's heart is working very hard, pumping 24 litres (6 gallons) of blood per day, and the liver has started producing bile. The bladder fills and empties itself into the amniotic fluid approximately once every 40 minutes. If your baby is a girl, her ovaries have formed and contain primordial follicles.

By week 16, your baby is fully formed: no new structures will be created from this point on. Growth and refining of the existing systems will be the focus from now on.

Weeks 19 to 22

Your baby's growth will slow down this month—weight will edge up to between 250 and 450 grams (9 and 16 ounces), and height between 15 and 19 centimetres (6 and 7.5 inches). Hair is starting to appear on Baby's head and eyebrows, as well as on the skin. Downy lanugo holds a protective layer of vernix caseosa—a greasy white coating you may discover if your baby is born a bit early—on the skin. Underneath that skin, brown fat is being laid down mainly around the neck, the breastbone, and the area surrounding the kidneys. This special type of fat keeps newborns warm when they're still too young to shiver to generate their own heat.

Baby's limbs are now in proportion with the rest of his or her body, and when those limbs move, you can feel it. (If you've been pregnant before or you're extremely slim, you may have felt the movements a week or two earlier.) Soon other people will be able to feel your baby's movements, too. And by weeks 20 to 22, your baby's breathing movements can be detected on an ultrasound. Non-nutritive sucking begins in this period, as your baby trains for the real world when he or she will rely on the sucking reflex for comfort and to obtain nutrition.

By week 20, the ovaries in female babies contain the maximum number of egg cells they will ever have. Even by the time she is born, much of a baby girl's reproductive stash will have dwindled away.

Also by week 20, the top of your uterus will reach your belly button. (This is when you may experience one of the weirdest pregnancy symptoms: belly button pain.) Inside, the placenta is exchanging amniotic fluid every three hours.

Weeks 23 to 27

Baby is gaining weight again, and will weigh between 500 and 820 grams (17.5 and 30 ounces) this month. Length will be between 20 and 23 centimetres (8 and 9 inches) from head to rump, and approximately 30 centimetres (12 inches) head to toe. With expert care in a neonatal intensive care unit, a baby born at week 24 may survive.

Rapid eye movements, which affect sleep patterns, brain development, memory, and learning, begin at 23 weeks. The eyebrows and eyelashes are well formed, and by 22 to 24 weeks, the eyelids are no longer fused together. Baby can now differentiate between light and dark, and will exhibit a blink-startle response to noise. As your pregnancy progresses, your baby will become increasingly sensitive to an increased range of sound frequencies. Your baby's movements become vigorous enough that other people can enjoy them, too.

Fingernails appear during this time. By now the skin is wrinkled and translucent, making Baby appear very red-pink. At this stage of development, your baby's skin water content is close to 100 per cent. It will be 92 per cent at term (compared to the 77 per cent water content in adult skin).

Alveoli are forming in the lungs, and the lungs begin to secrete surfactant, a detergent-like material composed of lipids (fats) and proteins that prevents the lungs from collapsing and also protects them from injuries and infection. Your baby's respiratory system is still very immature, however. By 22 to 26 weeks, digestive enzymes are present, except for lactase, which aids in the digestion of dairy products.

A baby boy's testicles will start to descend into the inguinal canal this month.

The Third Trimester: Your Incredible Growing Belly

The final sprint

Weeks 28 to 31

Your baby will weigh about 900 to 1,300 grams (32 to 46 ounces) this month, and will measure 24 to 27 centimetres (9.5 to 10.5 inches) long from head to rump. Head to toe, Baby will measure about 38 centimetres (15 inches) long. Much will happen during this month, which is a period of rapid brain development:

- Baby's central nervous system is capable of controlling some functions.
- Baby's eyelids open and close.
- Baby can distinguish between the sound of Mom's voice and the voices of other people.
- Baby is capable of mouthing. Ultrasounds have picked up images of babies with their thumbs in their mouths.
- During weeks 28 to 31, layers of fat (3.5 per cent of body weight) are deposited underneath the skin, giving Baby a less wrinkled and red appearance.
- Your baby's sweat glands are fully developed, but they aren't ready to start functioning yet.
- Fingerprints are present.
- Toenails are visible.
- By week 30, red blood cell production shifts from the liver and the spleen to the bone marrow.
- In male babies, the testes begin to descend into the scrotum by week 30.

approaching term

The closer a baby gets to term (37 completed weeks of pregnancy), the greater his odds of survival. Almost 30 per cent of babies born at 23 weeks of pregnancy survive, as compared to about 50 to 60 per cent of babies born at 24 weeks, about 75 per cent born at 25 weeks, and more than 90 per cent born at 27 to 28 weeks. But survival is only part of the picture. Babies born at less than 32 weeks of pregnancy (and weighing less than 3.3 pounds, or 1.5 kilograms) are at increased risk of developing such serious complications as respiratory distress syndrome (breathing problems), an intraventricular hemorrhage (bleeding in the brain), necrotizing enterocolitis (a serious inflammation of the bowel), and infections such as pneumonia, sepsis, and meningitis.

Baby's movements are slow, uncoordinated, and flailing since muscle tone, one of the criteria used to estimate gestational age, is limited before 28 weeks. Your baby becomes increasingly coordinated as your pregnancy progresses.

The lungs are now capable of breathing air and the central nervous system is capable of controlling breathing. However, a few more weeks in the womb will do wonders for your baby's respiratory system. Production of surfactant increases significantly after 34 weeks.

By the start of the third trimester, Baby is able to detect and respond to the scent and flavour of foods Mom has eaten. The amniotic fluid carries these scents and flavours. Fetal nutrition experts believe that early exposure to particular foods may play a role in programming dietary preferences after birth. They have also discovered that babies exhibit a preference for sweet substances even before they are born: while injecting a sweet substance into amniotic fluid increases fetal swallowing, injecting a bitter substance leads to a decrease.

Weeks 32 to 36

Baby is going through another period of rapid growth—gaining about 230 grams (half a pound) each week from weeks 31 to 35. By week 34, Baby will weigh between 1,400 and 2,100 grams (49.5 and 74 ounces) and will measure 28 to 30 centimetres (11 to 12 inches) long from head to rump. Your baby is behaving like a newborn in many ways: getting the hiccups (those rhythmic, jerky motions you feel from time to time), thumb-sucking, and crying. Baby has distinct periods of sleep and wakefulness, and now responds to sound, light, and taste (sampling what you're eating by swallowing amniotic fluid), already preferring sweet over sour. Babies born at or after week 34 have very good odds of survival.

Fetal movements increase in frequency until 34 weeks, then become less frequent. Contrary to popular belief, it's not cramped space or a reduction in amniotic fluid that causes your baby to kick less often. Baby's preoccupied with other things—like building a better brain. In other words, once the developmental focus shifts from fetal growth and movement to brain development, Baby becomes less active. Your baby will react to light, but the visual attention span is what you'd expect it to be at this stage: fleeting. Baby is also acquiring increased control over his or her body: movements are smoother and muscle tone is improving, particularly in the lower extremities (around week 32). Control over the upper extremities will come about two weeks later.

A pedicure is in order—the toenails now reach the ends of the toes. Your baby's skin is pink and smooth and the limbs are chubby. White fat now makes up 8 per cent of body weight. Underneath the skin, stores of important nutrients, including iron, calcium, and phosphorous, are building up, and by the end of week 33, the organs are almost fully developed. Fetal breathing movements occur 30 to 40 per cent of the time during the last 10 weeks of pregnancy—Baby is practicing for his or her first breath after birth.

A lot is going on in your body, too. The fundus reaches the height of your sternum by eight months of pregnancy. Your Braxton Hicks (pre-labour) contractions are much more common at night (occurring at a rate of five to six contractions per hour) than they are during the day (two to three contractions per hour)—no wonder sleep is hard to come by. By the time you reach term, the nerve cells in your uterus will be primed for instant communication. All of the muscles in your uterus can be activated within two to three seconds, resulting in an almost simultaneous contraction of an entire muscle layer. And as you approach term, biochemical changes cause the muscle tissue in your cervix to disappear, leaving your cervix stretchy and spongy.

Weeks 37 to 40

You've reached the home stretch, your ninth month of pregnancy. Your baby is getting bigger—by week 38, weight will be between 2,200 and 2,900 grams (77.5 and 102 ounces) and length will be between 31 and 34 centimetres (12 and 13 inches) from head to rump; by week 40, weight will be around 3,400 grams (7.5 pounds), and length from head to rump will be approximately 36 centimetres (14 inches). (Head-to-toe length at term averages 48 to 53 centimetres or 19 to 21 inches.) The distance around Baby's head and abdomen are roughly equal. Your baby is storing fat at a rate of 14 grams (0.5 ounces) per day. Baby's legs and arms are chubby—white fat now makes up approximately 16 per cent of body weight. The brown adipose tissue (BAT) that has been depositing under the skin since week 32 will continue to be deposited after delivery. In fact, the quantity of BAT, which generates heat for your newborn, increases by 150 per cent between the third and fifth week of life.

At the start of the ninth month, Baby's skin appears pink and smooth, and at full term it will appear bluish-pink. The mucous membranes also appear pink. Starting at week 37, the fine layer of hair (lanugo) that has covered Baby's body starts to disappear. Fingernails now reach the end of the fingertips. Small breast buds are present in all babies, and in most male babies, the testes now descend into the scrotum. (In some babies, the testes descend after birth but before the first birthday.)

You won't sense as much activity from your baby now. Typical movements at this stage of pregnancy include bumping or buzzing against your cervix (as your baby's head bobs up and down) or jabs from hands or feet underneath your rib cage. By week 37, your baby is test-driving some newborn reflexes—Baby has a firm grasp, and will turn his or her head toward light.

Your baby's heart will double in size between birth and the first birthday. And it will be four times the size it was at birth by the time Baby turns five. Perhaps Dr. Seuss took his inspiration for his not-so-grinchy Grinch from the incredible growing heart of a baby.

Baby's intestines are full of meconium, which is made up of cells shed from the lining of the gut. This sticky black-green substance will be your baby's first bowel movement.

At some point, the moment you've been waiting for will arrive: you'll finally get to meet your baby. It may be before 40 weeks or it may be after 40 weeks—or it may be right on your due date, although that's rather unlikely (only about 5 per cent of babies arrive when they're due). You've been supplying your baby with antibodies against disease, and now you'll get to give additional antibodies to your baby face-to-face (or, more accurately, face-to-nipple) through colostrum, the precursor to breast milk, when breastfeeding begins shortly after birth.

CHAPTER 7

The Pregnancy Road Map

"I found pregnancy to be a state of constant training. I would just get used to one symptom when another symptom would appear. It was nine months of gradually slowing down, becoming more and more focused on the baby, and setting new priorities. It's the most wonderful and amazing and exhilarating and exasperating time."

—LYNN, 41, MOTHER OF ONE

There may be days when you feel like you're venturing into uncharted territory: a place where no pregnant body has ever gone before. It can be reassuring to know that other mothers have, in fact, experienced that strange twinge or drive-you-crazy itch; that what you're experiencing is actually standard pregnancy fare.

That's the purpose of this chapter: to give you a mom's-eye view of what pregnancy is all about. After providing mom-proven advice on coping with a smorgasbord of pregnancy complaints, the next chapter will zero in on the amazing changes your baby and your body undergo between conception and birth.

The Complaints Department

We all know at least one woman who managed to breeze through pregnancy without so much as a single ache or pain. You know the kind of person I'm talking about: one of those Ms. Perfect Pregnancies who asks the prenatal instructor if it's normal to have so much energy, to feel so sexy and alive! Most of us mere mortals don't end up getting off quite that easily. We find ourselves battling an ever-changing parade of symptoms—everything from morning sickness to leg cramps to insomnia.

What's normal and what's not

Over the course of your pregnancy, you're likely to experience a variety of different complaints—everything from fatigue to round ligament pain to pre-labour contractions. Because these symptoms tend to randomly appear and disappear, it can be difficult to get a handle on whether a particular complaint falls into the "harmless but annoying" category or whether it could indicate a possible problem with your pregnancy.

As a rule, you should call your caregiver immediately or proceed to the hospital emergency department if you experience one or more of the symptoms listed in Table 7.1. (Have a chat with your caregiver about when she'd like you to call and when she'd prefer that you head to emergency first.) Also, become familiar with the signs of preterm labour in Chapter 9.

Pregnancy Complaints from A to Z

First, I'll cover all the scary stuff in Table 7.1 (I figured we'd get that over with right away so that it wouldn't be hanging over your head), then we can talk about the garden-variety complaints that you may experience at some point during your pregnancy.

To make it easier for you to access this information in a hurry (when you are about to hit the panic button), I've organized the list of complaints in alphabetical order. I've also included a chart that indicates when each symptom is most likely to occur (see Table 7.2). Just do me a favour and take this table with a grain of salt. Who knows? You could very well be the first pregnant woman ever to experience belly button soreness during the first or third trimester. Every pregnancy is unique, after all.

So let's head off to the Complaints Department.

Abdominal muscle separation

You don't have to be a rocket scientist to figure out why abdominal muscle separation (*diastasis recti*) tends to occur during almost one-third of pregnancies. As your uterus grows, it stretches and pushes apart the two large bands of muscle tissue that run down the middle of your abdomen between your ribs and your pelvic bone. The condition is generally painless, although some women will experience a bit of tenderness in the belly button region. In fact, the only way you'll know that it's occurred is if you notice a loss of abdominal tone in the

7.1   When to Call Your Caregiver

Type of Symptom	What It May Indicate
Heavy vaginal bleeding or clotting, or the passage of tissue from the vagina	You may be experiencing a miscarriage. If this happens later in pregnancy (e.g., during the second or third trimesters), you may be experiencing placenta previa or a placental abruption.
Vaginal bleeding that lasts for more than one day, or that is accompanied by pain, fever, or chills	You may be experiencing a miscarriage. If this happens later in pregnancy (e.g., during the second or third trimesters), you may be experiencing placenta previa or a placental abruption. What's more, if there's bleeding behind the placenta, you could be developing chorioamnionitis (an infection).
Severe abdominal or shoulder pain that may be accompanied by spotting or bleeding or the passage of tissue	Your pregnancy may be ectopic (i.e., the embryo may have implanted somewhere other than in the uterus) and you may be experiencing internal bleeding as a result. This typically occurs at six to eight weeks of pregnancy, but can also occur when your pregnancy is a little further along.
A severe or persistent headache (particularly one accompanied by dizziness, faintness, or blurry vision)	You may be developing high blood pressure or pre-eclampsia (a serious medical condition characterized by high blood pressure).
New vision problems (particularly dimness or blurring of your vision)	You may be developing high blood pressure or pre-eclampsia.
Dehydration (dry mouth, thirst, reduced urine output, frontal headache, low-grade fever)	You may be becoming dehydrated, which puts you at risk of experiencing premature contractions.
A fever of more than 38.0°C (100.4°F)	You may have an infection that requires treatment. Even if you don't, your caregiver will want to bring your temperature down because an elevated core body temperature during the first trimester can be harmful to the developing baby and, if experienced later in pregnancy, may trigger premature labour.

Painful urination	You may have developed a urinary tract infection, which can trigger premature labour and/or lead to a kidney infection.
A watery discharge or sudden release of fluid from the vagina	Your membranes may have ruptured.
Sudden swelling of the face, hands, or feet	You may be developing pre-eclampsia.
The symptoms of premature labour (uterine contractions, vaginal bleeding or discharge, vaginal pressure or pressure in the pelvic area, menstrual-like cramping, a dull backache or low back pain that doesn't go away, stomach or intestinal cramping with or without diarrhea and gas pains, generally feeling unwell)	You may be experiencing premature labour.
A significant decrease in fetal movement after the 24th week of pregnancy (see Chapter 10 for information about fetal movement counting)	Your baby's health may be suffering. Or your baby may simply be having a quieter day. Don't ignore this symptom however. Touch base with your doctor or midwife if you're concerned.

TABLE 7. 2 **The Complaints Department**

Pregnancy-Related Complaint	Month of Pregnancy When It's Most Likely to Be a Problem								
	1	2	3	4	5	6	7	8	9
Abdominal muscle separation				X	X	X	X	X	X
Acne	X	X	X	X	X	X	X	X	X
Backache							X	X	X	X
Belly button soreness					X				
Bleeding gums (pregnancy gingivitis)	X	X	X	X	X	X	X	X	X
Bleeding or spotting	X	X	X						
Braxton Hicks contractions							X	X	X	X
Breast enlargement	X	X	X	X	X	X	X	X	X
Breast tenderness	X	X	X						
Breathlessness								X	X
Carpal tunnel syndrome				X	X	X	X	X	X
Constipation	X	X	X	X	X	X	X	X	X
Cramping (abdominal)	X								
Cravings	X	X	X						
Ear changes				X	X	X	X	X	X
Eye changes (dryness and vision changes)	X	X	X	X	X	X	X	X	X
Faintness and dizziness	X	X	X	X	X	X	X	X	X
Fatigue	X	X	X				X	X	X
Food aversions	X	X	X	X	X	X	X	X	X
Gassiness and bloating	X	X	X	X	X	X	X	X	X
Headaches	X	X	X	X	X	X	X	X	X
Heartburn							X	X	X
Hemorrhoids				X	X	X	X	X	X
Hiatal hernia							X	X	X
Hip soreness				X	X	X	X	X	X
Insomnia	X	X	X	X	X	X	X	X	X
Itchiness (abdominal)							X	X	X
Laryngitis and voice changes				X	X	X	X	X	X
Leg cramps							X	X	X

Pregnancy-Related Complaint	Month of Pregnancy When It's Most Likely to Be a Problem								
	1	2	3	4	5	6	7	8	9
Linea nigra (vertical line down centre of abdomen)				X	X	X	X	X	X
Mask of pregnancy (chloasma)				X	X	X	X	X	X
Morning sickness	X	X	X						
Nasal changes	X	X	X	X	X	X	X	X	X
Perineal aching									X
Pubic-bone pain					X	X	X	X	X
Rashes							X	X	X
Restless leg syndrome					X	X	X	X	X
Rhinitis	X	X	X	X	X	X	X	X	X
Round ligament pain				X	X				
Sciatica							X	X	X
Skin changes	X	X	X	X	X	X	X	X	X
Smell, heightened sense of	X	X	X						
Stretch marks							X	X	X
Sweating, increased				X	X	X	X	X	X
Swelling and edema (fluid retention)							X	X	X
Thirstiness	X	X	X	X	X	X	X	X	X
Urinary incontinence (leaking of urine)							X	X	X
Urination, increased frequency of	X	X	X				X	X	X
Vagina, changes to the	X	X	X	X	X	X	X	X	X
Vaginal discharge, increased	X	X	X	X	X	X	X	X	X
Varicose veins							X	X	X
Weepiness	X	X	X	X	X	X	X	X	X
Yeast infections	X	X	X	X	X	X	X	X	X

middle of your belly or if you make a conscious effort to check for muscle separation by poking around in the middle of your abdomen. (If you try to do a sit-up, there will be a bulge in the middle between the two muscles.) Once it's occurred during one pregnancy, it becomes progressively worse in subsequent ones. Fortunately, it is possible to correct it after each pregnancy.

To minimize the amount of abdominal muscle separation you experience, you'll want to learn how to maintain good posture (avoid the swayback position, which pushes the tummy and the hips forward). And you'll want to avoid exercises that cause your abdominal wall to bulge out when you exert yourself. Your muscles are working hard enough as it is! Instead, do exercises that are designed to strengthen your transverse abdominis muscle (for example, abdominal compressions and pelvic tilts performed in a standing position against a wall).

If you develop abdominal muscle separation (something that happens in approximately 30% of pregnancies), avoid carrying very heavy objects (something you should be avoiding anyway) and coughing without supporting your belly (hold the two sides of your belly together during coughing episodes).

Acne

Think your problem-skin days are a thing of the past? Unfortunately, the hormonal cocktail of pregnancy can cause skin eruptions that you haven't experienced since your teenage years. Fortunately, pregnancy-related acne doesn't last nearly as long as the adolescent variety. It will disappear shortly after the delivery. In the meantime, you can minimize its severity by using an oatmeal-based facial scrub to help unplug oily pores. Note: Certain types of acne medications can cause serious birth defects and should not be used by pregnant women or women who have any possibility of becoming pregnant. Talk to your healthcare provider about any oral or topical acne medications that have been prescribed to you to find out whether they are safe for use during pregnancy.

hair	Your skin may be going to pot, but chances are you've got great hair. Pregnancy hormones reduce the rate at which your hair falls out, and can leave you looking positively hair-model like (at least until a few months after the delivery).

Backache

Approximately 70 per cent of pregnant women experience backache, typically after the fifth month of pregnancy. (If it is experienced prior to this point, it is generally the result of breast changes. And, yes, pregnancy breast changes can be that dramatic.) Backache is the result of the stretching of the ligaments in your back (caused by both the mechanical and hormonal changes of pregnancy), breast changes, the overstretching of your abdominal muscles, and changes to both your posture and the curvature of your spine, all of which create additional work for the muscles in your back.

Back pain during pregnancy is more common in older mothers, in mothers with pre-existing back pain, and in mothers who have experienced back pain during previous pregnancies. Despite what you might think (or what other people might suggest), it is not linked to weight gain during pregnancy, maternal obesity, your height, or infant birth weight.

You can minimize the amount of back pain you experience during pregnancy by taking steps to protect your back. Here are a few tips:

- Be aware that the weight of your pregnant uterus changes your centre of gravity, and that increased joint flexibility in the pelvic region (to open up the pelvis for childbirth) leaves you more susceptible to muscle and ligament strain and injury.
- Pay attention to good posture (stand upright, tuck in your pelvis, and rotate your shoulders) and do what you can to minimize your risk of injury (exercise caution when you're bending, lifting, or otherwise changing positions, and steer clear of high heels).
- Let someone else do the heavy lifting. If you have to haul your baby shower gifts into the house by yourself, lift with your legs, not your back.
- Rather than trying to sit up when you're lying on your back, roll over onto your side and then push up with your hands.
- Avoid standing or sitting in one position for long periods of time, as this places an added strain on your back. If you can't change positions as often as your body would like you to, put one foot on a stool while you're sitting or standing.
- Exercise to build up strength in your lower back and abdominal muscles, starting in early pregnancy. Take prenatal and postnatal fitness classes taught by a qualified instructor so that you can get your body ready for birth and then back in shape after baby. (I'm not talking about "super model" back in shape, by the way: I'm talking about "healthy for motherhood" back in shape.)
- Avoid high-impact sports that may be jarring to your spine. There are plenty of low-impact ways to be active during pregnancy.
- Back pain tends to be at its worst at night. Make sure you're sleeping on a firm mattress that provides solid back support. Get in the habit of tucking a pillow between your knees and another under your abdomen when you're sleeping on your side. (Sleeping on your left side maximizes blood flow to the baby, but you'll probably find that you flip from side to side during the night, for the sake of comfort.) Having

these extra pillows to support you while you're sleeping on your side will help to take some of the pressure off your lower back.

- Consider scheduling an appointment with a chiropractor or massage therapist who has experience in working with pregnant women. You may also want to try applying heat or ice to the affected area (whichever your health-care provider recommends).
- If you're experiencing unusual or acute back pain, get in touch with your health-care provider right away. It's important to distinguish between more standard pregnancy aches and pains and worrisome concerns like preterm labour.

Belly button soreness

I know, I know. It sounds like the most ridiculous complaint in the world. But just wait until it happens to you! Around the 20th week of pregnancy, you may experience some extreme tenderness in the belly button area. This is caused by the pressure of your expanding uterus on your belly button. The tenderness tends to subside as your belly grows, so this is one thing you can strike off the complaint list sooner rather than later.

Bleeding gums

Even if you're not usually a card-carrying member of the International Order of Compulsive Flossers, you might want to think about taking out a membership for at least the duration of your pregnancy. Between the second and seventh months of pregnancy, 30 to 80 per cent of pregnant women develop a condition called pregnancy gingivitis, which is characterized by inflamed and sensitive gums that bleed more easily than usual. In addition to flossing daily and brushing your teeth after every meal using a gentle-bristled toothbrush, you should plan to take the following steps to minimize symptoms of pregnancy gingivitis:

- See your dentist at least once during your pregnancy, ideally at a time when you won't be feeling too nauseated. Having the buildup of plaque that collects at the bottom of your teeth scraped off can help to reduce the severity of your symptoms.
- Rinse your mouth with antiseptic mouthwash several times a day. That will help to keep your mouth sparkling clean.
- Choose foods such as fruit and vegetables that are rich in vitamin C— something that helps to promote healthy gums.

Note: Don't be alarmed if you develop tiny nodules on your gums that tend to bleed easily. These nodules—known as pyogenic granulomas (pregnancy tumours)—are harmless, non-cancerous growths. They usually disappear on their own after you give birth, but if they're causing you a lot of grief in the meantime, your dentist can remove them.

> *dental hygiene*
>
> It's important to pay attention to dental hygiene during pregnancy, but if you find yourself gagging to the point of vomiting each time you try to brush your tongue, you might want to ask your dentist if there are other ways you can keep your mouth clean, like swishing thoroughly with a fluoride rinse, until you're feeling less queasy. And here's something else you should know: you shouldn't brush your teeth within 30 minutes of vomiting. The stomach acid combined with the brushing action can damage the enamel on your teeth. Instead, rinse your mouth with water or fluoride rinse to freshen your breath and protect your teeth.

Bleeding and spotting, vaginal

Any type of vaginal bleeding can be worrisome during pregnancy and should be assessed by your health-care provider, but sometimes the light bleeding or spotting you experience is completely harmless and not a symptom of an impending miscarriage. About seven days after conception (when you're three weeks pregnant, counting from the first day of your last menstrual period), you may experience a bit of spotting or very light bleeding as the fertilized embryo first implants itself in the uterine wall ("implantation bleeding"). Light spotting or very light bleeding can also occur if the cervix happens to get bumped during intercourse or accidentally grazed during a pelvic exam. While you should always report any vaginal bleeding or spotting to your caregiver, there's generally less cause for concern if the bleeding is very light (unless, of course, you're experiencing cramping at the same time, in which case you could be experiencing a miscarriage or placental abruption; or if you have developed placenta previa). (See Chapter 9 for more details on bleeding during pregnancy.)

Braxton Hicks contractions

This is the name given to the irregular contractions that occur during the last half of pregnancy. (Just a quick bit of pregnancy trivia: the contractions are named after John Braxton Hicks, MD, the British doctor who first described them back in 1872.)

While these contractions happen from early pregnancy onward as your uterus begins to train for the main event (labour!), you generally can't feel them until the mid-second or early third trimester. Typically lasting for 45 seconds or less, they feel as if someone has momentarily put a blood pressure cuff around your abdomen and then pumped it up. They are usually irregular and subside quickly, and they may be relieved if you move around. While they can be quite worrying, the cocktail of early pregnancy hormones helps to prevent these harmless contractions from progressing into full-blown labour.

Toward the end of pregnancy, these contractions become increasingly uncomfortable and sometimes even painful. In fact, some women have such powerful Braxton Hicks contractions that they have a hard time distinguishing them from bona fide labour contractions. They're more likely to be bothersome during subsequent pregnancies, although, like everything else pregnancy-related, that rule isn't necessarily carved in stone.

Note: Some childbirth educators are now treating a contraction as a contraction as a contraction, and only differentiating between (1) those contractions that result in the birth of a baby and (2) those contractions that do not. So don't be disappointed (or freaked out) if you don't hear about Dr. Braxton Hicks and the contractions he made famous. When your childbirth instructor is talking about practice contractions or, further on in your pregnancy, pre-labour contractions, she's talking about the same thing.

Breast tenderness and enlargement

Your breasts begin to undergo a dramatic metamorphosis starting as soon as the hormones of early pregnancy begin to kick in. Here's a quick snapshot:

- **Bigger.** The changes that a woman's breasts undergo during pregnancy have to be seen to be believed. One minute you're a woman with an average-sized bosom. The next, you're doing a darned good impression of Pamela Anderson. Okay, I'm exaggerating a little. But be forewarned: you're in for a few surprises in the breast department over the next nine months—you can expect your breasts to grow by one full cup size by the end of your first trimester and by another full cup size by the time you give birth.
- **Bolder.** You'll also notice some changes to the appearance of your breasts. The areola—the flat area around the nipple—begins to darken; the tiny glands on the areola begin to enlarge and start excreting a lubricating, antibacterial oil; your nipples become more erect; and you may notice bluish veins showing through your skin due to increased

blood flow to your breasts. (Blood flow to your breasts doubles during pregnancy.) It almost looks as if someone has taken a blue pen and drawn a map of river and lake country on your chest. You'll hold on to the map effect until after you give birth.

- **Super-sensitive.** Soon after the pregnancy test becomes positive, your breasts may become sore and swollen, particularly if you're pregnant for the first time. They may feel fuller, tingly, and more sensitive (even taking a shower may become excruciating), and you may find yourself experiencing the odd throbbing or shooting pain. The thought of sleeping on your stomach may simply be out of the question. The tenderness will ease up as your pregnancy continues (to be replaced by itchiness as your breasts continue to enlarge), but by then your growing belly will be well on its way to making tummy sleeping a virtual impossibility. To cope with your discomfort in the meantime, you may want to wear a well-fitting, supportive bra, even when you're sleeping, and talk to your doctor about pain relief options.

- **Lumpy and leaky.** And the list of changes goes on. You may notice that your breasts feel slightly lumpy (like you have a small beanbag stashed in each breast). This is because your breasts are putting in place all the factories and transportation networks (glands and duct work, actually) needed to manufacture and carry breast milk. And as for the leaky bit, your body secretes small amounts of a clear type of colostrum during pregnancy. (This isn't the same type of colostrum that your breasts will have on tap when your newborn arrives. That nutrient- and immune-factor-rich colostrum will be a creamy yellow: the result of being jam-packed with beta carotene.) Prolactin levels increase during pregnancy, reaching their maximum at term. High progesterone levels during pregnancy suppress colostrum and milk production until that time.

Soap is not a pregnant or lactating breast's best friend. Soap can wash away breast secretions designed to lubricate and protect the breast from infections. There's no need to wash your nipples or areola (consider them self-cleaning, like an oven). Wash the rest of your breast with a mild soap as often as you need to for hygiene purposes (no more than once per day), but don't go crazy. Itchiness tends to be a problem for most pregnant women (your skin is getting stretched, stretched, and then stretched some more). Soap will only make the itchiness worse.

Breathlessness

It's like that Jerry Lee Lewis song: "You leave me breathless, oh, baby!" But in this case it actually *is* a baby that's causing your breathlessness. Over the course of your pregnancy, your rib cage becomes a few inches wider than usual in order to accommodate the added capacity of your lungs. Your diaphragm shifts upward by four centimetres in early pregnancy to make room for your ever-expanding uterus. But, despite this bit of pre-planning on Mother Nature's part, pressure from your growing uterus makes it increasingly difficult for you to breathe easily. Shortness of breath (experienced by 60 to 70 per cent of pregnant women) is at its worst between 28 weeks and term, when moms-to-be complain of such symptoms as reduced exercise tolerance (your oxygen needs are 15 times greater when you exercise during pregnancy: you're not out of shape, you just need more oxygen) and increased hoarseness (like you're auditioning for the part of an obscene telephone caller). You get a bit of relief when your baby's head begins to descend into your pelvis (during the last month of pregnancy). You can ease the discomfort in the meantime by using an extra pillow when you're sleeping. (For some reason, breathlessness tends to be particularly annoying at night— yet another tool that Mother Nature uses to prepare you for the sleepless nights of early parenthood!) To make matters worse, high levels of progesterone leave you feeling short of breath, something that triggers the desire to breathe more deeply. (Is it any wonder that most women heave a sigh of relief when the nine months of pregnancy finally come to an end?!)

Carpal tunnel syndrome

This condition is characterized by swelling, numbness, or tingling in the hands (either "pins and needles" or an outright burning sensation); pain in the wrist that can shoot all the way up to the shoulder; cramping or stiffness in the hands; weakness in the thumb; and a tendency to drop things. Carpal tunnel syndrome is relatively common during pregnancy and results from a pinched nerve in the wrist. (Just as your entire body tends to retain fluid when you're pregnant, you have more fluid in your wrist area. This can cause the median nerve that runs through the carpal tunnel to become compressed.)

In most cases, carpal tunnel syndrome disappears on its own shortly after you give birth. A few moms do require surgery to correct the problem, however. While you're waiting for delivery day to roll around you can minimize the discomfort by elevating the affected hand, wearing a plastic splint at night, and investing in keyboard and mouse wrist supports if you're on the computer a lot.

Constipation

It's hardly surprising that so many women have trouble with constipation during pregnancy (up to one-third of pregnant women during the first and third trimesters). High levels of progesterone cause the muscles of the intestine to function far less efficiently than normal, and the increasing size of your uterus can interfere with the passage of stool, resulting in bloating and abdominal distention, increased flatulence (gas), dry, hard stools, and infrequent bowel movements. Looking on the bright side, scientists believe there may a benefit to having a sluggish intestine during pregnancy. After all, the longer the food remains in your intestine, the more nutrients (iron, calcium, glucose, amino acids, water, sodium, and chloride, in particular) your body is able to absorb.

Fortunately, there's plenty you can do to alleviate this particular complaint. Most pregnant women find the problem takes care of itself if they drink plenty of water, consume large quantities of high-fibre foods (fruits and vegetables, whole grains), exercise regularly, and use the bathroom as soon as the need arises. If you've tried all these natural remedies and you're still experiencing the misery that is constipation, talk to your health-care provider. She may recommend a stool softener or other medicinal solution. Note: Laxatives are not generally recommended for use during pregnancy, due to side effects such as fluid accumulation, sodium retention, edema (swelling), and cramping.

If you're taking an iron supplement, it may be adding to your constipation problems. Try taking it on a full stomach and washing it down with plenty of liquid. If that doesn't work, you might want to fall back on the anti-constipation remedy that worked for your grandmother: two tablespoons of unsulphured blackstrap molasses dissolved in a glass of warm water. Another solution is to treat yourself to a fruit compote once or twice a day: add a splash of water to three or four pieces of dried fruit and microwave for 15 to 20 seconds.

Taking mineral oil (or a laxative that relies on mineral oil) to get your bowels moving is not a good idea during pregnancy. Mineral oil absorbs vitamin K and other fat-soluble vitamins—nutrients your body and your baby are counting on right now.

Cramping

It's not unusual to experience period-like cramping (but without any accompanying bleeding) around the time your first menstrual period is due. The cramping is caused by the hormonal changes of early pregnancy and your body's response to the stretching of the uterine muscle, and is considered harmless unless it's accompanied by heavy bleeding (a possible symptom of miscarriage) or a sharp pain on one side of your abdomen (a possible sign of an ectopic pregnancy).

Note: Severe abdominal pain can also be caused by appendicitis, a gallbladder attack, the stretching of adhesions from previous abdominal surgery, or preterm labour, so it's important to get in touch with your caregiver immediately if the pain you're experiencing is severe or long-lasting.

Cravings

Some experts pooh-pooh the whole idea of cravings during pregnancy, claiming that they're all in a woman's head. Others argue that they're actually Mother Nature's way of ensuring you get the nutrients you need. (Of course, this particular argument doesn't do much to explain why some women develop cravings for road salt, coal, soap, disinfectant, mothballs, starch, clay, chalk, and other inedible substances during pregnancy—a disorder known as pica.)

What we do know is that estrogen suppresses appetite while progesterone and leptin stimulate it; that appetite and thirst increase during the early part of pregnancy and decrease toward the end of pregnancy; and that you may experience powerful cravings for fruit or foods with strong flavours, such as pickles (possibly because the sensitivity of your taste buds is dulled during pregnancy), as well as food aversions (often to tea and coffee, meat, fried foods, eggs, alcohol, and/or cigarette smoke) as your taste buds and sense of smell are affected by the hormonal changes of pregnancy, including hCG levels.

One thing the experts *do* agree on, however, is that cravings can get you into a lot of trouble if you use them as an excuse for overeating during pregnancy—something to bear in mind the next time a truckload of Timbits starts calling your name.

Ear changes

Some women experience ear stuffiness or blockage during pregnancy (the kind of sensation you experience when you're on an airplane). This is the result of the effects of estrogen on the mucous membranes or Eustachian tubes in the ears as well as fluid changes and extra water in other parts of the ear. The net result can be mild temporary hearing loss. The problem will resolve itself after you give birth. In the meantime, it can be very annoying, particularly because you can't get rid of the full-ears feeling by swallowing like you can when you're flying.

Eye changes

You already know that the changes triggered by pregnancy are rather far-reaching. What you might not realize, however, is that even your eyes can be affected.

Here's why:

- Pregnancy affects the amount of fluid in your eyes. This changes the shape of your eyeballs, which may result in vision changes (you become more near-sighted).
- If you use contact lenses, you may find that you have to stop wearing them for the duration of your pregnancy because your eyes can no longer tolerate them or because changes to the composition of your tears result in increased blurring.
- Progesterone, relaxin, and hCG affect pressure levels in the eye, which drop by about 10 per cent. This is good news if you happen to suffer from glaucoma.
- Rising levels of estrogen can lead to a condition called dry eye, characterized by dryness and burning, blurred vision, and increased sensitivity to light. (If you find yourself suffering from this latter condition, you'll have to use an artificial-tears product to restore moisture to your eyes and you'll need to wear sunglasses whenever you're out in bright light.) Fortunately, both conditions correct themselves after you give birth, but that can be small solace if eye problems are driving you crazy and you're not even out of your first trimester yet.

Note: Vision problems can also be an indicator of diabetes, so be sure to report any symptoms to your caregiver.

Faintness and dizziness

While the soap opera scriptwriters typically have the heroine fainting long before the pregnancy test comes back positive, real pregnant women don't tend to experience much fainting and dizziness until they're well into the second or third trimester, when their rapidly increased blood volume (your blood volume increases by 30 to 50 per cent during pregnancy, and by 70 per cent if you're pregnant with twins) can lead to a decrease in blood pressure. Then, to make matters worse, pressure from the uterus on the major blood vessels in the abdomen during the third trimester can slow the rate of the return of blood to the upper half of the body, leading to feelings of light-headedness.

You're less likely to have problems with faintness and dizziness if you

- avoid standing in one position for a prolonged period of time (the blood pools in the lower part of the body, away from your brain);
- don't allow yourself to become overheated;

- get up slowly if you've had a warm bath or if you've been sitting or lying down (your cardiovascular system doesn't react as quickly when you're pregnant);
- avoid hypoglycemia and its resulting dizziness by eating at least every two hours and by limiting the number of sugary foods you consume;
- stay well hydrated, which will help keep your blood pressure up.

Fatigue

Fatigue is Mother Nature's way of reminding you that you're pregnant. If you didn't slow down a little, your body would have a hard time directing your energy to where it's needed most—growing a baby. You feel tired because of the increased production of progesterone (which acts as a natural sedative) and the increase in your body's metabolic rate (your body's way of making sure it can provide for the needs of your growing baby).

Some women are shocked by how exhausted they feel during the early weeks of pregnancy. That was certainly the case for Jennifer, a 32-year-old mother of one: "Being so drop-dead tired took me by surprise and reduced me to tears at first. Once I realized and accepted that this was my body's way of dealing with the massive task ahead, I was okay. I lessened my work schedule where I could and gave myself permission to be tired. I also allowed myself to fall asleep whenever I wanted, provided, of course, I wasn't driving or in public!"

The best way to cope with fatigue is to get the rest your body is craving. Hit the hay an hour or two earlier at night and try to squeeze in a nap at some point during the day—either during your lunch hour or afternoon break, or after you arrive home from work.

Anemia (low iron) can be another cause of fatigue. Iron levels tend to be at their lowest levels between weeks 16 and 22 of pregnancy. Your health-care provider will be monitoring your iron levels throughout your pregnancy. If your test results indicate that you are low in iron, talk to your health-care provider about ways of getting more iron in your diet and whether you should be taking an iron supplement (in either liquid or pill form).

Food aversions

Don't be surprised if the hormones of early pregnancy end up affecting your taste buds. You may experience a mildly metallic taste in your mouth that can make your morning cup of tea or coffee taste downright repulsive. (Maybe it's a sign that you should kick your caffeine habit.)

Unfortunately, these food aversions are often accompanied by a heightened sensitivity to odours and increased salivation, something that can add to your misery.

Gassiness and bloating

The increased levels of progesterone in your body make your intestines more sluggish during pregnancy, which can cause both gassiness and bloating. The problem tends to be aggravated during the first trimester by the tendency to swallow air as a means of relieving nausea.

Here are tips on minimizing the amount of gassiness and bloating you experience during pregnancy:

- Keep your bowels moving. Drink plenty of liquids, eat a variety of high-fibre foods, and make exercise part of your regular routine. Your body has to push food through your 22-foot-long intestines, so it needs all the help it can get.
- Eat slowly and avoid sipping hot beverages and soup in order to minimize the amount of air you swallow.
- Choose your food wisely. Avoid carbonated beverages and fried and greasy foods. (High-fat foods are harder to digest, so they stay in your intestines longer, adding to your gas problems.)
- Eat your veggies, but watch how you do it. Cook fruits and vegetables instead of eating them raw, and limit your consumption of gas-producing vegetables such as cabbage, broccoli, cauliflower, Brussels sprouts, and green peppers.
- Try papaya (either fresh or in papaya enzyme tablets) and ginger (in tea or capsules), which help with digestion and make for fewer tummy problems.

Headaches

Headaches are another common pregnancy-related complaint. Some women, like Lori, consider them to be the worst aspect of being pregnant. "They were so severe and I suffered from them every single day from about my third month to about my seventh or eighth month, when they would ease up but not go away completely," the 29-year-old mother of four recalls. "They were just horrible."

While the only true cure for what ails you is giving birth, there are a few things you can do in the meantime to minimize the pain:

- Try to avoid getting headaches in the first place. Little things like changing your position slowly, eating every couple of hours so that you keep your blood sugar stable, drinking lots of fluids, and getting plenty of fresh air can help to prevent headaches.

- If you feel a tension headache coming on (a headache caused by muscular contractions or tension, and which is characterized by a vise-like pain from the base of the neck to the forehead), apply an ice pack to your forehead right away. This will cause the blood vessels to contract, which will generally help to eliminate your headache within about 20 minutes—roughly the same amount of time it takes a typical painkiller to kick in.
- Put a hot water bottle on your feet. This will cause the blood vessels in your feet to dilate, drawing the blood toward your feet and away from your head.
- Have your partner massage your feet. Since the big toe is the acupuncture point for the head, this can help to relieve your headache. If you can feel a lot of tension in your neck and shoulder muscles, you might also ask your partner to massage these areas as well.
- If you need to take a painkiller, avoid any product containing acetylsalicylic acid (ASA), such as Aspirin, and other non-steroidal anti-inflammatories, such as Advil and Anaprox. When taken in large doses close to term, ASA can lead to blood clotting problems that can cause excessive bleeding in the mother or the baby or both. ASA use during pregnancy is also thought to be linked to low birth weight, prolonged gestation and labour, and cardiac problems in the newborn. Note: There are certain conditions that are treated with ASA during pregnancy. See Chapter 9 for details.

If you experience a severe headache, particularly one that's accompanied by blurry vision, get in touch with your caregiver immediately. You could be developing high blood pressure or pre-eclampsia.

Heartburn (a.k.a. reflux)

The hormonal changes of pregnancy are to blame for yet another common complaint—heartburn (experienced by 30 to 70 per cent of pregnant women). High levels of progesterone in the body cause the valve at the entrance to the stomach to relax, which can allow stomach acid to pass back up into the esophagus (the tube leading into your stomach) and cause a strong burning sensation in the centre of your chest as well as increased burping.

You can minimize your heartburn problems by

- eating smaller, more frequent meals;
- avoiding spicy or fried foods, chocolate, and coffee;
- drinking a glass of milk before you eat (coating your stomach may reduce the amount of acid burn you experience);
- not eating too close to bedtime (avoid lying down for one to three hours after meals);
- keeping your head well elevated while you're sleeping and avoiding positions that make regurgitation more likely (for example, bending forward);
- chewing gum, especially if the gum contains pepsin, which aids in digestion;
- asking your doctor or midwife to recommend a medication that's safe for use during pregnancy. Note: Certain types of antacids may have undesirable side effects such as diarrhea, constipation, cramping, and so on. A calcium-magnesium–based antacid consumed after meals and at bedtime is probably your best bet.

Hernia, hiatal

About 15 to 20 per cent of pregnant women develop a hiatal hernia, starting at seven to eight months of pregnancy. This condition is caused by alternations in the muscle tone that occur as a result of changes to the widening esophageal hiatus, the opening in the diaphragm through which the esophagus passes into the stomach.

If you have been diagnosed with a hiatal hernia and you experience nausea, vomiting, severe pain in the chest or abdomen, and are unable to have a bowel movement or pass gas, you may have a strangulated hernia or an obstruction, which are medical emergencies. Get in touch with your healthcare provider immediately.

Hemorrhoids

Hemorrhoids—itching, soreness, and pain or bleeding in the tissue around your anus when you empty your bowels—are yet another common pregnancy complaint. They occur when pressure from your increasingly heavy uterus, combined with increased blood flow to the region, results in a pooling of blood in the veins around your anus and causes the veins to become engorged and swollen. They can also arise during labour, as a result of all the pushing and straining.

Hemorrhoids can be downright unpleasant, particularly if they rupture and start to bleed (something they're more apt to do if you strain during bowel movements, sit or stand for long periods of time, or if you're carrying a lot of extra weight).

The best way to deal with hemorrhoids is to prevent them from occurring in the first place. That means eating foods that are fibre-rich, drinking plenty of fluids, exercising regularly, avoiding constipation, keeping your pregnancy weight gain in the recommended range, and avoiding prolonged periods of sitting or standing.

While mild hemorrhoids tend to go away on their own after the baby is born, more severe hemorrhoids may require minor surgery to repair. Thrombosed or prolapsed hemorrhoids are not usually treated with surgery until after the pregnancy is over.

Here are some tips on coping with the discomfort of hemorrhoids during pregnancy:

- Avoid straining when you're having a bowel movement, standing for long periods of time, or sitting for long stretches on hard surfaces. Each of these situations can cause your hemorrhoids to worsen.
- Keep the area around your anus clean and dry. Gently wash it after each bowel movement by using either soft, undyed, unscented toilet paper (to avoid irritation), alcohol-free baby wipes, or hygienic witch hazel pads, or by gently swabbing the area with lemon juice or vinegar. Put a dry cotton ball on your anus before putting on your underpants.
- Gently tucking the protruding vein (hemorrhoid) back into your anus so that it is not exposed may provide relief.

You can relieve the itching of hemorrhoids by applying an ice pack to the affected area or by using an ointment that's been prescribed by your doctor.

Hip soreness

It's also not unusual to experience some soreness in your hips during pregnancy, particularly when you're sleeping on your side at night. The ligaments in your hips stretch and the cartilage softens in preparation for the birth of your baby, which can cause minor hip pain and contribute to that classic pregnancy "waddle." There's no real remedy for this particular complaint other than changing position frequently while you sleep and using pillows to help you to maintain the most comfortable position possible.

Insomnia

Sleeping problems are extremely common during pregnancy—the one time in your life when you could really use a good night's sleep! Whether it's anxiety about the upcoming birth, the nighttime trips to the bathroom, your baby's nocturnal gymnastics routine, or the physical challenges of finding a comfortable sleeping position when you've got a watermelon strapped to your belly, you're likely to encounter at least a few sleeping problems at some point during your pregnancy.

You can help to minimize your sleep problems by

- practising good "sleep hygiene" (going to bed at a regular time, getting up at a regular time, and watching the number of naps you sneak in during the day);
- limiting your caffeine intake or kicking your caffeine habit altogether;
- enjoying a mug of warm milk (with cinnamon and honey or sugar, if it tastes too bland on its own) or a cup of herbal tea before you go to bed (milk contains an amino acid that can make you sleepy, and herbal teas like chamomile can help you to unwind);
- exercising regularly (sleep experts have found that 20 to 30 minutes of exercise five days a week can really help to reduce the severity of insomnia);
- not consuming large quantities of liquids within two hours of going to bed (to help minimize the number of middle-of-the-night treks to the bathroom);
- skipping that late-evening snack (eating right before bed boosts your metabolism, which can keep you awake);
- taking time to relax and unwind before you go to bed (listening to soothing music, reading a book, or taking a warm bath);
- keeping your room at a comfortable temperature—neither too hot nor too cold;
- surrounding yourself with pillows (tuck one under your belly and one between your legs when you're sleeping on your side to minimize hip and back soreness).

Itchiness (abdominal)

When you consider how much the skin on your abdomen has to stretch during pregnancy, it's hardly surprising that so many pregnant women have problems

"Toward the end of my pregnancy, sometimes my tummy would itch like crazy. I used to warm some olive oil in the microwave and slowly rub it on my tummy while talking and singing to the baby. It felt absolutely wonderful and the baby seemed to enjoy the massage. These were powerful bonding moments between mother and child."

—ALEXANDRA, 33, MOTHER OF TWO

with abdominal itching. While the problem tends to correct itself shortly after you give birth and your abdomen returns to its normal size, it can drive you crazy in the meantime. You can reduce the severity of any itching you're experiencing by avoiding strong soaps and rubbing cocoa butter cream or other natural moisturizers like grapeseed or olive oil (rather than petroleum-based ones) on the affected areas of your belly.

Just one quick word of caution before you reach for the cocoa butter: don't slather on the creams and lotions right before your prenatal checkup. These substances can interfere with sound transmission when your caregiver is trying to detect your baby's heartbeat—something that can cause your own heart to skip a beat or two!

Laryngitis and voice changes

The hormonal changes of pregnancy can play all kinds of crazy tricks on your voice. You may find that you end up with a hoarse, sexy voice, or that your voice cracks like that of a teenage boy going through puberty (Mother Nature's idea of a hilarious joke, no doubt, on a woman who is pregnant out to here). Or you could sound like yourself with a really bad case of laryngitis. These voice changes aren't permanent. You'll lose your husky or teen boy sound after you give birth.

Leg cramps

Leg cramps are those painful muscle contractions (typically in the calves and feet) that up to 30 per cent of moms-to-be experience in the middle of the night or upon awakening.

Leg cramps are most common after 26 weeks of pregnancy. They're more likely to be a problem for sedentary as opposed to active women due to the reduced circulation these women experience. Leg cramps can be totally excruciating, so you'll want to do whatever you can to avoid them: alter your calcium intake (some experts think the cramps are triggered by a calcium-phosphate imbalance, and this may mean increasing or decreasing your milk consumption or even trying calcium supplements) and soak in a warm tub and stretch out your calf muscles before going to bed (pull your toes up toward your knees while pushing your heels away from you).

If you feel a cramp coming on, point your toes upward toward your knees while pushing your heels downward. Whatever you do, don't make the mistake of pointing your toes outward (as if you were going to stand on your toes, like a ballerina) or you'll be hit with a massive cramp in the back of your calf.

If the cramp does set in, massage the affected area and then walk around on it to improve circulation to the area.

Just in case you feel like turning this particular lemon into lemonade, leg cramps are similar in intensity to uterine cramps, so you could take this opportunity to practise your breathing techniques for labour.

Morning sickness (a.k.a. nausea and vomiting of pregnancy)

What pregnancy book would be complete without a detailed discussion of morning sickness? After all, morning sickness is one of the best-known, most annoying, and most common pregnancy-related conditions.

Morning sickness (a.k.a. nausea and vomiting of pregnancy or NVP) affects approximately 75 per cent of pregnant women, with 50 per cent experiencing both nausea and vomiting, 25 per cent experiencing nausea only, and 25 per cent remaining completely symptom-free. It typically sets in at around six weeks of pregnancy, peaking by around eight to twelve weeks of pregnancy. And 80 per cent of women who develop morning sickness can expect their symptoms to subside by the end of the first trimester. (As for the other 20 per cent of morning sickness sufferers, their symptoms may subside anytime thereafter. An unfortunate few will still be feeling miserable right up until baby makes his grand entrance, according to the Society of Obstetricians and Gynaecologists of Canada.)

Before we get into a detailed discussion of morning sickness, however, let's talk a bit about the name. While morning sickness does tend to be most severe in the morning, some women experience nausea and vomiting at other times of the day, too—which helps to explain why a growing number of health authorities and moms-to-be are ditching the term *morning sickness* and choosing to go with the more medically accurate term *nausea and vomiting of pregnancy* instead.

Bevin, a 27-year-old mother of one, supports the name change: "Morning sickness: who came up with that term anyway? I was sick morning, noon, and night—sometimes even in the middle of the night when I was sleeping—for the first three months."

So what causes morning sickness? No one knows for sure, but most scientists believe that skyrocketing levels of human chorionic gonadotropin—the hormone that makes the pregnancy test turn positive—may overstimulate the part of the brain that keeps nausea and vomiting in check. Others suggest that an enhanced sense of smell, excess acid in the stomach, or the sensations associated with the stretching of the uterine muscles could trigger the nausea and the vomiting. There's even a theory to suggest that morning sickness may have a purpose—turning you off foods that have strong odours or tastes (indications that food has gone "off").

While morning sickness can be a sign that your pregnancy is progressing well, there's no need to panic if you're not experiencing morning sickness. A study conducted at the Motherisk Clinic at the Hospital for Sick Children in Toronto dispels the long-standing theory that a lack of morning sickness is linked to an increased risk of miscarriage. "This provides a reassuring result to women who may have worried about their pregnancies because they *weren't* experiencing morning sickness," notes Gideon Koren, MD, Director of the Motherisk Clinic.

Surviving it

Enough theory. If you're suffering from morning sickness, you want survival strategies. Here are some that have worked for countless queasy moms and that are recommended by leading health authorities.

Get plenty of sleep. Excess fatigue will only make morning sickness worse. However, don't lie down right after a meal. That will only add to your nausea.

Start your day gradually. Sit up in bed and nibble on a few crackers before you get up. Yes, you have a licence to eat crackers in bed.

Think mini-meals. A too-full or too-empty stomach triggers nausea, so aim for five or six small meals per day, starting with a couple of crackers on the bedside table before you get out of bed in the morning.

Switch to "morning sickness cuisine." You can move on to more exciting menus once your stomach settles down, but for now, keep these basic tips in mind:

Don't force yourself to eat foods that make you gag (see Table 7.3) just because they're good for you. It's better to survive on crackers and rice cakes alone than to upchuck all the nutrient-rich veggies you forced yourself to knock back at dinnertime. ("One week, I lived primarily on McDonald's french fries and Kraft

> "At different times, different 'remedies' would calm my stomach. I'd keep cycling through my bag of tricks until something worked: crackers, potato chips, ginger ale, wristbands, walking in fresh air, getting plenty of rest."
>
> —LYNN, 41, MOTHER OF ONE

Dinner," confesses Jennifer, a 32-year-old mother of one. "That shot my Canada's Food Guide plan all to hell, but those were the only two foods that seemed to calm the queasies and leave me feeling satisfied.") You'll have plenty of time to reach for those nutrient-rich foods later in your pregnancy. In the meantime, your baby is drawing upon the stores that you built up before you conceived— the stockpile that Mother Nature saw to in anticipation of just such a "famine."

Choose foods that are bland and easy on the stomach (for example, soda crackers, mashed potatoes, yogourt), as opposed to anything spicy, fried, or fatty—and serve foods cold (rather than hot) to minimize cooking odours. You may discover that certain categories of foods (salty, tart/sweet, earthy, crunchy, bland, soft, sweet, fruity, liquid, or dry, for example) have particular appeal right now. (See Table 7.3 for suggestions.)

Avoid consuming fluids within 30 minutes of a meal. This will only add to your nausea. Just remember to make a point of consuming lots of liquids at other times of day so that you don't become dehydrated. Dehydration will only add to your nausea as well, and it could land you in the hospital to boot.

Shake up your vitamin routine. Having a vitamin on an empty stomach can leave you feeling queasy. Try having your vitamin with food or right before bed. If that doesn't work, talk to your doctor or midwife about switching to a lower-iron formulation (sometimes that helps) or a lactose- or gluten-free type (if food intolerances or allergies could be contributing to your misery), or about taking folic acid on its own until you start feeling better. Don't worry about depriving your body or your baby: "You don't need much extra iron until the start of the third trimester, unless you're anemic," explains Gideon Koren.

Avoid unpleasant odours as much as possible. Run a fan at your desk or sit near an open window. Sniff slices of lemon, grated ginger, or sprigs of mint. And hand over the smelly cooking duties to someone else.

Wear loose-fitting clothing. Anything that puts pressure on your abdomen (such as belts and tight-fitting waistbands) contributes to nausea. You may even find brief-style underwear too uncomfortable, in which case switch to bikini style or hip-huggers instead.

Try something new. Acupuncture, acupressure (via wristbands that apply constant pressure to the acupuncture pressure points on the wrist that

7.3   Bite-Sized Solutions: Foods That Decrease or Increase Nausea

You may have to do a bit of experimenting to figure out which foods appeal to you right now and help to minimize your nausea. Some moms-to-be find that zeroing in on foods by considering their taste or texture works well; others prefer to consider food groups. You can, of course, combine or alternate strategies. Just do what works for you.

Strategy 1: Choose Foods by Taste and Texture

Salty	Chips, pretzels
Tart and Sweet	Pickles, lemonade
Wholesome and Earthy	Brown rice, mushroom soup, peanut butter
Bland	Mashed potatoes, gelatin, broth
Soft	Bread, noodles
Sweet	Cake, sugary cereals
Fruity	Fruity popsicles, watermelon
Liquid	Juice, seltzer, sparkling water, ginger ale
Dry	Crackers

Strategy 2: Choose Foods by Food Group

Food Group	Stomach-Friendly Food Choices	Foods That Tend to Aggravate Morning Sickness
Grain products	Rice cakes, soda crackers, bagels, pasta, cereal, oatmeal	Spicy, high-fat crackers
Fruits and vegetables	Lemons (for sucking on or sniffing), bananas, applesauce, rhubarb, grapes, watermelon, pears, papaya juice, potatoes (baked, boiled, or mashed), avocados, celery sticks, carrot sticks, zucchini, tomatoes	Onions, cabbage, cauliflower
Milk products	Yogourt smoothies, frozen yogourt, puddings	High-fat cheeses
Meat and alternatives	Sunflower seeds	Fried meats, greasy foods, high-fat meats (e.g., sausages), fried eggs, spicy foods, foods containing monosodium glutamate (MSG)
Other foods	Ginger (root extract, fresh-ground, capsules, tea, sticks, crystals, pickled, and in other forms), mints (especially peppermint), lemon drops, licorice, potato chips, chewing gum, pickles, chamomile tea, lemonade, carbonated mineral water with a twist of lemon, sherbet	High-fat foods (e.g., French fries), fried foods (e.g., onion rings), spicy foods (e.g., corn chips), and beverages containing caffeine (e.g., coffee and cola)

control nausea), and hypnosis are other options to consider. Your doctor or midwife can advise you about the benefits of the various treatment options. You might also want to get in touch with the Motherisk Nausea and Vomiting of Pregnancy Helpline at 1–800–436–8477 or check out the NVP forum on their website, www.motherisk.org.

Add some spice to your life. A study reported in the *Annals of Pharmacotherapy* in August 2005 noted that ginger appears to be a fairly low-risk and effective treatment for NVP and may be appropriate in low doses for patients not responding to traditional drug therapies. Note: Ask your doctor or midwife for guidance before using any herbal product during pregnancy.

Make sure your doctor or midwife is aware of how you're feeling. You should seek medical attention *immediately* if you suspect that you are becoming dehydrated or seriously ill (you're urinating less frequently and your urine is dark yellow, you can't keep liquids down, you're feeling faint or dizzy, you're vomiting up blood). Hyperemesis gravidarum is a particularly severe form of nausea and vomiting of pregnancy that occurs in approximately 1 per cent of pregnant women. It is diagnosed when vomiting becomes so severe that a pregnant woman becomes dehydrated, develops an imbalance of the electrolytes in the blood, or loses more than 5 per cent of her pre-pregnancy weight, or all three. Hospitalization may be required in order to treat this condition.

Hyperemesis gravidarum tends to ease after the first trimester—and typically disappears before 20 weeks—but 10 to 20 per cent of women with this condition will experience symptoms throughout their entire pregnancy. If you've experienced hyperemesis gravidarum during a previous pregnancy, your doctor may suggest taking a medication sooner during your next pregnancy.

think pink

Women who experience severe nausea and vomiting during the first trimester are more likely to give birth to a girl. Researchers in Sweden found that 55.7 per cent of women admitted to hospital for severe morning sickness were carrying female babies. They believe that high levels of human chorionic gonadotropin (a hormone found in larger concentrations in female babies) may help to explain why these women are more likely to have such severe morning sickness. Of course, before you paint the nursery pink, you'll want to keep in mind that not all scientists subscribe to this theory.

Here's something else to bear in mind when you're planning your next pregnancy: your odds of developing a severe case of NVP decrease if you are taking a multivitamin regularly at the time you conceive.

Talk to your doctor or midwife about pharmacological treatments for morning sickness. Don't play the martyr unnecessarily. If you're suffering from a severe case of morning sickness, talk to your health-care provider about the advisability of taking an anti-nausea medication such as Diclectin (a combination of vitamin B6 and an antihistamine). There are other treatments available as well.

Try not to worry too much about the effects of morning sickness on your baby. There is no evidence that the baby suffers from the temporary malnutrition brought on by morning sickness, even when it is fairly severe.

Nasal changes

Increased blood flow to the mucous membranes can trigger all kinds of annoying (but temporary) pregnancy side effects, including rhinitis, sinusitis (swelling of the sinuses), and nosebleeds. It also increases the likelihood that you'll snore at night. See the section on sleep in Chapter 5 for more about breathing-related sleep problems.

Rhinitis. Feel like you've had a runny nose since the moment the pregnancy test came back positive? You're probably suffering from rhinitis—a swelling of the mucous membranes in the nose that's triggered by both your increased blood volume and all the pregnancy-related hormones raging through your body. (Cool cocktail-party fact: placental growth hormone is believed to be responsible for the ramp up in nasal mucus production.) If your stuffy nose is driving you crazy, you can get temporary relief by doing nasal washings with a saline solution or steaming your face and nose area with a facial steamer. Tips: Nasal sprays should be avoided because they can cause rebound congestion. If you're still smoking, quit: pregnancy rhinitis is more common in moms-to-be who smoke. Talk to your doctor before taking any type of antihistamine.

The best cure of all for pregnancy rhinitis is having your baby: the 30 per cent of pregnant women who are afflicted by pregnancy rhinitis find that their symptoms disappear shortly after they give birth.

Nosebleeds. Some women also experience nosebleeds during pregnancy. They're typically caused by increased blood flow but can also be a symptom of high blood pressure, so you'll definitely want to let your caregiver know if you're experiencing these.

Perineal aching

Feel like you're carrying a bowling ball with your perineum, that previously ignored area between the vagina and anus that suddenly becomes an acceptable topic of conversation once you're pregnant? You're not alone. It's not at all unusual to experience aching, pressure, or sharp twinges in the perineal area during late pregnancy. Perineal aching tends to occur during the last month of pregnancy, once the baby's head has descended into the pelvis.

Those Kegel exercises that your prenatal instructor likes to rave about can help to strengthen your perineal muscles, readying them for the challenges of labour. Just make sure you have your Kegeling technique down pat. A physiotherapist who specializes in women's health can check your technique and provide you with other tips on preparing your body for birth.

How to do Kegels:

1. **Find the right muscles.** The easiest way to do this if you've never done Kegels before is to insert a finger inside your vagina and then try to squeeze your finger using the muscles in your vagina and pelvic floor region. Practise tightening and relaxing these muscles until you know exactly what to do to control them.
2. **Work them.** Now that you've found those muscles, use 'em. Contract your pelvic floor muscles for a count of five and then relax for a count of five. Repeat. Eventually you want to work up to sets of ten repetitions of ten seconds each. And you want to do three sets of ten repetitions each day.
3. **Pay attention to your technique.** For maximum impact, only contract your pelvic floor muscles, not the muscles in your abdomen, thighs, or buttocks. And don't hold your breath.

Note: It's not a good idea to do Kegels by stopping and starting the flow of urine. Doing Kegels with a full bladder can weaken your muscles and lead to poor bladder emptying (which, in turn, will increase your risk of developing a urinary tract infection).

Pubic-bone pain (osteitis pubis)

While pubic-bone pain (inflammation of symphysis pubis) is a seldom-mentioned pregnancy-related complaint, it's troublesome to some women nonetheless. The pain is caused by the loosening of the cartilage that joins the two pubic bones together in the middle of your pelvic area. (A maternity belt may provide some relief.) Consider what Chris, a 36-year-old mother of three, has to say about what she experienced during her last pregnancy: "I had excruciating pain at the front of my pubic bone that got worse with each pregnancy. With my second, I could hardly walk after the birth."

While pubic-bone pain tends to disappear on its own after you give birth, sometimes it doesn't disappear quite as quickly as you'd like, so be prepared for some continued tenderness during the first few weeks postpartum. If your symptoms continue, your doctor may suggest a physical exam to evaluate the extent of your discomfort and to test your range of motion. Imaging tests may also be ordered. Treatment options may include avoiding activities that could further irritate the area, going for physical therapy, and taking medications that reduce pain and inflammation. In cases that do not respond to treatment, surgery may be recommended.

Rashes

Some women develop rashes during pregnancy. These rashes—which are particularly common in overweight women—are most likely to occur in the sweaty skin folds under the breasts or in the groin area and are caused by a fungal infection known as intertrigo. The best way to cope with intertrigo is by wearing loose-fitting cotton clothing (to reduce sweating), washing and drying the affected areas frequently (using non-perfumed soap to minimize irritation), and applying calamine lotion or zinc oxide powder to the affected areas. This will both relieve the itching and help to decrease some of the moisture in the area. Note: It's important to treat intertrigo early. Left untreated, it can become superinfected with yeast and will require treatment with a specific antifungal cream.

Approximately 1 in every 150 pregnant women will develop a particularly miserable rash known as pruritic urticarial papules and plaques of pregnancy (PUPPP)—a condition characterized by itchy, reddish, raised patches on the skin. The condition tends to run in families and is more common in first pregnancies. It can be treated with oral medications, anti-itching creams, oatmeal or baking-soda baths, cold compresses, Noxzema (it contains cooling agents), and, in particularly severe cases, cortisone or prednisone. But, the most effective cure for this condition is giving birth.

Approximately 1 in every 500 to 1,000 pregnant women will develop a potentially serious condition called intrahepatic cholestasis of pregnancy.

Women with this condition experience severe itchiness caused by a buildup of bile acids in the liver and bloodstream. If you experience this type of itching, your caregiver will want to monitor you closely for the duration of your pregnancy, because some studies have shown a link between intrahepatic cholestasis of pregnancy and stillbirth, preterm labour, fetal distress, and postpartum hemorrhage. Researchers at the University of Birmingham in the UK believe the disorder is underdiagnosed and that it may be responsible for as many as 4 to 5 per cent of unexplained stillbirths.

Restless leg syndrome (RLS)

The term *restless leg syndrome* (RLS) describes a variety of unpleasant sensations in the legs: creeping, crawling, tingling, burning, or aching in the calves, thighs, feet, or in the upper portions of the legs. The symptoms occur approximately 10 to 20 minutes after going to bed. Nighttime leg twitching may also be a problem. The symptoms of RLS tend to last from week 20 until the baby is born.

RLS—which affects up to 26 per cent of pregnant women—may be genetic in origin or it may be related to the hormonal changes of pregnancy. There also appear to be some nutritional links: it may be associated with anemia. Treating anemia reduces the symptoms of RLS. And women who are taking folic acid are less likely to develop RLS.

The best way to cope with the discomforts of restless leg syndrome is by exercising early in the day, avoiding caffeine, and taking a warm bath and massaging your legs before you go to bed. There are some medicinal treatments available, but these are only considered in situations where the symptoms of RLS are particularly severe. (The potential risk to the baby has to be balanced against the benefits to the mother.)

Another source of leg discomfort can occur when the legs become swollen with fluids, which leaves the veins and arteries poorly supported, causing vascular fatigue. The discomfort is more noted at bedtime when you have stopped moving and are lying down. You can get some relief from this during pregnancy by wearing prescription-strength compression hose. The problem tends to go away after the pregnancy ends and the excess fluid has dissipated.

Round ligament pain

Round ligament pain tends to be one of the more alarming (although absolutely harmless) pregnancy-related complaints. Round ligament pain is the name given to that awful ripping sensation you experience if you roll over in bed or otherwise change your position too suddenly (or that sore and achy sensation you may experience after a day of being particularly active). Caused by the sudden stretching of the ligaments and muscles that support the uterus, it tends to be at its worst during the first half of the second trimester, when the uterus is large enough to exert pressure on the ligaments, but not yet large enough to rest some of its weight on the nearby pelvic bones.

The best way to cope with round ligament pain is by supporting your belly and moving slowly and carefully when you're changing positions. If you do end up experiencing pain, you'll find that soaking in a warm tub can help to ease some of the discomfort.

Don't be afraid to check in with your doctor or midwife if you're not sure if what you've experienced is round ligament pain or if it's another sort of abdominal pain. It's always best to seek answers and reassurance when you're not sure.

maternity support belt

Wish you could tote that heavy uterus around in a sling? A maternity support belt could be the solution. Although cumbersome and expensive, these "abdominal bras" help to provide much-needed support if your abdominal muscles are having a tough time doing the job on their own. They're ideal for women with oversized uteruses—women who are carrying more than one baby, or who have fibroids, for example—but they can also provide welcome relief to mothers whose abdominal muscles may have long since given up the ghost (for example, some women who are giving birth for the third or subsequent time).

Saliva, excessive (ptyalism)

Ptyalism (excessive saliva) is most likely to occur in women who are struggling with hyperemesis gravidarum (the most extreme form of nausea and vomiting of pregnancy). It is likely triggered by hormonal changes and made worse by the tendency of anyone who is struggling with nausea to minimize the amount of swallowing that they do (a strategy that causes saliva to build up in the mouth). Couple that with the fact that heartburn and nausea can trigger the salivary glands to produce extra saliva (to coat the esophagus and protect the mouth and throat against the irritation that occurs with frequent vomiting), and you can see why ptyalism is more of a problem for some moms-to-be than others.

To cope with it, you may want to try brushing your teeth regularly, sipping water, chewing sugarless gum, or sucking on hard, sugarless candy to get rid of any bad taste in your mouth. These strategies don't work for everyone, however. Some moms-to-be find that they have to resort to spitting out their saliva or removing it manually using cloths or paper tissues in order to avoid the nausea that can accompany swallowing excessive or thickened saliva.

Sciatica

Sciatica is the name given to the shooting pain, tingling, or numbness that many women experience in their lower backs, buttocks, outer thighs, and legs during pregnancy. (Typically, you'll experience a pain that shoots down your leg to a point below your knee.) It occurs when the baby's head, the enlarging uterus, or the relaxed pelvic joints press down on the major nerves that run from the backbone through the pelvis and toward each leg. Once it flares up it can be aggravated by lifting, bending, and even walking.

If you're having trouble with sciatica, you might want to start seeing a chiropractor or physiotherapist on a regular basis. Chiropractic treatments can help to relieve some of the pain and discomfort. The only catch is that you have to keep going on a regular basis in order to keep your sciatica under control. Still, if you're hobbling around, unable to put your full weight on your affected leg, trekking off to the chiropractor a few times a week seems like a small price to pay for becoming mobile again.

You can also eliminate a lot of the discomfort of sciatica by changing positions regularly during the day (for example, getting up and moving around at least once an hour) and by hitting the swimming pool. Floating around in the pool helps to temporarily take the weight of your uterus off your sciatic nerve, a source of much-welcome relief.

Skin changes

We've already talked about a few skin-related problems that you may experience during pregnancy: acne, itchiness, and rashes. Something else you need to know: it's not unusual for moles, birthmarks, recent scars, and freckles to darken. Ninety per cent of pregnant women experience pigmentation changes, with these changes occurring gradually over the course of pregnancy. Pigment changes occur to the areola (the circular area around the nipple),

---

hot mama

Increased blood flow to your skin helps your body to get rid of excess heat. (Can you imagine what a hot mama you'd be if your blood stream *wasn't* carrying away excess heat on a constant basis?) There's also an additional, unexpected payoff: the increased blood flow stimulates the growth of your hair and nails, so you end up with lush hair and longer nails, you gorgeous thing, you.

genital skin, axillae (armpits), inner thighs, and along the linea alba (the vertical white line on the abdomen that turns into the linea nigra during pregnancy). Pigmentation changes tend to fade after the birth in fair-skinned women, but some pigmentation changes may remain in dark-skinned women.

Here are a few other surprising skin changes you may notice during pregnancy:

Palmar erythema. The palms of your hands and the soles of your feet may take on a reddish hue at some time during the first or second trimester. These skin changes are triggered by elevated levels of estrogen and increased blood flow to the skin, and disappear spontaneously within a week of the birth. Palmar erythema tends to run in families and is twice as likely to occur in Caucasian women (occurring in two-thirds of women) as in African-American women (occurring in one-third of women).

Spider nevi, spider angiomas, spider telangiectasias, nevus araneuses. All names for red spider web–like clusters of dilated blood vessels that can occur during pregnancy thanks to hormonal changes and increased blood volume. They are more common in Caucasian women (60 to 70 per cent develop them by term) than in black women (10 per cent develop them by term). They are most likely to occur in the parts of your body that are drained by the vena cava (the eyes, neck, throat, and arms), and they are most likely to appear between months two and five. Spider nevi can pop out on your face or in the whites of your eye following an intense pushing stage. These conditions usually become less prominent after the delivery (approximately seven weeks to three months after the birth), but if they don't fade enough that you can live with them as is or with a dab of cosmetic cover-up cream, a dermatologist can treat them. Unfortunately, your provincial or territorial health plan may not cover the cost of this cosmetic procedure. What's more, the spider veins may recur if you become pregnant again, if you gain weight, or as you grow older.

Cutis marmorata. Cutis marmorata refers to bluish mottling of the legs that becomes more prominent when your legs are exposed to the cold. It occurs during pregnancy because elevated levels of estrogen lead to changes to your vascular system. The condition should disappear after the birth. Other related effects include flushing to your face (that much-talked-about pregnancy glow) and sudden temperature swings (hot and cold flashes—but, of course, the term cold is relative when you're pregnant and you have a placenta, a baby, and extra weight to keep you warm).

Other skin conditions related to vascular changes include hemangiomas (birthmark-like non-malignant vascular tumours) and varicosities (achy, bulging veins). Decreased capillary strength can lead to purpura (bruise-like blood spots) and scattered petechiae (small, flat red or purple blood spots), which can appear on legs. These conditions usually resolve postpartum.

Skin tags. You may develop a series of skin tags (tiny polyps that occur in areas of the body where the skin rubs against your clothing or against itself—in the folds of your neck, along your bra lines, and so on). While these skin tags may disappear a few months after you give birth, they can be annoying in the meantime. If they're causing you a lot of discomfort, you might want to talk to your doctor about the possibility of having them removed. (Once again, you may be on the hook for the cost of this procedure, since most provincial and territorial health plans don't pay for skin tag removal.)

Linea nigra. This is one of those pregnancy complaints that you swear should make it into the pages of *Ripley's Believe It or Not*. I'm referring to the brown crayon-like mark down the centre of the belly that some moms-to-be develop during pregnancy. It runs from your belly button to your pubic area. If this isn't a "tattoo" you would have chosen for yourself, don't stress about it: it's not permanent. It generally disappears within a few months of giving birth.

Mask of pregnancy. The term *mask of pregnancy* (chloasma) is used to describe the irregular, blotchy areas of pigmentation (light to dark brown) that occur on the cheeks, chin, and nose in 45 to 70 per cent of pregnant women. There are three different patterns of chloasma: centrofacial (cheeks, forehead, upper lip, nose, and chin: the pattern exhibited 63 per cent of the time when chloasma occurs), malar (cheeks and nose: the pattern exhibited 21 per cent of the time), and mandibular (in the lower jaw area: the pattern exhibited 16 per cent of the time). Like the linea nigra, chloasma is caused by skin pigmentation changes and tends to disappear shortly after the birth. You can minimize the extent of these changes by reducing your exposure to the sun. (Wear a non-allergenic sunscreen of SPF 15 or greater or non-allergenic cover-up of SPF 15 or greater when you head outdoors.)

Smell, heightened sense of

Find yourself being hit by a wave of nausea each time you smell coffee, cigarette smoke, or strong perfume? That's because most women develop a heightened sense of smell during pregnancy. Janis, 31, remembers this as one of the most annoying things she experienced during her pregnancy: "Odours drove me around the bend. I could barely stand to walk down my apartment hall and smell various foods cooking. I was also sensitive to my husband's breath, which seemed so unbearable some nights I felt like sleeping on the couch!"

You'll probably find that your heightened sense of smell is less likely to trigger nausea once the peak period of morning sickness passes (around the end of the first trimester, for most women). In the meantime, you might want to try an old trick: carrying around a handkerchief that's been dipped in lemon juice. Not only does the powerful lemon scent help to block other offending odours, it can also help to relieve nausea.

Stretch marks

Stretch marks (the medical term is *striae gravidarum*) occur whenever your skin is forced to stretch more than it's designed to. (Your skin has a certain amount of elasticity, but it has limits.) Stretch marks appear as pink or purple wrinkled streaks on various parts of your body—most commonly your thighs, abdomen, groin area, and breasts. While they typically fade away to white or silvery streaks over time, stretch marks seldom disappear entirely.

Stretch marks are more likely to occur in Caucasian women (90 per cent incidence rate), tend to run in families, and are more common in younger women who experience a greater total weight gain. There is some speculation that women who develop stretch marks have less elastin in their skin than those who don't, which means that their skin will separate rather than sag when stressed. You can reduce your chances of developing stretch marks by not gaining an excessive amount of weight. As for using special creams and lotions to avoid or get rid of stretch marks, don't waste your money. Studies have yet to prove the effectiveness of cocoa butter, vitamin E, tretinoin, olive oil, or massage oil in preventing stretch marks. That's because the marks are believed to be triggered by hormonal changes or hormonal changes combined with stretching. And nothing you rub on the surface of your skin is going to do a thing about your hormones. If only.

Sweating

Feeling like you're sweating more than usual? It's not all in your head. High levels of progesterone and increased blood flow boost your body temperature by a full degree Fahrenheit. While your body will do its best to keep you cool by causing you to perspire, there are a few things you can do to help the cause. Wear loose-fitting clothing that breathes (cotton is ideal), dress in layers so that you can peel off a layer or two at a time if you start to feel overheated, and drink plenty of extra fluids to replace those you're losing through perspiration.

Don't be surprised if you end up driving your partner a little crazy with this whole temperature thing. You may get looked at like you've lost your mind when you insist on turning on the car air conditioner in the middle of November because you're feeling too hot—or when you refuse to sleep in a bed that has anything warmer on it than a lightweight cotton sheet, even though there's a snowstorm outside.

Swelling and fluid retention

Swelling (edema) is another common pregnancy-related complaint—and one that tends to become more bothersome as your pregnancy progresses. It occurs because your body retains extra fluid during pregnancy. (Your body needs that extra fluid because your blood volume increases by an astounding 40 per cent when you're pregnant.) It's not unusual to have slightly swollen ankles, particularly during warm weather or after spending a day on your feet, but you shouldn't feel any pain or discomfort as a result of this swelling. If you experience sudden or extreme swelling, particularly in your hands or in your face in the area around your eyes, and especially if these symptoms are accompanied with one or more of the following symptoms—a severe headache, blurred vision, dizziness, or abdominal pain—you could be developing pre-eclampsia (a potentially life-threatening condition characterized by swelling and high blood pressure).

You can help your body rid itself of extra fluids by lying on your side or sitting with your feet elevated above the level of your heart, soaking in a warm (not hot!) tub, increasing your fluid intake (becoming dehydrated can actually make your fluid retention problems worse), and limiting (but not eliminating entirely) your salt intake.

Wondering why your feet are feeling so swollen? Not only does progesterone encourage your body to retain fluid, your uterus puts pressure on the veins that carry blood back from your lower extremities, which can encourage fluid to pool in your feet and ankles. If your feet are visibly swollen, you are probably retaining about 2 litres (70 ounces) of extra fluid. If you notice swelling throughout your entire body, your body tissues are probably retaining 4.5 litres (150 ounces) of extra fluid.

To minimize symptoms, put your feet up—literally. Elevating your legs and feet will help to improve your circulation and minimize fluid retention. Lie down on your left side to give your circulation a boost. And keep yourself cool. Becoming overheated will only make the swelling worse.

Thirstiness

Don't be surprised if you find yourself feeling thirstier than normal while you're pregnant. Your increased fluid intake helps your kidneys get rid of the waste products that are being produced by your baby. What's more, your body needs extra fluids to replenish the supply of amniotic fluid and to maintain your increased blood volume. You should plan to drink at least eight glasses a day of water or other hydrating beverages. (Don't count coffee, tea, or other caffeinated beverages—which function as diuretics, removing fluid from your body—or sugary drinks and juices, since sugar is a desiccant, meaning it causes dryness.)

Urinary incontinence

Urinary incontinence is a common complaint toward the end of pregnancy (experienced by 30 to 50 per cent of pregnant women versus 8 per cent of non-pregnant women). You may find that you leak a small amount of urine when you run, cough, sneeze, or laugh. The problem is caused by weak pelvic floor muscles and the weight of your growing baby pressing against your bladder. Once it starts, it tends to get progressively worse during pregnancy and it is likely to recur during subsequent pregnancies. To strengthen your pelvic floor muscles, do Kegel exercises (see the How to do Kegels steps earlier in this chapter). And, to prevent yourself from straining those muscles any further, avoid constipation and heavy lifting. (You're not supposed to be doing any heavy lifting anyway, remember?)

Since you're likely to be leaking only a small amount of fluid, you can probably get away with using sanitary pads rather than special incontinence products to contain any leaks that occur.

Urination, increased frequency of

While we're talking about the waterworks department, let's deal with the issue of increased frequency of urination. Given that there's a baby camped out on your bladder for much of your pregnancy, an increased need to urinate (60 per cent of pregnant women need to urinate more than seven times each day, and that only accounts for their bathroom breaks during daytime hours) is hardly surprising. What's more, long before your uterus starts encroaching on your bladder's territory, increased blood flow to the kidneys triggers the need to urinate more frequently. (This is your body's way of flushing waste products from your system more efficiently.)

To minimize those annoying middle-of-the-night treks to the bathroom, don't overdo it with the liquids right before bedtime, and make a point of leaning forward a bit when you're making one of those middle-of-the-night bathroom pit stops to ensure that you empty your bladder completely.

It's normal to spend your pregnancy scouting out the location of the nearest washroom. It's not normal to feel pain during urination. If you experience any sort of pain or burning, or if you feel the urge to urinate again immediately after urination, get in touch with your caregiver: you may have a urinary tract infection. It's important to seek treatment promptly because these infections, if left untreated, can lead to premature labour.

You are more susceptible to urinary tract infections during pregnancy than when you aren't pregnant. Increased levels of progesterone decrease the tone of your bladder, making it more difficult for you to empty your bladder fully. And your glucose- and amino acid–rich pregnant urine allows bacteria to multiply at a rapid rate.

Vagina, changes to the

Increased blood flow to the vagina during pregnancy causes the tissues in your vagina to become softer and more sensitive. This can result in increased sexual arousal (the good news), but it can also cause your cervix to bleed a little more easily than usual if it happens to get bumped during lovemaking. This can result in much angst on everyone's part if you don't know what's going on. (You might notice some light pinkish spotting when you head to the bathroom after sex or some brownish spotting a day or two later.) Changing your position slightly is generally all that's required to prevent the problem from recurring (and causing needless stress for everyone). If this experience has you freaking out about sex during pregnancy, period, stay tuned. We'll be having a (pregnant) facts of life talk in Chapter 8.

Increased blood flow to the vagina causes the cervix to become softened and lilac-tinged during the early weeks of pregnancy. This is known as Jacquemier's or Chadwick's sign.

Vaginal secretions, increased

Don't assume that you've developed a vaginal infection if your vaginal secretions become wetter or more abundant. It's normal to experience an increase in the amount of leukorrhea (the odourless clear or white mucus discharge produced by the female body) during pregnancy. Increased estrogen levels cause an increase in the quantity of leukorrhea as well as changes to its composition (it tends to become thicker and white). You can deal with your more abundant discharge by wearing a light sanitary pad, if necessary. What you shouldn't do, however, is use douching products, vaginal deodorants, or any sort of perfumed soap—all of which could be irritating to your vaginal tissues. (Douching also poses some additional risks, something we talked about back in Chapter 2.)

There could be cause for concern if you experience soreness or pain in your vagina or vulva, or if your discharge becomes greenish-yellow, foul smelling, or watery. These symptoms could indicate an infection or premature rupturing of your membranes. (If in doubt, check things out with your health-care provider.)

It's particularly important to report any increased vaginal discharge if you've just had amniocentesis performed, since it's possible that you may have experienced an amniotic fluid leak. Try not to panic, however—these types of leaks frequently repair themselves. Your caregiver will likely recommend that you rest for a day or two to see if the problem resolves itself. (You can find out more about amniocentesis in Table 9.2, starting on page 296.)

If you're diagnosed with trichomoniasis (a vaginal infection characterized by a yellowish-green discharge with a fishy odour), your infection will be treated with an oral medication or a vaginal gel or suppository. To reduce the risk of re-infection, your partner will be treated with an oral medication at the same time.

Varicose veins

Varicose veins are caused by an accumulation of extra blood in and around the valves of the veins. They're more likely to flare up during pregnancy, and are more likely to be a problem if your mother or other female relatives have had them.

Varicose veins tend to occur in the legs (both the calves and thighs) and, less commonly, in the labial region. In both cases, the affected area can become painful and swollen.

If your legs are affected, your caregiver will likely suggest that you elevate your feet whenever you're sitting or lying down. (You can raise the foot of your bed by putting pillows under your mattress.) He or she might also recommend that you do leg exercises if you have to sit for any prolonged period of time, and that you get in the habit of wearing support stockings (although, to derive any real benefit from them, you have to put them on first thing in the morning, before you hop out of bed or have your morning shower). Your caregiver will also likely suggest that you avoid wearing any tight-fitting clothing that restricts your circulation, especially knee-high pantyhose and tight calf-height socks.

You should never knead or vigorously massage your varicose veins. Doing so can damage your veins further and may cause a blood clot. And if you happen to notice a red, swollen, tender area that appears to have become infected, elevate your leg and contact your caregiver immediately. You may have developed thrombophlebitis (when a blood clot leads to swelling in one or more of your veins).

Weepiness

Don't be surprised if you find yourself feeling extra weepy while you're pregnant, even for no particular reason. That wacky, pregnancy-related hormonal cocktail can cause your emotions to fluctuate wildly. "The hormonal ebbs and flows did me in," admits Chris, a 36-year-old mother of three. "I'd be sobbing one minute, laughing the next. Suddenly any bad news, especially if it had to do with babies or children, brought me to tears. There were also very high highs: feeling the baby move always brought a smile to my face."

While it's normal to have weepy moments—to find yourself with tears streaming down your face because you're just so darned touched by the latest long-distance phone commercial—it's not normal to experience extreme depression. If you find yourself feeling hopeless and overwhelmed, you could be suffering from prenatal depression or perinatal anxiety—a problem that afflicts more women than most people realize. Be sure to let your caregiver know about the difficulty you're having so that he or she can recommend a possible treatment (individual counselling, group therapy, or medication). See Chapter 5 for more on perinatal mood disorders (mood disorders such as depression and anxiety during pregnancy and postpartum).

> "Throughout my pregnancy, I really found myself at odds with society's perspective on being pregnant and having a baby. I just found it very difficult to talk about my fears and my negative feelings with anyone except Scott and my doctor. I think I must have gone through my 'postpartum depression' before I had Norah, but I think a lot of it was because of all the pressure to be happy, to be blissful, and not to question things so much."
>
> —MYRNA, 32, MOTHER OF ONE

Yeast infections

It isn't hard to figure out why so many pregnant women end up developing yeast infections, since the accompanying hormonal changes practically open the door to these. Not only is your vaginal environment less acidic and your immune system less effective, there's an increased amount of sugar stored in the cell walls of the vagina. (And, as we all know, yeast *loves* sugar.)

You should suspect that you have a yeast infection if you've developed a thick, cheese curd-like white vaginal discharge accompanied by severe itching, if you develop a very red rash that is surrounded by red spots, or if you experience pain and soreness when you urinate.

You can minimize the misery of a yeast infection and reduce the chance of a recurrence by keeping the genital area as dry as possible; wiping from front to back when you use the bathroom; ensuring that your vagina is well lubricated before you have intercourse; wearing cotton or cotton-crotch underwear and avoiding pantyhose, tight jeans, perfumed soaps, and vaginal deodorants; cutting down on the amount of refined sugar in your diet; eating yogourt with acidophilus (active cultures) or taking acidophilus supplements; not spending too much time sitting on vinyl seats in your car, home, or office; and soaking in a warm tub to which one cup of cornstarch and a half cup of baking soda have been added. Your doctor may also recommend over-the-counter medications for treating your yeast infection.

CHAPTER 8

This Is Your (Soon-to-Be) Life

"Pregnancy ends the illusion of autonomy. You are housing somebody else, a living presence . . . [Your partner] may sing to the baby and converse with your belly, but it's still just an idea, until the baby is born. For the woman, it's already the root, the core around which she walks and dreams."

—MARNI JACKSON, *THE MOTHER ZONE*

Feel like you're living two different lives: your pregnant life and your soon-to-be life? Sure, you're spending a lot of time thinking about being pregnant—but you're also spending an increasing amount of time focusing on what your life will be like after your baby is born.

It only makes sense that your brain keeps taking side trips to the future. After all, you're about to venture into previously uncharted territory (or at least territory that's yet to be charted by you if this is your first pregnancy). As Daniel N. Stern, Nadia Bruschweiler-Stern, and Alison Freeland note in their book *The Birth of a Mother: How the Motherhood Experience Changes You Forever,* "The mind during pregnancy is a workspace where the future is assembled and worked over like an invention in progress."

That's what this chapter is all about: your soon-to-be life. We'll be talking about some of the decisions you'll be asked to make over the next few months, practical things that you can do ahead of time to make the early days of parenthood a little less stressful, how becoming parents is likely to affect the relationship between you and your partner (and what your partner is likely to be worrying about right now), and why this is the perfect time to start thinking about the parent you want to be and the family you hope to create.

Decisions, Decisions . . .

You've spent the time since your pregnancy test came back positive making decisions, frantically flipping through pregnancy books so that you can arm yourself with the facts on a variety of different issues. You'd think that at this stage of the game your homework would all be finished and you'd be able to coast from here to delivery day; but, a pregnant woman's work is never done— or so it would seem. You still need to decide which maternity clothes to buy and when, whether or not to sign up for prenatal classes (early bird prenatal classes, childbirth classes, or both), whether to bank your baby's umbilical cord blood, what to do about the circumcision issue (assuming, of course, that you give birth to a baby boy), whether to breastfeed your baby (about 90 per cent of Canadian babies are breastfed for some duration of time), and how to go about choosing your baby's name. In the remainder of this chapter, I'll arm you with the facts you need to make up your mind about each of these important issues.

Pregnant and chic

Gone are the days when dressing in maternity clothing meant dressing in A-frame dresses emblazoned with bunnies or butterflies. The fashion industry has finally clued in to the fact that pregnant women want to look chic while they're sporting a baby bump. And you don't have to go broke to look fab. Here's some tips:

Don't hit the stores too soon. Rather than blowing your entire maternity clothing budget in one go (and too early on in your pregnancy), only buy what you need when you actually start to need it. You will probably be able to get away with wearing most of your regular clothes until at least the start of the second trimester, although you may have to bid a fond farewell to your dress pants and fitted skirts a little sooner than that. Ideally, you'd like to be able to treat yourself to a new piece every now and again throughout your pregnancy to add some variety to your wardrobe.

Look for bargains and freebies. "Get hand-me-downs from friends and relatives, shop consignment stores, and make a point of hitting the sale racks," suggests Carolin, a 34-year-old mother of three. "Used maternity clothes are usually in really good condition because they're worn for such a short time."

As well as checking out the sale racks at the big maternity stores, be sure to visit the maternity-wear sections of the major department stores. And don't forget to search the discount racks at plus-sized retailers as well.

Look for clothes that will grow with you. The more flexible the garment is, the more wear you'll get out of it. And look for high-quality pieces that can be combined to create the maximum number of outfits. "I bought only the basics: black pants, two vests, and a skirt and sweater/cardigan set," says Alexandra, a 33-year-old mother of two. "I mixed and matched along with my 'regular' turtlenecks and blouses."

When in doubt, buy large. If you're torn between two sizes of maternity clothes, buy the larger one. It's difficult to anticipate just how much you'll grow during the months ahead and it can be more than a little disheartening to outgrow your maternity wardrobe when you've got another two months of pregnancy still ahead.

Allow room for cleavage expansion. Choose clothes that have plenty of room across the chest and under the arms. By the time you're ready to give birth, your breasts will each be up to a full pound heavier. And treat yourself to some decent bras—ones with wide, padded straps that won't dig into your shoulders as the weight of your breasts increases.

Don't skimp on underwear. Choose loose-fitting cotton underwear that breathes and that won't irritate your increasingly sensitive skin. Since pregnant women are notoriously susceptible to yeast infections, spending nine months in polyester underwear is a recipe for disaster. It's up to you, however, whether you go with bikini underwear or traditional maternity briefs. Let comfort be your guide.

Invest in some good basics—a nice pair of maternity jeans, a good skirt or dress in basic black—just like what you might do with your regular wardrobe. This is a good idea especially if you're planning on having more than one child. If you choose timeless classics you'll be able to wear them during subsequent pregnancies.

Don't skimp on that maternity or nursing bra. Not only do you deserve to look and feel your best during every stage of pregnancy and motherhood, you can also damage the ligaments that support your breasts if your bra isn't up to the task. And with your breasts each gaining up to an extra pound during pregnancy, it's time to tuck your regular bra away for the foreseeable future. It's particularly important to purchase a well-designed sports bra before you hit the gym. Researchers from the Department of Sports and Exercise Science at the University of Portsmouth in the UK recently discovered that breasts are capable of moving up to 21 centimetres (8 inches) in any direction during exercise—and yet a typical bra is only designed to provide vertical support.

Raid your partner's side of the closet for casual wear. "Large-size men's shirts can be worn over leggings, slacks, tailored skirts, and so on," says Marguerite, a 36-year-old mother of two.

Don't waste your time looking for outfits that you can wear after baby. Choose clothes that look good and feel great now. While you might think you'll be happy to wear that smart-looking maternity suit long after delivery day, chances are you'll be sick to death of it by the time your baby arrives. Besides, there's always the off-chance that someone will see you wearing it and assume you're pregnant again—reason enough to banish it to the back of the closet.

Beat the heat. Your body's thermostat is cranked up when you're pregnant, so choose lightweight clothing made of cotton or other natural fibres. Try to choose garments that can be layered so that you can add or remove them to keep your body at a comfortable temperature. "I was pregnant in the winter and was hot the whole time," recalls Jenny, a 31-year-old mother of one. "I bought lots of coloured T-shirts and wore maternity vests over them so that I could look reasonable at work, but not be sweltering."

Think comfort and joy. While we're talking comfort, here's another important point to remember: anything that binds at the waist or restricts blood flow in your legs (for example, knee-highs) isn't going to be particularly comfortable during pregnancy.

Don't fall into the trap of buying gimmicky products just because you think you might need them. "Combined maternity shirts/nursing shirts seem like a wonderful idea, but in reality they aren't worth the money," insists Maria, a 31-year-old mother of two. "I felt funny wearing a 'nursing shirt' when I was still pregnant, and yet it didn't fit right when I was no longer pregnant but nursing. The shirt hangs lower in the front when you don't have the belly to support it."

Put your best foot forward. Choose low-heeled comfortable shoes that won't pinch your feet if they begin to swell. Believe it or not, your feet may grow as much as a full size during pregnancy. If all else fails, think slip-ons.

Look for clothes that will do double duty. "Business casual is a good category to aim for, as it will allow you to dress for work and for your leisure time without turning to two different wardrobes," says Janet, a 32-year-old mother of one.

Treat thyself. Pregnancy is, after all, a time for indulgence. "Splurge on a few things that make you feel good, like a special sundress or a formal dress to wear to a wedding," suggests 25-year-old Christina, who is currently pregnant with her third child. If you don't want to spend a small fortune on a drop-dead-gorgeous ball gown for New Year's Eve, consider renting it instead. Maternity clothing rental boutiques are springing up in a growing number of large cities.

Buy proper maternity clothes—especially pantyhose. It will be a relief to slip into a pair of maternity pantyhose after wearing queen-size, which can be about eight inches too long.

Prenatal classes: Who needs them?

Prenatal classes were once a rite of passage for most pregnant women; but these days only one-third to one-half of women attend public or private prenatal classes. Depending on what's available in your community, you may have the chance to attend one or more of the following types of prenatal classes:

- first- or second-trimester classes that cover such topics as nutrition and exercise during pregnancy;
- third-trimester childbirth classes designed to prepare you for the birth (most include a tour of the birthing suite at the hospital where you'll be delivering your baby);
- breastfeeding classes designed to give you a preview of what you can do to get breastfeeding off to the best possible start;
- a fathers-only (or partners-only) class designed to address the specific worries and concerns of partners.

Prenatal classes have a lot to offer a pregnant woman and her partner in terms of education and support. (If your pregnancy hasn't felt real up until now, it will when you find yourself in a room full of pregnant women.) Classes can give you

- a sneak preview of what to expect during both a vaginal and Caesarean delivery. (Be sure to pay attention during the Caesarean part of the birth movie, by the way. Not all Caesareans are planned.)
- the facts you need about your various birth options (for example, the pros and cons of using different types of pain relief during labour—both medicinal and non-medicinal) so that you can make informed decisions.
- the opportunity to ask any questions you may have about pregnancy, labour, birth, breastfeeding, and newborn care.
- the chance to connect with others who are due at roughly the same time you are—contacts that can be pure gold if you find yourself housebound in February with a new baby.

"I can honestly say I didn't learn much from the prenatal classes, but I'm so glad we went because they made it all seem so much more real. I remember the instructors had these round name tags on and they explained to us that these were 10 centimetres in diameter—the exact size our cervixes would have to dilate to in order to give birth. You should have seen the shocked expressions on everyone's face. It certainly put things into perspective!"

–MARIA, 35, MOTHER OF TWO

Some couples find prenatal classes to be highly beneficial—one of the highlights of being pregnant. "We had a wonderful experience at our prenatal class," says Nicole, a 29-year-old mother of one. "The group of parents was fun and the instructor was a wealth of information. We came away with a package of information as well as a phone number we could call if we ever had any questions or needed any advice."

Maria and her husband had a similarly positive experience. "I think the classes were very beneficial for my husband," the 35-year-old mother of two explains. "He learned a lot and the classes really helped to demystify the birthing process for him."

Jennifer, a 32-year-old mother of one, enjoyed the opportunity to get to know other pregnant couples—something that made for a fun reunion class a couple of months down the road. "It was amazing to see everyone with flattened bellies and real little people in their laps, and to see everyone casually feeding or changing when a few months earlier most of us didn't have the first clue about how to care for an infant."

Other couples, however, are considerably less enthralled with the whole prenatal class experience. Jennifer, 27, who's about to give birth to her first child, found that the prenatal classes she took left her feeling anxious. "It didn't help that the instructor liked to tell scary stories," she remarks.

Carole, a 33-year-old mother of two, thought the classes she took didn't do an adequate job of preparing her for anything other than a medication-free delivery: "I found the classes a little misleading in that they gave the impression that if you used proper breathing, you wouldn't need medical intervention. That wasn't the case for me. I did require an epidural during my first birth, and because of the class I felt like somewhat of a failure."

When you're shopping around for prenatal classes, make sure that the instructor and the childbirth class philosophy seem like a good fit. If you are less than impressed by the prenatal classes offered by the hospital, health unit, or childbirth association in your community, there is an alternative. Depending on where you live, you may be able to arrange for a childbirth educator to conduct private classes for you and your partner. You can either ask your doctor or midwife to pass along the names of childbirth instructors in your community who provide this type of service or you can contact the Childbirth and Postpartum Professional Association of Canada (CAPPA Canada) through its website (www.cappacanada.ca) or by phoning 1–866–CDN–BIRTH (236–2478). A number of childbirth instructors now offer childbirth classes on-line, so that is another option to consider, too.

Umbilical cord blood banking

To bank or not to bank? That is the question. A couple of decades ago, umbilical cord blood banking was the stuff of which science fiction novels were made. But now that the procedure is widely available, it's an issue that most prospective parents are being forced to grapple with. Here's what you need to know.

Umbilical cord blood contains a very high concentration of stem cells (cells that can develop into any other type of cell the body needs). This makes cord blood an ideal product for use in bone marrow transplants. If your child were to require a bone marrow transplant in the future and you had banked his cord blood, you would be able to turn to the blood that you had stored on his behalf instead of searching frantically for a suitable donor. Likewise, if your child's sibling were to require such a transplant, it's highly likely that the cord blood banked from his or her sibling would provide a close enough match to allow for such a transplant. (Of course, if you made the decision to bank one child's cord blood, you might make the decision to bank the cord blood for all of your children, in which case a sibling donation would be a moot point.) Some parents consider banking their baby's umbilical cord blood to be tantamount to taking out biological insurance on their child: they want to know that their baby's cord blood will be available if their baby or another family member ends up needing a bone marrow transplant.

Of course, not all parents who decide to bank their baby's cord blood decide to store that blood specifically for their own family's use. Some parents donate the cord blood to public cord blood banks, which provide blood products to people who need them (for example, people who've undergone radiation therapy or chemotherapy, or who suffer from certain types of blood, immune, or metabolic disorders). Because the stem cells in the umbilical cord blood have not had the opportunity to build up antibodies, they are less likely to trigger the kind of blood incompatibility problems that can result from standard bone marrow transplants, thereby allowing for a less precise donor match.

Based on what you've read so far, you're probably thinking that cord blood banking is an absolute no-brainer: who *wouldn't* want to store their child's umbilical cord blood for possible use in years to come? Unfortunately, the issue isn't nearly that black and white—in fact, it's positively steeped in grey! For one thing, the jury's still out on the benefits of umbilical cord blood banking. Some medical authorities have argued that the odds that you will actually need to access the stored cord blood are very slim. In fact, according to figures cited in the Society of Obstetricians and Gynaecologists of Canada's (SOGC's) March 2005 clinical practice guideline on *Umbilical Cord Blood Banking*, less than 5 per cent of privately stored cord blood has been used clinically. Furthermore, it has been estimated that the use of umbilical cord blood on the original donor only occurs in 1 in every 20,000 collections. An earlier article, published in the *Washington Post,* found that only 10 out of the 18,000 units of cord blood stored by a cord blood bank in San Bruno, California, had been retrieved to date and, in each case, they were used by a family with a history of medical problems requiring transplants— in other words, not your typical low-risk family. What's more, in almost every case in the United States for which cord blood was needed for a transplant, a cord blood match was found at a public blood bank, a fact that basically nullifies the benefits of storing umbilical cord blood privately for the use of individual donors. Add to that the fact that there are concerns about the shelf life of cord blood ("At present, it is not certain how long frozen cord blood will remain viable," the SOGC notes in its clinical practice guideline), and you can see why the whole issue of cord blood banking continues to be highly controversial.

Does this mean that you should forget the whole idea of banking your baby's umbilical cord blood? Not at all. It's an issue that you'll want to research further so that you can make the best decision for your family. Some parents feel that the roughly $900 to $2,000 in upfront charges and $100 to $150 per year in storage costs is a small price to pay for the added peace of mind that comes from knowing that their baby's umbilical cord blood is sitting in a warehouse somewhere, accessible to that child should he ever need it. Others feel that private cord blood banks are simply preying on parents' fears at a time when they are particularly vulnerable—during the emotionally charged weeks leading up to the birth.

If you decide to store your baby's blood in a private bank or to donate your baby's cord blood to a public bank (what the SOGC recommends when cord blood banking is being considered), you will need to make suitable arrangements prior to the birth. This is because cord blood must be collected at the time of delivery (after the baby has been born, but before the delivery of the placenta). Obviously, this is one of those issues that you'll definitely want to discuss with your doctor or midwife as early on in your pregnancy as possible, just in case Baby decides to make his grand entrance a little sooner than planned, catching everyone off guard.

blood banks	"Commercial cord blood banks should be carefully regulated to ensure that promotion and pricing practices are fair, financial relationships are transparent, banked cord blood is stored and used according to approved standards, and parents and care providers understand the differences between autologous [cord blood reserved for the original donor] versus allogeneic [compatible cord blood] donations and private versus public banks." —FROM THE SOCIETY OF OBSTETRICIANS AND GYNAECOLOGISTS OF CANADA'S CLINICAL PRACTICE GUIDELINE: *UMBILICAL CORD BLOOD BANKING: IMPLICATIONS FOR PERINATAL CARE PROVIDERS*, MARCH 2005

The circumcision decision

Think the cord blood decision was a tough one? We're about to wade into even murkier and more emotionally treacherous waters. The subject at hand? Circumcision!

If circumcision has been discussed at your prenatal classes, you already know just how hot this particular topic tends to be. People don't often have lukewarm opinions when it comes to circumcision: they're usually passionately for or against it. Not surprisingly, many couples find that this becomes a source of conflict in their own relationship as they try to decide whether to circumcise their sons.

Jennifer and her partner found themselves at a total impasse on the issue until they came up with a creative solution that worked for their family. The

35-year-old mother of one explains: "We got into a long negotiation over whether or not to circumcise our baby if we had a boy. I was very much against circumcision. So my husband said that he would agree not to do it if, in exchange, he could choose the middle name for any daughter we might have. I agreed and now we have an uncircumcised son. However, if we have a daughter next, she is going to have a very strange middle name that, due to our agreement, I must live with. If she ever asks me why she has such an odd name, I will have to tell her that it was in order to save her brother's foreskin!"

What makes the circumcision decision so challenging is the fact that there's no obvious right or wrong answer (although people in both the pro and con camps would certainly have you believe otherwise). Even the Canadian Paediatric Society acknowledges that the arguments for and against the procedure (see Table 8.1) are pretty much on par—although new evidence showing that rates of urinary tract infection, penile cancer, and HIV transmission are lower in circumcised men is causing health authorities around the world to re-examine their position on infant circumcision. While the CPS remains opposed to routine circumcision, it acknowledges that parents have to make up their own minds about the issue, taking into account personal, religious, or cultural factors. The CPS also notes that circumcision is a surgical procedure and, as such, is not entirely without risk (although the incidence of complications such as bleeding, infection, inflammation and tightening at the end of the penis is low.)

This is where the waters become increasingly murky. Some couples feel that they want to circumcise their sons because it's traditional for religious or cultural reasons, or because the father was circumcised and one or both parents feel that both father and son should have "matching" penises. Of course, some couples faced with the intergenerational penis dilemma decide it's really a non-issue. "No small boy could look at his penis and his father's and think they looked the same," noted one couple. These parents decide to take a pragmatic approach with their sons, if and when the problem arises, explaining that while doctors used to routinely recommend circumcision a generation ago, that's simply not the case today, which explains why many fathers and sons have different "equipment."

If you take a step back from the religious, cultural, and physical factors for a moment and look at the procedure from a purely medical standpoint, you'll see that the pros and cons are fairly equally balanced.

You might also find it useful to know exactly what's involved in a circumcision. The operation, which takes roughly five to ten minutes, is usually done within a baby boy's first few days of life. The purpose of the procedure is to

8.1 The Pros and Cons of Circumcision

Pros	Cons
Reduced risk of balanoposthitis (inflammation of the skin of the penis caused by either trauma or poor hygiene), urinary tract infections and sexually transmitted diseases.	The procedure is both painful and stressful for the newborn and has been shown to affect the baby's behaviour for up to 24 hours after.
Reduced risk of penile cancer. (A study found that only 2 out of 89 men who developed invasive penile cancer over a 43-year period had been circumcised.) Note: Penile cancer is extremely rare, only occurring in 1 out of 100,000 men.	Complications occur in approximately one in a thousand circumcisions, and infection, hemorrhaging, and improper healing occur in 2 to 10 per cent of cases. In rare situations, severe penile damage can occur. Note: Circumcision is not recommended for infants who are sick, premature, or have any type of penile abnormality.
Prevents paraphimosis (an emergency situation that occurs if the foreskin gets stuck when it's first retracted). Note: Many cases of balanoposthitis and paraphimosis are believed to be caused by well-meaning caregivers who try to forcibly pull the foreskin back. If the foreskin is generally left alone, the combination of spontaneous erections and masturbation are generally enough to loosen it.	In most cases, circumcision is not medically indicated.
Greater ease of hygiene.	The procedure is no longer covered by provincial or territorial health insurance.
Newborn circumcision is less risky than circumcision later in life.	Note: While circumcision has long been touted as an effective way of lowering the risk of urinary tract infections, the odds of an uncircumcised baby developing such an infection are low. One study found that uncircumcised boys were only 3.7 times as likely to develop a urinary tract infection as circumcised boys. (Earlier studies had indicated that the risk was 39 times.)
The transferral of sexually transmitted infections is lower in heterosexual circumcised men. A recent study published in the *New England Journal of Medicine* reported a 25 per cent reduction in the prevalence of herpes and a 34 per cent reduction in the prevalence of HPV among heterosexual circumcised men. HPV is the most common sexually transmitted infection in the world. It causes cervical cancer (which kills 300,000 women annually) as well as anal and penile cancers. That's not to say that circumcision prevents infection, however. Only safe sexual practices can do that.	
A study of African males found that heterosexual males who had been circumcised were 60 per cent less likely to contract HIV than uncircumcised heterosexual males.	

remove the foreskin that covers the end of the penis, thereby exposing the tip of the penis (the glans). Here's a brief description of what happens:

- The baby is placed on a restraining board. His arms and legs are strapped into place to keep him from moving around during the procedure.
- Pain relief is administered before the procedure begins. (Contrary to traditional belief, newborns can and do feel pain.) Depending on the medical practitioner's preference, a local anaesthetic or a painkiller such as acetaminophen may be given to the baby. If a local anaesthetic is used, it is injected into the base of the penis to block the major sensory nerves entering the penis.
- A medical instrument is used to separate the tight adhesions between the foreskin and the penis. The foreskin is then held in place with a metal clamp.
- A metal or plastic cap is placed over the tip of the penis and the fore-skin is pulled up over this cap and cut. Approximately one-third to one-half of the skin of the penis is removed.
- A protective lubricant such as petroleum jelly is applied to the circum-cision site and the site is then wrapped in gauze. It takes approximately one week for the circumcision site to heal.

If you'd like to find out more about circumcision, you might want to con-sider visiting the Canadian Paediatric Society website at www.cps.ca, where you'll find a copy of the society's official position paper on circumcision.

Deciding to breastfeed

You've no doubt heard that breastfeeding is a good thing. What you might not know is exactly why. Here's a laundry list of the reasons why breastfeeding makes sense for mothers and babies:

- Breast milk is the perfect food for babies, serving up all the nutrients a baby needs at any given stage of life in exactly the right proportions. A toddler may be drinking from the same breast that he drank from as an infant, but there's an entirely different beverage on tap.
- Breast milk is higher in cholesterol than formula. This may not sound like a good thing—after all, isn't cholesterol supposed to be bad for you? But studies of animals have indicated that early exposure to cho-lesterol may help prepare a baby's body to process cholesterol more efficiently during adulthood, thereby providing some measure of pro-tection against heart disease.

- Colostrum and breast milk are packed with antibodies—something that no artificial baby formula can deliver. This is because they contain immunoglobulin A proteins, which line the baby's respiratory and intestinal surfaces, thereby protecting him against certain types of viral and bacterial agents during the period in his life when he needs such protection most—while his own immune system is still very immature. Not surprisingly, studies have shown that breastfed babies are less likely than bottle-fed babies to develop gastrointestinal infections, respiratory infections, middle ear infections, food allergies, tooth decay, pneumonia, and meningitis. Breastfeeding even improves the effectiveness of vaccines, which helps to ensure that your baby will get the ultimate boost from each of his booster shots.

- Breastfed babies are less susceptible than bottle-fed babies are to sudden infant death syndrome (SIDS). They also enjoy added protection against intestinal disease, eczema, certain types of heart disease, allergies, and cancer—health benefits that last long after weaning.

- Breastfeeding appears to be helpful in reducing the risk of childhood obesity and type 1 diabetes. Breastfeeding may program babies to regulate their appetite better and it may result in more optimal fat deposition patterns.

- Breastfeeding helps to promote normal development of the jaw and facial muscles. Breastfed babies are less likely to require orthodontic work than their bottle-fed counterparts are.

- Breast milk contains DHA, a fatty acid that positively affects cognitive development and eye development. Breastfeeding is linked to earlier mastery of motor skills in infants and fewer emotional and behavioural problems in older children.

- Breastfeeding helps mothers and babies to connect. Physical contact is important to newborns and can help them feel secure, warm, and comforted.

- Breastfeeding helps your uterus to contract after the birth, which reduces the amount of blood lost after delivery and helps you to regain your pre-pregnancy shape more quickly.

- Breastfeeding helps to suppress ovulation and consequently your menstrual periods. If you breastfeed exclusively, you probably won't menstruate for about six months after giving birth, and possibly even longer. In addition to avoiding the inconvenience of getting your period (to say nothing of the cost of all those tampons and pads), you will have the chance to build up your iron reserves once again since you won't be losing the same amount of iron that you normally do when you're menstruating. The one benefit that you shouldn't count on, however, is built-in birth control. Breastfeeding is not a reliable method of contraception.

- Breastfeeding can help you to lose your pregnancy weight because breastfeeding a baby requires about 500 calories' worth of energy per day.
- Breastfeeding may help to reduce your risk of developing breast or ovarian cancer later in life. It may also protect you from osteoporosis, heart disease, and type 2 diabetes, all the while potentially decreasing myopia and reducing the incidence of postpartum depression (as long as breastfeeding is going well).
- Breastfeeding is convenient. You don't have to purchase or measure anything, there is no best-before date to worry about, and your baby's food is always ready to serve.
- Breastfeeding forces you to take regular breaks throughout the day— the very thing that a new mother should be doing. As Marvin S. Eiger, MD, and Sally Wendkos Olds wisely note in their book *The Complete Book of Breastfeeding*, "When you breastfeed, you're forced to relax during your baby's feeding times, since you cannot prop a bottle or turn the baby over to someone else while you run around doing chores. Your baby's feeding times are your enforced rest times."
- Breastfeeding is green. There's no packaging to worry about. In fact, the containers are reusable *and* multi-functional. (Mother Nature is so smart.)

Worried about the news stories you've heard discussing contaminants in breast milk? It's important to put those concerns in perspective. Concern about contaminants in breast milk must be balanced against the proven health benefits of breast milk and the risks associated with the use of commercial infant feeding products. The use of infant feeding products, including formula, is sometimes necessary and there are standards in place to minimize public health risks. However, the manufacture, preparation, and use of these products provide opportunities for contamination with bacteria (if the formula is made up with microbiologically contaminated water) and potentially toxic substances. What's more, infant formula, like any food, contains trace levels of contaminants. For example, metals such as lead, aluminum, and cadmium and other contaminants, including PCBs, dioxins, and phthalates, have been found in infant feeding products. According to the Natural Resources Defense Council, a U.S. environmental group, levels of organic contaminants tend to be higher in the breast milk of first-time mothers and during the early months of breastfeeding, *breast milk banking*

The Canadian Paediatric Society (CPS) is calling for an expansion of Canada's breast milk banking system.

"The most vulnerable babies should receive human milk," said Dr. Sharon Unger, principal author of the CPS's October 2010 statement on human milk banking and member of the CPS Nutrition and Gastroenterology Committee. "Only about half of the mothers of these babies will have an adequate milk supply, sometimes because they are sick themselves, or due to the stress of having a very sick baby or from being separated from their baby."

Canadian mothers would also like to see breast milk banks expand across the country. Many are participating in informal woman-to-woman milk-sharing networks. The CPS does not, however, endorse the sharing of unprocessed breast milk: "Human milk must be pasteurized before being made available, and milk that has not been processed should not be shared," says Unger.

You can learn more about the origins of the Canadian breast milk sharing movement and find out how breast milk sharing is handled in other countries (and how it is viewed by organizations such as the World Health Organization) by visiting the website of the INFACT Feeding Action Coalition (INFACT Canada): www.infactcanada.ca.

but they can be lower in mothers who breastfeed for a long period of time or who breastfeed more than one child.

As you can see, the benefits of breastfeeding are indisputable. Breastfeeding is the best possible way to feed a baby, period. (It's the way babies were designed to be fed, after all.) But that's only half of the story. What women who are pregnant for the first time have no way of knowing is that breastfeeding is much more than a method of feeding a baby. It's a whole way of mothering. It fosters a special bond between you and your baby, and it can increase your confidence in your mothering abilities. As Marni Jackson notes in her book *The Mother Zone*, "Breastfeeding is an unsentimental metaphor for how love works, in a way. You don't decide how much or how deeply to love—you respond to the beloved and give with joy exactly as much as they want."

How long should you breastfeed?

Health Canada, the Canadian Paediatric Society, Dietitians of Canada, and the Breastfeeding Committee for Canada updated *Nutrition for a Healthy Term Infant,* Canada's infant feeding guidelines, in 2012. The revised guidelines recommend breastfeeding "exclusively for the first six months, and continued up to two years or longer with appropriate complementary feeding" (for example, introducing iron-rich foods to prevent iron deficiency). Supplemental vitamin D is recommended for all breastfed infants and children. You can find a copy of the revised guidelines on the Health Canada website: www.hc-sc.gc.ca.

Of course, that's not to say that breastfeeding is necessarily the right choice for everyone, or that it always works out perfectly for every mother and baby. Nor does breastfeeding always come as easily or as naturally as some people would have you believe.

Sometimes it's hard to decide if breastfeeding is for you. My advice? If in doubt, give breastfeeding a try. That way, you won't be tempted to second-guess your decision after the fact and wonder if you missed out on something really special. If you try breastfeeding your baby and decide that it's not for you, you can always stop. Consider these wise words from Marvin S. Eiger, MD, and Sally Wendkos Olds, co-authors of *The Complete Book of Breastfeeding*: "The regrets we have in life are less often for the things we have done than for those missed opportunities that will never come again. This priceless chance to nurse your baby comes only once in each baby's lifetime. Make the most of it. You may count these nursing days among the most beautiful and fulfilling of your entire life."

You can increase your odds of success by learning as much as you can about breastfeeding before your baby is born. (I know it sounds a bit like putting the cart before the horse but trust me, it can be done.) Sign up for a breastfeeding class, sit in on a La Leche League meeting, watch on-line videos, or load up on books and DVDs designed to teach you the ins and outs of this supposedly instinctive process. (I say "supposedly" because I can tell you from personal experience that things don't always go like clockwork. My first three babies were natural-born nursers who made breastfeeding an absolute breeze, but it took my youngest almost 24 hours to master the art of latching on—and he had a highly experienced breastfeeding mom working with him!) Bottom line? The more you can learn upfront, the more confident you'll feel about your ability to breastfeed your baby.

What if you try breastfeeding your baby and it doesn't work out? Does that mean that you're a failure as a mother, or that your relationship with your baby is doomed right from the start? Of course not. There's more to being a mother than breastfeeding. You will find other ways to connect with and form a loving bond with your baby. If you're feeling disappointed or angry about the way things went when you tried to breastfeed your baby, talk to someone you trust. It's important to obtain support for those feelings. Society puts a lot of pressure on mothers to breastfeed their babies, but doesn't always come through with the necessary support when a mother and baby are struggling to make breastfeeding work. What we need is more hands-on support when it's needed most—and less judging after the fact.

The name game

What's in a name? Plenty if you're the poor unfortunate tyke whose clueless parents saddle him with a name like Hubert Oswald—or if you're one of eight little girls named Amelia who end up in the same kindergarten class!

Yes, choosing a name for your child is an awesome responsibility—one that will no doubt have you clicking your way from baby name site to baby name site.

If you're lucky, you might already have a few names in mind—names that have caught your fancy over the years and somehow stuck in your head. That was certainly how things worked for first-time parents Molly and Paul: "Years before we even conceived, we talked about names and decided that Aurora was a beautiful name for a little girl," recalls Molly, 36. "We wanted something different. I briefly changed my mind about the name, but Paul was set on Aurora, so Aurora it was."

Not all prospective parents are fortunate enough to have had their baby's name picked out since long before the pregnancy test came back positive. Many couples find that there's considerably more work involved in zeroing in on the perfect name (or if not the perfect name, at least a name that both parents can live with). Here are some practical tips if you happen to find yourself in the undecided camp:

- Be clear about what you're looking for in a name. Do you want a name that's long or short? Traditional or modern? Plain or flowery? Easy to spell or something a bit fancier? The clearer you are about your criteria from the beginning, the easier it will be for you to make your final decision.
- Avoid names that are too pretentious. Carol McD. Wallace, author of *The Greatest Baby Name Book Ever*, suggests giving any potential name the playground test: "If you call the name across a crowded playground, do you feel foolish? Do heads whip around to stare at you? ('Who would name a child Everest?')."
- Consider naming your child after someone who is special to you if you feel confident that the person in question will remain near and dear to you in years to come and keep his or her nose clean. After all, you don't want your precious baby to end up being named after an ex-friend of the family who goes on to become a career criminal.
- Look for a name that will grow with your child. "What's cute for a baby may not be so cute when the baby is 35," explains Lisa, a 36-year-old

mother of three. "That's what I liked about Kaitlyn's name. Right now, as a teenager, she goes by Kaity and later, when she's older and is starting a career, she can opt to go back to Kaitlyn or start using Kate."

- Stick to names that will work well with your last name. "Keep in mind how the first name and the last name sound together, as well as any short forms of the first name. Also, look at the initials and make sure they don't spell anything you don't like. We have an unusual surname, so we wanted first names that the boys wouldn't have to spell their entire lives!" explains Susan, a 36-year-old mother of two.

- Keep the spelling simple. "Think of the poor teachers down the road who won't be able to pronounce the name!" says Mary Ann, a 31-year-old mother of one.

- When in doubt, err on the side of caution. "Don't saddle your poor child with a weird, trendy name that she will forever have to explain to people," insists Jennifer, a 35-year-old mother of one. "The same goes for made-up names and names of soap opera characters."

- Go back to the drawing board if it becomes obvious that the name you picked out is becoming too common, suggests Carole, a 34-year-old mother of two. "We initially picked the name Caitlin, but by the time our daughter was born, the world was—pardon the pun—crawling with Caitlins!"

Don't be surprised if you and your partner don't initially agree about names. Most couples find that there's a bit of give and take involved in coming up with a name that both parties can live with. "We both kept throwing out names that we liked and the other person kept vetoing them," recalls Dee, a 33-year-old mother of one. "Fortunately, we did eventually agree on some of the choices."

Kathryn, a 33-year-old mother of two, remembers feeling similarly surprised by how much back-and-forthing was involved in the baby name negotiation process: "My husband could always come up with some kid he knew in school who had a runny nose or who wasn't a team player, so most of the boys' names I came up with were vetoed right away!"

Althea hit a roadblock when she was trying to sell her husband on the merits of the name Aquinnah—a name he couldn't seem to wrap his head around. Then the 30-year-old mother of one had a moment of inspiration: "I told him we could call her Quinn for short. He loved that name." Althea admits to being tremendously relieved that the baby she was carrying ended up being a girl. She and her husband never did manage to agree on a boy's name!

Carolin and her husband had difficulty coming to a negotiated agreement when it came to choosing a name for their middle child. In the end, they decided to flip a coin. The 35-year-old mother of three explains: "With our first and third children, we were in agreement. For our middle daughter, we could not decide between two names: Hannah and Emma. We both liked both names, although he preferred Hannah and I preferred Emma. We decided to toss a coin to decide. He won the toss and our daughter's name is Hannah."

Sometimes negotiation becomes impossible because one of the parents has his or her heart set on a particular name and is simply unwilling to consider any other choices. Kimberlee, a 28-year-old mother of two, freely admits to having forced her husband to go along with her decision to name their first child Heaven. Her rationale? She was the one going through pregnancy and birth. "My first child's name was a headstrong decision on my part that was not of mutual consent," she confesses. "I decided that because I was the one donning stretch marks and bearing labour, I could name the child whatever I pleased." It's a decision she's come to regret, not because she regrets the choice of name but because she wishes she'd involved her partner more in the decision. "I now realize that the enduring of pregnancy may well be more my husband's burden than mine!" she jokes.

Some couples have an additional decision to make—what last name to give the baby. Dee, who kept her own last name when she got married, still wonders if giving her daughter her husband's last name was the right thing to do. Lynn and her partner found this an equally challenging situation to deal with. Their solution? To give each of their two children a different last name. "The first child has my last name and the second child has my husband's last name," the 35-year-old mother explains. "So far, it has worked fine for us, but friends of ours who did the same thing got a lot of grief from both sets of grandparents. We'll see how it goes down the road."

Once you've both agreed on names for your baby, you'll have to decide when to share those names with the world, a decision that may, in part, be determined by how this is handled in your culture. If you know the sex of your baby before birth, you might wish to start calling your baby by her "real" name while you're still pregnant; but if the sex is going to be a surprise until after the birth, you might want to keep the name that you've chosen under wraps until after baby makes her grand entrance. The downside to sharing the baby's name too early is that you may find that people want to weigh in with unwelcome comments about the name you and your partner have agreed upon. They're far less likely to criticize your choice once the baby has been formally named. And there's always the chance that the cousin who is due the month before you are might love your baby's name so much that she decides to give it to her baby. Family feuds have erupted over much less.

Planning for your maternity leave

You've still got one big discussion ahead of you as you head down the home stretch of pregnancy: planning for your maternity leave. In addition to planning the details of your maternity leave—researching your rights to government benefits (visit the Service Canada website for starters: www.servicecanada .gc.ca) and finding out if your company offers any extras, as well as deciding when you'd like to start your maternity leave—you'll also want to do what you can to help smooth the transition for the person who is replacing you on the job. That means keeping your records well organized so that anyone filling in for you while you're on leave can access key documents quickly and easily, and providing your replacement with a list of key contacts so that he or she will know whom to turn to within the organization for support and assistance.

maternity and parental leave benefits	Not every new mom is able to take advantage of the maternity and parental benefits available under the Employment Insurance Act. The moms who don't qualify for benefits typically miss out on a paid maternity leave because they are already providing full-time care to other children, they haven't worked enough EI-insurable hours to qualify for benefits, or they are self-employed and didn't sign up for or start contributing to the voluntary EI program for self-employed workers at least 12 months before becoming pregnant. What's more, some new moms who do qualify for benefits can't afford to take leave from their jobs because their full paycheque is required to pay the family's bills. (EI pays 55 per cent of insurable earnings.)

At some point before you leave, you'll want to have a frank discussion with your employer about how much contact you are likely to want to have with the company while you're off on maternity leave. If you feel quite strongly that you want to stay in the loop while you're away, then you should be given that option, as well as the option to change your mind if motherhood proves to be more demanding—or more enchanting—than you had anticipated. Just remember: you should be the one calling the shots. It's your maternity leave.

While most women try to schedule their maternity leave so that they have as much time as possible to spend with their babies after the birth, there's a lot to be said for taking a bit of time off before the baby arrives. The last thing you want, after all, is to head for labour and delivery after putting in a 12-hour day at the office! If you don't want to stop working entirely during the last few weeks of your pregnancy, why not see if your employer would be willing to have you work on a part-time basis? That way, you could help to train your replacement and still have time to rest and prepare for your baby's arrival.

There's just one small problem with this particular game plan that you need to know about: working part-time hours will diminish your maternity benefits. If you can afford to take the financial hit, then working part-time hours may be the solution for you during those last few weeks. If you can't, then you may have little choice but to drag your weary bones into work five days a week.

Here's something else to keep in mind when you're scheduling your maternity leave: no matter how carefully you map out your plans, they're not carved in stone. Pregnancy can be a rather uncertain business. If you develop complications during the final weeks that require you to leave work early, you and your employer will have to rethink your maternity leave game plan.

Before you sit down with your employer to work out the details of your maternity leave, make sure you take the time to bring yourself up to speed on your rights as a pregnant worker. Unfortunately, this is sometimes easier said than done. With each province or territory setting its own leave-related policies, and federal workers being covered by yet another body of legislation, you practically need a degree in labour law to make sense of all the legislation. That said, here's what you need to know to plan your maternity leave:

Pregnancy leave, parental leave, sick leave, etc. Pregnancy leave, parental leave, sick leave, and other types of family-related leave are administered by the various provincial and territorial ministries of labour. Federal government employees and workers in certain federally regulated industries are covered by a separate body of legislation. This means there are 14 separate jurisdictions in Canada, each with their own legislation covering employment leave. Because of the number of different jurisdictions involved and the sheer complexity of this legislation, you'll want to get in touch with the government department responsible for administering labour law in your jurisdiction to learn about the specifics that apply to you.

Maternity benefits, parental benefits, and sickness benefits. The federal government is responsible for setting policy and issuing payments for maternity benefits, parental benefits, or sickness benefits (something pregnant women experiencing complications may have to draw upon). You have to register with your local Service Canada office in order to qualify for such

benefits. The benefit rate is 55 per cent of your average weekly insurable earn-
ings, up to a maximum of $514 per week (as of January 1, 2014). The number
of hours of insured employment required to qualify for such benefits is 600.
Only one parent is required to serve the two-week waiting period without
benefits. The Canada Labour Code ensures that the jobs of pregnant workers
are protected for the full duration of their parental leave.

- *Maternity benefits* are payable to the birth mother or surrogate mother
  for a maximum of 15 weeks. The mother can start collecting maternity benefits either up to eight weeks before she is expected to give
  birth or at the week she gives birth. Maternity benefits can be collected
  within 17 weeks of the actual or expected week of the birth, whichever is later. If your baby is hospitalized, then the 17 week limit can be
  extended for every week your child is in the hospital up to 52 weeks
  following the week of the child's birth. You will still receive benefits
  for a maximum of 15 weeks, but payments can be delayed until your
  child comes home. If you received maternity benefits prior to the birth
  and wanted to receive the remaining benefits when your child comes
  home from the hospital, get in touch with your local benefits office to
  arrange to put your benefits on hold in the meantime.
- *Parental benefits* are payable either to the biological or adoptive parents
  while they are caring for a newborn or an adopted child, up to a maximum of 35 weeks. Parental benefits can be claimed by one parent or
  shared between the two parents. To receive parental benefits you are
  required to have worked for 600 hours in the last 52 weeks or since your
  last claim. Parental benefits for biological parents and their partners are
  payable from the child's birth date, and for adoptive parents and their partners from the date the child is placed with you. Note: If your newborn
  or newly adopted child is hospitalized, you can choose to claim parental benefits immediately following the child's birth/placement or when
  he/she comes home from the hospital. In either case, you could receive
  35 weeks of parental benefits. Each week that your child is hospitalized
  extends the period in which you can claim parental benefits, up to a maximum of 104 weeks. You must provide proof of the child's hospitalization.
- *Sickness benefits* may be paid for up to 15 weeks to a person who is unable
  to work because of sickness, injury, or quarantine. Note: Sickness benefits may be paid when a pregnancy ends during the first 19 weeks of
  pregnancy, as long as the qualifying conditions for sickness benefits

are met. If the pregnancy ends in the 20th week or later, the claim for benefits can be considered for maternity benefits if the qualifying conditions for maternity benefits are met.

Government policies and procedures are constantly changing. To obtain the most up-to-date information about applying for maternity and parental leave, registering your baby's birth, obtaining a birth certificate and a social insurance number, obtaining a health-care provider for your baby, and registering your child for the Canada Child Tax Benefit, the Universal Child Care Benefit, a Registered Education Savings Plan, and/or the Child Disability Benefit, visit the Having a Baby section of the Service Canada website: www.servicecanada .gc.ca/eng/lifeevents/baby.shtml. You can also call 1–800–206–7218 or visit your nearest Service Canada Centre to obtain answers to specific questions.

There's some additional fine print you should know about as well, so you aren't caught off guard down the road:

- If you are self-employed and you wish to apply for maternity leave, parental leave, or sickness benefits, you must have entered into an agreement with the Canada Employment Insurance Commission at least 12 months before you make a claim for EI special benefits. And once you receive benefits, you will be committed to paying into the EI program for self-employed workers for the rest of your life as a self-employed worker. (It's important to know that up front.)
- You may receive up to 50 weeks of benefits when regular EI benefits are combined with maternity, parental, and sickness benefits.
- You are able to collect maternity and parental benefits while you are outside Canada. However, you must advise your Service Canada Centre if you leave the country.
- When you file your income tax return, if you received maternity, parental, or sickness benefits during the taxation year, you will be exempted from benefit repayment no matter what your income is. But, if you received either maternity, parental, or sickness benefits and regular benefits within the same taxation year, you may be required to repay some or all of the regular benefits.

Planning your "babymoon"

Everyone expects a newly married couple to take some time to themselves after the wedding: it's widely recognized that they need to be given some space so that they can become comfortable in their new roles (to say nothing of beginning to recover from the sheer insanity of those stress-filled weeks leading up to the wedding). But when couples who've just had a baby ask to be given a few days to themselves before the visitors start arriving in droves, they're sometimes made to feel as if they're being unreasonably selfish in depriving other people of the chance to sneak a peek at the new arrival.

There's certainly a strong case to be made for taking what renowned anthropologist and childbirth educator Sheila Kitzinger has dubbed a "babymoon"— time alone as a family during a baby's first few days of life. Not only do new mothers need to physically recover from the rigours of giving birth and adjust to the hormonal changes that are triggered as they move from a pregnant to a non-pregnant state, but both parents also need a chance to regain their bearings and to get used to the fact that from this point forward they're going to be someone's mom or dad. As Kitzinger notes in her book, *Homebirth*, "The time immediately following birth is precious . . . A child is born and for a moment the wheeling planets stop in their tracks, as past, present, and future meet."

"In the sheltered simplicity of the first days after a baby is born, one sees again the magical sense of two people existing only for each other."

—ANNE MORROW LINDBERGH

People in other parts of the world would no doubt be amused to hear about Western society's supposed "invention" of the babymoon. In many cultures, it's been a long-standing tradition to give mothers and babies the time and space required to get to know one another better. One tribe in Brazil, for example, routinely grants a mother and her baby a month of seclusion, while in India, it's traditional for new mothers to focus solely on meeting the new baby's needs during the first 22 days after the birth. These cultures have long known what we're just now discovering: that it's only natural to want to drink in everything about your new baby—the softness of her skin, the vulnerability of her cry, the irresistible smell of the top of her head, and those soulful stares that tell you there's a lot more going on inside her head than you might otherwise have suspected.

Marguerite, 37, feels fortunate that she and her husband, David, were able to enjoy some quiet time as a family after the births of their two children. Marguerite's father was on hand to celebrate the arrival of each of his grandchildren but managed to give the new parents the breathing space they needed to settle into their new routines. "With both of my children, my dad came up the day they were born to help us get settled in at home, but then left soon after to give us some time alone for a few days," she recalls. "Then he returned several days later for another short visit. This was the perfect amount of intervention. He helped when we needed it, but left us alone to sleep and babymoon."

"We had a few days alone after the baby was born, but it was no babymoon! My husband was so freaked out about being a dad that he could barely string two words together. He was a master at bringing me cups of tea and then fleeing! Then some out-of-country relatives showed up when the baby was nine days old and stayed in my home. I ended up waiting on them, offering support to my husband, and caring for the baby—all the while dealing with some physical complications from the birth. Looking back, I should have said that there was no way I could take all this on, but I didn't know how I could do that: I was too busy being superwoman. Everyone wanted something from me, and I felt obliged to say yes. It was disastrous. I wasn't able to get my energy back until the baby was a year old. Next time I have a baby, I'm going to climb into bed with puzzles and games for the toddler and a pile of cloth diapers for the baby—and I'm not getting out of bed for at least six weeks!"

—MARY, 35, MOTHER OF ONE

Like Marguerite, Althea was fortunate to have a very supportive family—so supportive, in fact, that she chose to include them in her babymoon circle. "While I can see how some people might want total solitude during the first few days, I really enjoyed having our immediate families around us during that time," the 30-year-old mother of one recalls. "We're very close to our parents and usually spend a lot of time with them. I found that it made me feel more 'normal' to go out and visit them in the first few days, when everything else seemed so out of whack."

Jane had a similar experience: "My mother moved in immediately after the baby was born—and it was a godsend," the 32-year-old mother of one recalls. "I was totally unprepared for motherhood, even though I had read every book going."

Lisa, 35, also felt that she benefited from inviting selected family members to participate in her family's babymoon last year. "We had a couple of days with just the four of us and my sister, who was present at Keeghan's birth. She was part of our babymoon family. Then my mom and my other sister arrived two days into his life. Other than that, we were on our own for the first week or two."

Don't make the mistake of assuming that you don't need a babymoon if this is your second or subsequent baby, Lisa adds. Contrary to popular belief, babymoons aren't just for first-time parents. "Having a babymoon is even more important the next time around," she insists. "Life seems to go back to its normal pace sooner than you want it to, and people aren't as generous with you when it's not the first baby. There seems to be an assumption that this is all old hat and you don't need the support as much."

Like Lisa, third-time mother Chonee, 36, agrees that a babymoon is as important for veteran parents as it is for first-timers: "I believe that whether it is the first or the second or even the third child, there needs to be a quiet time to adjust and get settled. I think the exact period of time needed differs for everyone, but what is most important is that new moms and dads not feel guilty about saying no to visitors during that period of time. We found that people readily accepted it when we said, "We'd love to see you, but not until next week. We need this week just to get back to normal."

Unfortunately, it can sometimes be quite difficult to get this time alone as a family without unwanted intrusions. Vicky, a 28-year-old mother of one, found that the parade of visitors began even before she had left the hospital: "It was hard to control the visits in the hospital from my husband's family because his sister and mother both work there," she recalls. "I actually had to snap at one of them and point out how often they were in my room! Once we arrived home, it wasn't so much the dropping in as the phone calls—again from my in-laws. The calls got to be such a problem that we had to record a message about how the baby was doing and place it on our answering machine. Unfortunately, this only made my mother-in-law hang up and redial until one of us answered the phone."

> "Everyone seemed to be particularly eager to help me out because they knew I was a single mom. They didn't seem to realize that they could have helped me out most by simply leaving me alone with my baby for a couple of days. The constant phone calls and visits—while made with the best of intentions—prevented me from bonding with my baby and made it difficult for me to sleep when he slept, something that added further strain."
>
> —KELLI, 34, MOTHER OF ONE

Other mothers have experienced similar intrusions from well-meaning but nonetheless annoying relatives and friends. "I had visitors all day and all night during my first week home," recalls Jane, a 32-year-old mother of one. "No wonder I was exhausted and suffering from the postpartum blues!" Darci, a

29-year-old first-time mother, found that the steady flow of visitors during the early days of her baby's life left her feeling totally drained: "I was so overwhelmed by visitors that at one point I left the room and cried, and when my husband came in to see how I was, I told him to send everyone home."

Dee, a 32-year-old mother of one, enjoyed having family members around but wished that they had given her a bit more space so that she could gain greater confidence in her mothering abilities. "There are good and bad sides to having people constantly around in the beginning," she explains. "I was able to get some much-needed rest, but I soon discovered that you don't get the chance to develop confidence in your ability to care for your baby if someone is always taking him away from you to comfort or change him."

As these veteran moms have indicated, the payoffs of spending some time alone with your baby during the first few days of his or her life can be tremendous. The trick is to figure out how to pull it off when friends and neighbours are literally banging at your door, begging to see the new arrival. Here are some practical tips on defending your right to a babymoon without alienating those around you:

- Talk to your partner about your plans for the babymoon. It's important to be upfront about your expectations so that there won't be any crossed wires or hurt feelings down the road. It's also important to be prepared to compromise with regard to your partner's involvement: while you might want him or her to participate wholeheartedly in the babymoon experience, you have to be prepared to respect your partner's feelings if he or she isn't willing or able to hang out with you and the baby 24 hours a day. Forcing the issue will only lead to stress and conflict at the time in your life when you most need to feel in sync with your partner. Molly, a 36-year-old mother of one, is still dealing with the fallout from this type of conflict three years after the fact. "I really wanted a babymoon," she recalls. "I had this vision of the three of us (my husband, our baby, and I), lying together in bed for hours at a time, just getting to know one another as a family. Unfortunately, my husband did not understand why I wanted this and had no interest in participating. He felt that there were many things that needed to be done—cleaning, shopping for groceries, and so on—and he spent the entire first week (the only time he had off from work) running errands. Aurora wanted to nurse nearly all the time and, as a result, we spent most of our time sitting in the living room together, cuddling and nursing. She and I babymooned alone."

- Communicate your wishes to friends and family. Once you and your partner have agreed about how you intend to handle your babymoon, be sure to get the word out to friends and family members. You'll find that people will be more accepting of your need for privacy during the early days if you reassure them that there will be ample opportunities for visiting down the road. Another way to handle this situation is to let the baby addicts in the crowd pay a quick visit shortly after the birth: with any luck, they'll back off a little once they've had an initial baby fix.
- Put technology to work for you. Don't allow those precious daytime naps to be interrupted by the incessant ringing of the telephone. Let voice mail pick up the calls so that you can get back to people at a more convenient time—including a short update in your voice mail message might even be enough to appease some callers. Better still, post a daily Baby Bulletin on your Facebook page to keep well-meaning friends and relatives updated on the latest news at your house while eliminating the need to return dozens of calls each day. It can get a little tedious to spend all your free time on the phone when there are a million and one other tasks demanding your attention (including sleeping and getting to know your baby).
- If all else fails, consider establishing visiting hours. If you're convinced that your mother or mother-in-law will self-destruct if she doesn't have daily access to her new grandchild, set limits on the frequency and duration of visits. Just don't fall into the all-too-common trap of assuming that you need to play host each time she drops by. This is one time in your life when you can get away with not offering visitors so much as a cup of tea or a store-bought cookie.

With any luck, those around you will respect your need for privacy during this momentous time in your life, but even if they don't, stick to your guns. A babymoon comes around just once in each baby's lifetime. Don't deny yourself or your baby this very special experience.

Other Things You Can Do to Make the Early Weeks Less Stressful

You've no doubt heard the horror stories about the first few weeks of parenthood—hair-raising tales about exhausted parents stumbling around in a zombie-like state.

While these accounts tend to be a little bit exaggerated, there's still a grain of truth to them: the early weeks of parenthood can be both physically and emotionally overwhelming. Even though you may luck out and coast through the entire postpartum period without hitting as much as a single road bump, it only makes sense to do as much as possible beforehand to minimize the stress of the early weeks. Here are a few things you can do before the birth to make the transition to parenthood a little easier.

Put your support team in place

Until you've been through it, it's hard to imagine just how much time and energy go into caring for a single 8-pound (3.5-kilogram) infant. (Trust me, that tiny baby can zap the energy of two adults in practically no time flat!) Because you don't know what to expect, it's easy to underestimate the amount of help you may require after your baby arrives. If you pride yourself on being well organized, you may naively assume that it will be business as usual within a couple of days of the birth. But that's seldom the case.

While new mothers in generations past could count on enjoying a one- to two-week "holiday" in the hospital, most new moms today are discharged within 24 to 48 hours of giving birth (unless, of course, they have a Caesarean section or experience a lot of delivery-related complications, in which case they might end up staying in the hospital for three to five days, or even longer). While there are a lot of good things to be said about leaving the hospital sooner rather than later (there are much nicer places to hang out with your new baby than in a hospital, after all), the downside is that you don't have access to the same hospital-based support services your mother enjoyed during her much lengthier hospital stay. The moral of the story? You owe it to yourself and your baby to line up as much support as possible for after you go home.

Since you're going to be on your own almost immediately after the birth (and, in many cases, you'll be miles away from members of your extended family, too), it's important to find out ahead of time what types of postpartum support services will be available to you in your community. Here are some of the questions you'll want to ask your doctor or midwife.

- What is the postpartum appointment schedule (for Baby and for you)? Will these visits take place in my home (likely to be the case for the first week at least if you and your baby are under the care of a midwife) or in a medical office (the norm if you and your baby are being cared for by one or more doctors)?
- What other services are available in my community, both through health-care and family-service agencies, and non-profit community

groups like La Leche League (a group that offers support to breast-feeding mothers)?

- Does my local hospital or health unit offer a 24-hour parent information helpline that is staffed by a maternal infant nurse or other qualified health professional? (It can be reassuring to know that you can obtain answers to all your baby-related questions by simply picking up the phone and giving someone a call.)
- Does my health unit offer a breastfeeding support network that matches up experienced nursing mothers with first-timers? (A program like this can be a lifesaver if you don't know other mothers who have breastfed their babies.)
- Does my health unit or hospital provide home visits and/or telephone support from a public health nurse and/or a lactation consultant?

In addition to determining what's available to you in your community, you'll want to consider what types of support are available through family members and friends. Just make sure that the people you turn to will support rather than criticize you, build your confidence in your own mothering abilities rather than simply step in and take over, and decrease rather than add to your stress level.

Unfortunately, not all friends and relatives are necessarily cut out for the role of postpartum helper—a lesson that 33-year-old Maura learned the hard way shortly after her daughter was born. "My in-laws arrived the day after Trina's birth for a one-week visit, so they were at our house when we arrived home," she recalls. "My mother-in-law was wonderful: she baked, cooked, cleaned, and did her best to help out. My father-in-law acted like a bigger baby than Trina. He pestered my husband about inane little jobs that didn't need to be done immediately, he was annoyed with me because I didn't spend more time visiting in the evenings, and, worst of all, he had a huge temper tantrum on the morning of their departure, upsetting all of us and stressing us out for the next couple of weeks. I've never been so glad to see anyone's vehicle pull out of the yard as I was that morning. It's taken nearly two years for all of us to rebuild a relationship that was pretty good before that week. That experience still gives me the jitters!"

In addition to figuring out whom you'd like to have pitch in and help, give some thought to what you'd like these people to do. Chances are you'll want to spend as much time as possible enjoying your new baby, so rather than delegate baby-care tasks to other people, allow them to handle day-to-day chores that you don't mind handing over to someone else: dishwashing, laundry folding, vacuuming, and running errands, for example. You'll find it easier to delegate these types of tasks if you keep a to-do list on your refrigerator. That way, if people call or drop by and ask what they can do to help, you'll know exactly what to suggest.

If you can't line up enough help by calling in favours from family members and friends, then do the next best thing: pay for it. Consider hiring a high school or college student to help you with light chores around the house or arrange for a cleaning service to come through a week or two after the birth, just to get everything spic and span again. If you can't afford to pay for cleaning services because your budget has already been stretched to the max, let people know that you'd love to receive cleaning service gift certificates as baby gifts.

Whatever you do, don't make the mistake of assuming that your partner will be able to pick up the extra slack while you're recovering from the birth. Your partner is going to need some time to settle into this new role, to get to know the new baby, and to catch up on sleep, so it's not fair to dump a million and one additional responsibilities in his or her lap. Partners may not have to physically recover from the birth or figure out the ins and outs of breastfeeding, but they have a number of other postpartum adjustments to make. If you keep that in mind, you'll reduce the amount of conflict that you and your partner experience during what is likely to be one of the more challenging periods in your relationship.

Keep a running list of the names and phone numbers of people who've offered to help so that you'll be able to call in any and all favours after the baby arrives. If you're really organized, you might want to take things a step further and do what Lynn, a 35-year-old mother of two, did. She prepared a sign-up sheet for people who were willing to drop off prepared meals after the birth. "I had meals coming for about six weeks. It was fantastic!" she recalls.

Consider hiring a postpartum doula

You've no doubt heard the buzz about birthing doulas—labour assistants who offer support to a woman and her partner during and immediately after the birth. (You can find out more about them in Chapter 10.) You might not be quite as familiar with postpartum doulas, but they offer a similar service during the postpartum period, providing hands-on assistance to new parents during the first days or weeks of parenthood. Postpartum doulas are "Jills of all trades" who bring a range of different skills to the table. As Elisabeth Bing and Libby Colman note in their book, *Laughter and Tears: The Emotional Life of New Mothers*, "The postpartum doula is baby nurse, housekeeper, and experienced advice giver all in one."

If you don't have extended family members in the area who can provide you with this kind of hands-on help and emotional support, a postpartum doula might be just what you need. She can take care of light housekeeping tasks while you and Baby grab a nap and then answer any breastfeeding questions you might have when Baby wakes up hungry. She can pop dinner in the oven and see to that basket of laundry that's been sitting on the couch all day, waiting for someone to magically find enough time to fold it. In other words, she can offer both an extra set of hands and an eager listening ear—the two things a new mother needs most when she's trying to make her way through the first few weeks postpartum.

You can obtain referrals to doulas from your local midwifery practice, your local childbirth association, your family doctor, your local hospital or health unit, area lactation consultants, your local La Leche League chapter, DONA International (www.dona.org), and CAPPA Canada—the Canadian branch of the Childbirth and Postpartum Professional Association (www.cappacanada.ca).

Regardless of how you go about finding someone to provide you with support during the postpartum period, here are some questions that you'll want to ask before you agree to use that person's services:

- Do you provide both labour and postpartum support services?
- Are you likely to be available around the time of my due date?
- Do you have a backup person lined up in case I deliver sooner or later than anticipated, or if you are otherwise unavailable? Can we arrange to meet your backup person?
- What type of training have you had? Are you certified through DONA International, the Childbirth and Postpartum Professional Association (CAPPA), or some other accrediting body? What types of qualifications does your backup person have?
- Do you have any other related skills (such as certification as a lactation consultant or a registered massage therapist)?
- How many years of experience do you have?
- What are your philosophies about childbirth, breastfeeding, and parenting?
- How many children do you have and what are their ages? Did you breastfeed your own babies?
- What role would you see yourself playing if we were to hire you to provide us with support during the postpartum period?
- What types of tasks do you typically perform for the families that you work with?
- What hours are you available to work? Do you have minimum and maximum numbers of hours that you're willing to work in a day?
- What are your fees and what types of services are included in those fees?

You'll also want to check the postpartum doula or professional labour support person's references and to go with your gut instincts about her. Is she warm and reassuring—someone you'll want to have around during your baby's first few days or weeks of life? Do you and your partner both feel comfortable with her? Does she seem knowledgeable and experienced? These are perhaps the most important points of all to consider when you're making this all-important decision.

Stock your home with healthy, easy-to-prepare foods

Man cannot live by bread alone—and a postpartum woman certainly can't live on a tub of margarine, some prehistoric cheese slices, and whatever else happens to be living in the most remote corners of her refrigerator.

Since grocery shopping and cooking are likely to be low priorities for you during the early days and weeks postpartum, you could very easily find yourself falling prey to empty refrigerator syndrome or, even worse, being forced to play takeout roulette. ("It's Tuesday, so this must be pizza night!")

A smarter (and cheaper) alternative is to stock your home with a variety of healthy, easy-to-prepare foods before your baby is born. (You'll find a list of suggestions in Table 8.2.) Try to zero in on foods that can be pretty much eaten "as is." (Hint: Since peeling an orange may take too long if you've got an unhappy baby to deal with, an apple or a banana is probably a better bet. If necessary, you can peel a banana using one hand and your teeth!) That brings to mind another important point: you should look for foods that can be eaten with one hand since you're likely to have a baby in your arms while you're eating. A word to the wise: this pretty much rules out soup and other messy foods that tend to drip, unless you happen to be exceptionally coordinated. Otherwise, you could find yourself dripping noodles all over your baby's head—not exactly a way to score points with the new arrival!

Something else you can do ahead of time is to stock your freezer with a variety of precooked entrees. Your goal? To ensure that dinner preparation doesn't involve anything more mentally or physically draining than moving a dish from the freezer to the microwave and hitting the reheat button, while still including at least three out of four food groups in breakfast, lunch, and dinner, and at least two food groups in snacks. Molly, a 36-year-old mother of one, learned the hard way that meal preparation can be a tremendous challenge during the postpartum period: "I found it extremely difficult to get meals prepared during the first few weeks after the birth," she confesses. "If we had heeded people's advice and cooked and frozen extra dinners well in advance, it would have made life a lot easier for me."

8.2 Nutrition on the Run: Healthy Foods for Busy Moms

These foods have been chosen because they take just seconds to prepare and can be enjoyed with a baby in your arms. Best of all, they work equally well at mealtime and snack time and are all highly versatile.

Yogourt mixed with cereal and diced fruit	Chocolate milk or almond milk
Hard-boiled eggs	Fruit-and-yogourt shakes
Sliced meat	Low-fat cheese
English muffins, bagels, or pitas	Hummus, tzatziki, and
Whole-grain crackers	other spreads/dips
Fresh fruits	Bran muffins
Salads in bags (stuff the salad in a pita to make	Dried fruits and nuts
it easier to eat when you're holding a baby)	Fresh vegetables
Peanut butter or soy butter and banana on	Granola bars
whole-grain bread	Hearty soups with a stew-like consistency
	(full of good stuff; less likely to drip)

Carolin, a 35-year-old mother of three, agrees that preparing meals ahead of time can simplify life tremendously after the birth. "There were many days when dinner might have been cold cereal if it weren't for the pre-made meals I had stashed in the freezer ahead of time."

Fortunately, preparing extra meals doesn't have to mean chaining yourself to the stove for a three-day-long cooking marathon. If you simply get into the habit of making double portions of casseroles, hearty soups, sauces, and entrees like lasagna that freeze well, you'll soon end up with a freezer that's amply stocked with delicious home-cooked meals.

Don't be afraid to ask others to pitch in and help the cause. Chances are they'll be only too happy to roll up their sleeves and whip up a dinner or two. One of the best baby presents that Karen, a 30-year-old mother of three, received was a slow cooker full of stew: "All I had to do was to plug the slow cooker in and dinner was ready whenever we needed it." Just one quick word of caution if you decide to get other people involved in Operation Dinner (and, frankly, you've got little to lose and plenty to gain!): be sure to be upfront about your food preferences; otherwise, your seafood-loathing partner could find himself less than thrilled to discover that the "secret surprise" in Aunt Mildred's famous "secret surprise casserole" is shrimp!

Whether you decide to do all the cooking yourself or let others join you for kitchen duty, try to aim for as much variety as possible. That way, if your breastfeeding baby is bothered by traces of a particular food in your breast milk (such as onions, cabbage, or broccoli), you won't find yourself in the frustrating situation of knowing that every single entree that's tucked away in your freezer contains that very same food.

Keep on top of chores on the home front

Find yourself playing Martha Stewart? There's no need to hit the panic button. What you're experiencing is perfectly normal and *completely* reversible. You'll stop being this obsessive about housework soon after the baby arrives. I can practically guarantee it. After all, it's a whole lot more difficult to find the time to stencil walls when you have a baby who wants to eat every two to three hours. So I say go for it: succumb to that urge to clean out cupboards, reorganize your closets, and file your tax records neatly by year. You may never have this chance again. (Or at least not for a while.)

And while you're at it, channel some of that energy into taking care of tasks that will make life easier after your baby arrives. We've already talked about how helpful it can be to have a freezer full of healthy, easy-to-prepare meals. Here are some other things you can do ahead of time to reduce the stress of post-baby life:

- Stay on top of the laundry during your final weeks of pregnancy. Get in the habit of tossing a load in the washing machine first thing in the morning and last thing before you go to bed. This will help to ensure that you have at least one clean outfit to take with you to the hospital when the moment of truth arrives. And since you're going to be trekking to and from the laundry room on a regular basis anyway, you might as well get a head start on all the baby laundry. You don't have to tackle all of the baby clothes at once, of course. But if you launder all of the linens plus all the clothes in sizes 0 to 6 months, you'll avoid having to do all that baby-related laundry the moment your baby arrives.
- Keep the kitchen and bathroom reasonably clean. While you shouldn't expect either room to pass the white glove test, some basic hygiene is definitely in order. There are few things more depressing than discovering that you can't even make yourself a sandwich or a cup of tea because there's not a single clean dish in the house, or being unable to enjoy a long, leisurely soak in the tub because you can't remember when you last cleaned the bathroom! If you're too pooped to tackle these cleaning jobs yourself in your mega-pregnant state (and, frankly, that's likely to be the case at this stage of the game), hire someone to give your house a thorough cleaning the week before your baby is due, or—better yet—see

if you can talk a group of sympathetic girlfriends into tackling some of your housekeeping chores for you. (You'd be amazed at what women will do for another woman who's about to have a baby. As those '60s feminists liked to chant, "Sisterhood is powerful!")

- Reorganize your living space to make it mesh better with your post-baby lifestyle.

- Move the cordless phone into your family room and place it on the coffee table along with the TV remote, a box of tissues, and other items you're likely to need while you're curled up on the sofa cuddling your baby.

- If your sofa is light coloured or otherwise likely to stain, consider purchasing some sort of throw or sofa cover. The acid in baby spit-ups can bleach the colour out of certain fabrics almost instantly, so unless you're after some sort of performance art effect in your family room, you might want to protect your furniture until your baby outgrows the sofa-destroying stage. The same goes for carpets that could easily be damaged by a cascade of upchucked milk. You might want to purchase an inexpensive area rug and plonk it down in front of your sofa in an attempt to give the Persian rug underneath at least a fighting chance of surviving Baby's first year.

- Drag your glider rocker or rocking chair out of the spare bedroom and place it in your bedroom. You're likely to clock countless hours in this chair, particularly if your baby ends up being fussy, so you might as well ensure that it's as handy as possible for those middle-of-the-night feedings.

- Set up baby change stations on each floor of your house. You don't have to spring for a change table on each floor: all you really need is a change bag or other container stocked with a waterproof change pad and other diapering essentials.

- Reorganize your kitchen cupboards so the items that you need most often are all within easy reach. You don't want to have to climb on a stool, lean over a hot stove, or do other risky gymnastic manoeuvres while you're making your way around the kitchen with a baby in your arms. The same goes for the deep freeze in your basement, by the way: it's almost impossible to reach a pot roast in the bottom of the freezer when you have a baby strapped to your chest.

Get the rest of your life in order

Now that you have your physical surroundings in order, it's time to tackle the rest of your life. Here are some other tasks that you'll definitely want to tackle before the baby arrives:

Choose a doctor for your baby. Finding it hard to get your partner to agree on your choice of a doctor for your baby? Believe it or not, this is yet another arena where the Battle of the Sexes is being waged! Researchers at Penn State University in Pennsylvania discovered that women and men look for very different things in a doctor. While women feel that it's important to choose a doctor who is caring and easy to relate to, men are more concerned about the quality of the medical care they will receive.

If you intend to have your baby cared for by your regular family doctor, your job is already done. But if you're hoping to have your baby seen by a pediatrician, you should plan to start looking for Dr. Right long before your baby is born. When you're interviewing prospective pediatricians (assuming, of course, that you actually have the luxury of being able to choose your baby's doctor: not necessarily a given in all parts of Canada), you will want to find out

- how soon after the birth the doctor will arrange to see your baby, and whether the newborn check will be done by the pediatrician on call at the time your baby is born (as a rule of thumb, your baby should be seen within the first 24 hours of life—and sooner than that if there's been a complication with your pregnancy or the delivery);
- when your baby's subsequent checkups should be scheduled;
- what the doctor's office hours are and whether evening, early morning, or weekend appointments are available;
- whether certain days and times are set aside for various types of visits such as "well-baby" checkups, immunizations, or special consultations;
- whether the doctor replies to phone calls during the day from patients and, if so, how long it typically takes to get a call back;
- whether you'll actually hear back from the doctor himself or a member of his staff;
- whether the doctor takes emergency calls after hours, and if not, who does;
- who covers the practice when the doctor is unavailable.

Something else you might not think to ask is whether or not the doctor is also a parent. You may find it easier to relate to and accept advice from someone who's done some time in the parenting trenches as opposed to someone whose only experience with babies has occurred in a purely clinical setting.

Get your financial act together. Prepay as many bills as possible (especially the bills that are likely to come due around your due date). Otherwise they may get overlooked in all the excitement and chaos, and you may get hit with some heavy-duty interest charges as a result. This can be as simple as prepaying your bills on-line weeks—even months—ahead of time. If you rely on snail mail to pay your bills, you can postdate your cheques and either mail them immediately or sort them into piles according to the date on which they need to be mailed. (Just make sure that your partner is clear about your method of tackling the bills so that the appropriate bills end up in the mail at the appropriate time—and you don't end up with any duplicate or missed payments.)

Re-evaluate your life insurance needs. Few things change your financial situation more dramatically than giving birth to your first child. Rather than carrying a bargain-basement policy with just enough coverage to pay for the costs of your burial, you now need a policy that will cover the costs of raising your child until he's able to become self-supporting. Your life insurance agent or financial planner can help you to crunch the necessary numbers and make the life insurance decisions that are right for you.

---

choosing a guardian

Wondering who to name as your child's guardian? Here are a few points to consider as you make this crucial decision:

• Are the potential guardian's child-rearing philosophies similar to your own?
• Is the potential guardian youthful and energetic enough to assume responsibility for caring for a young child?
• Is the potential guardian actually willing to step in and assume responsibility for raising your child? Or has he or she agreed out of a sense of obligation alone?
• Is this person likely to outlive you and your partner or is he or she considerably older than you and/or in poor health?
• If you plan to choose a married couple to serve as your child's guardians, which party would you want to gain custody of your child if the couple were to separate or divorce?

Note: Be sure to name an alternative candidate just in case your first choice of a guardian falls through (for example, if the person you have designated is in poor health, dealing with a family emergency, or otherwise unable to assume the responsibility for caring for your child).

Write a will. While your own mortality is probably the last thing you want to think about as you're preparing to witness the miracle of birth, you've never needed a will more than you do right now. It's your responsibility as a parent to take steps to ensure that your child would be well taken care of if something were to happen to you or your partner. Don't let concerns about the costs of writing a will cause you to put off this all-important task. The costs are relatively low (a couple of hundred dollars to have a simple will prepared by your lawyer).

Pick up cards and gifts for any upcoming birthdays or anniversaries. You can take care of these simple tasks quickly and easily now—particularly if you shop on-line. This is one time in your life when you won't want to shop till you drop. If you're coming into the holiday season as your due date approaches, plan to wrap up your holiday preparations in advance just in case Junior decides to make an unanticipated early arrival. (It'll also save you the nightmare of weaving your increasingly bulky body down the department store aisles at the height of the holiday shopping season—just one of the many festive nightmares Nancy White describes in her hilarious song "It's So Chic to Be Pregnant at Christmas." You'll find that track—and other equally wonderful anthems of motherhood—on her album *Momnipotent*, required listening for all Canadian mothers, by the way.)

> "We had a get-together just before the birth of each baby and asked each of our friends to bring something that would symbolize a positive thought for the baby. I then used these items to make a mobile that was filled with heartfelt wishes and mementoes as well as some very humorous pieces."
>
> —LYNN, 35, MOTHER OF TWO

Get a head start on your baby announcements. Who says you have to wait until the baby arrives to get your baby announcements under way? Not Dawn, a 39-year-old mother of four who's pretty much got the baby announcement thing down to an art: "I prepare the birth announcement on the computer ahead of time. There is one announcement for a baby girl and another one for a baby boy. All my husband has to do is add the relevant information and print the announcements off. I also have mailing labels prepared and envelopes stamped and ready to go. That way, I can ensure that the baby announcements are taken care of before I leave the hospital, so I'll have one less thing hanging over my head."

Take care of as many routine appointments as possible now. It's a lot easier to get your teeth cleaned or your hair cut before your baby arrives than to try to set up these types of appointments when you have to fit them in between feedings and diaper changes. So if you're overdue for a haircut or any sort of medical appointment, try to schedule your appointment sooner rather than later.

Shop for essentials for yourself. These are some of the things you'll need:

- **The mother of all sanitary napkins.** You'll need at least two large boxes of the most absorbent sanitary napkins you can find—ideally ones designed specifically for postpartum or overnight use. Light pads won't cut it, even when bleeding tapers off, about 10 to 14 days postpartum. Avoid pads coated with wicking material, which can cause contact dermatitis that you may mistake for a yeast infection. Tampons are taboo during the postpartum period, and they'd be next to useless anyway, so forget about simply relying on any old tampons you might have kicking around in the back of your bathroom vanity.
- **Breast pads.** Washable cotton or wool breast pads are not only the most economical and the most environmentally friendly, they're also the most comfortable. (Unlike paper breast pads, they don't have the annoying habit of cementing themselves to your nipple—something that makes removing even the most stubborn of bandages seem like a picnic.)
- **A nursing bra or two.** You're going to need more than just one or two—particularly during the early days of nursing, when leaking is the norm—but you don't want to load up on too many nursing bras until you're reasonably confident that you can judge the final size of your postpartum breasts. In other words, don't blow the entire bra budget all at once.
- **A breast pump.** A breast pump is handy to have, even if you're not planning to spend much time away from your baby. It can help you to relieve engorgement during the early days (although you'll also want to learn how to hand-express milk, so that you're not totally reliant on your breast pump each time you need to get rid of a little excess milk) and allow you to stockpile some breast milk in the freezer so that you can enjoy an occasional baby-free outing. If you're intending to return to work, you might want to consider renting or purchasing a high-end breast pump—one that will allow you to pump quickly and efficiently with minimum noise and discomfort. Hospitals often have rental options, or if you'd like to try before you buy, many breastfeeding clinics will allow you to test drive them.
- **A bottle of witch hazel lotion or ointment.** There's no denying it: witch hazel is a hemorrhoid-suffering girl's best friend. (Hemorrhoids are a common by-product of both pregnancy and the pushing stage of labour.) Pick up a bottle at your pharmacy or health-food store and apply it to your tender parts with a cotton ball, or buy witch

hazel−soaked pads. It will help to reduce some of the itching and burn-ing. If you prefer, pick up alcohol-free baby wipes (ones that contain alcohol sting and can be drying to your skin) or hemorrhoid wipes instead—keep the container in the fridge to help put the fire out. While you're at it, why not splurge on some really good toilet paper?

- **A hemorrhoid cushion.** These doughnut-shaped pillows can make sit-ting a little more comfortable if you're dealing with a tender perineum and/or hemorrhoids. Be sure to have one on hand.
- **Prenatal vitamins.** It's a good idea to continue taking your prenatal vita-mins throughout the postpartum period (and even beyond that if you're nursing or planning to get pregnant again in the very near future).
- **A sports bottle and a hot beverage container.** You'll be unbelievably thirsty if you're breastfeeding, so you'll want to tote a container of liquid with you wherever you go. You can fill your sports bottle with ice-cold water and your hot beverage container with decaffeinated cof-fee or tea. It doesn't matter which type of beverage is on tap as long as you're getting plenty of fluids.

Shop for essentials for baby. While most new parents get a great deal of plea-sure shopping for the new arrival, there's no need to go overboard. The fact that baby superstores stock hundreds of different products doesn't necessarily mean that your baby needs one of each. Here are some points to keep in mind.

- **Don't hit the stores too soon.** If you do all your shopping while you're still pregnant, you're going to end up with doubles or triples of some things— great news if you're having multiples, but a bit overkill if you're having a single baby. Believe it or not, you're going to be deluged with baby gifts. People who barely gave you the time of day before you were pregnant will show up on your doorstep, baby gift in hand, hoping for a peek at the wee one. And, at the same time, friends and relatives will offer to loan you mountains of baby stuff. A better strategy is to ensure you've got the basics on hand, and then wait to see what else comes your way.
- **Learn to distinguish between frills and necessities.** The juvenile-product manufacturers are always coming up with new things that babies and their parents supposedly need, but some of these items are nothing more than costly extras. A car seat, a stroller, a baby carrier, and a safe place for your baby to sleep are the only true necessities for a newborn other than clothing and diapers and you.

8.3	**Clothing: What Your Newborn Needs**
12	sleepers in a seasonably suitable weight and fabric
2	hooded towel and washcloth sets
3	fitted crib sheets
12	extra-large receiving blankets
3	pairs of socks
3	sweaters (depending on the season)
2	cotton hats
1	snowsuit or bunting bag (depending on the season)
4	large bibs

Note: You'll need 1.5 times as many clothes for twins as you would for a single baby.

- **Pass on the designer togs when your baby is first born.** Rather than loading up on high-priced outfits, stick to basic newborn sleepers. Your baby will need at least a dozen outfits and at least as many receiving blankets, unless of course you're planning to do laundry every day. Your baby will grow at a phenomenal rate during the early weeks and months of life and will likely outgrow his entire newborn wardrobe before he's 6 weeks old! Note: A baby who weighs in at more than 9 pounds (4 kilograms) may have a hard time fitting into the 3-month size of clothing, let alone the newborn size. Be sure to have some 6-month-size clothing on hand, just in case you end up giving birth to a larger-than-average baby.
- **Look for clothing that will grow with your baby.** Certain brands of sleepers feature adjustable foot cuffs that allow them to be worn longer.
- **Stick to unisex clothing as much as possible.** That way, if you decide to have another baby, you won't have to go out and buy a whole new wardrobe if he or she happens to be the opposite sex.
- **Don't buy clothing more than a season in advance.** While you might be tempted to pick up that size-two snowsuit now while it's on sale, you have no way of telling whether it'll fit your baby during the right season—and, despite what some Americans believe, we Canadians don't have much use for snowsuits in July! That $30 "bargain" could end up being a $30 waste of money.
- **Put safety first.** A second-hand crib or car seat is no bargain if it results in injury or death. Check government safety sites for product recall information, avoid products that are overly worn, and turn down any

second-hand car seat unless you know for a fact that it's never been involved in a car accident. (Even minor fender-benders can twist the frame of the car seat, making it unfit for use.) Keep in mind that your insurance company may not insure second-hand seats. Car seats must have the Canadian National Safety Mark on them to be legal, so that cross-border bargain could actually get you in trouble.

- **Know what you're buying if you're hitting the garage sale circuit.** Before you buy any piece of second-hand equipment, make sure you know who manufactured it and when (this information is generally included on a sticker on the product or in an accompanying manual), what the model number is, how many families have used it (for example, did the person who's selling it buy it new or second-hand), whether it's ever been repaired, whether any of the parts are missing and, if so, whether replacement parts are still available, and whether the product conforms to current safety standards.

Sex and Relationships: Top Worries

Will being pregnant or having a baby affect our sex life? What about the other aspects of our relationship? Have we made a mistake by having another baby? (Our family is pretty perfect as it is.) These are some of the questions that tend to worry expectant parents, which is why I'm addressing them in this final section of this chapter.

Sex during pregnancy

A study conducted by researchers at Memorial University in Newfoundland confirmed what most doctors and midwives have known for years: more than half of couples believe that making love during pregnancy poses some sort of threat to the developing baby. Yet this is quite untrue. Sex during pregnancy is generally considered perfectly safe for couples who are experiencing low-risk pregnancies. Your doctor or midwife is likely to recommend that you forgo intercourse, orgasm, or both for all or part of your pregnancy only if

- you have a history of recurrent, first-trimester miscarriage or there is a threat of miscarrying this time around;
- you have been diagnosed with an incompetent cervix (a condition in which the cervix opens prematurely);
- you've been diagnosed with placenta previa (a condition in which the placenta blocks all or part of the cervix) or a placental abruption (a condition in which the placenta begins to separate from the uterine wall);

- you're carrying more than one baby;
- you have a history of premature labour or you're showing signs of going into premature labour during this pregnancy;
- you or your partner have an untreated sexually transmitted infection;
- your membranes have ruptured.

If your doctor or midwife tells you that sex is off-limits for now, make sure you're clear about what you can and can't do. Some couples are given the go-ahead to enjoy everything but intercourse, while others are told to avoid nipple stimulation and any form of sexual activity that could lead to orgasm. (Both activities cause the uterus to contract.)

spotting after sex	Try not to panic if you experience a small amount of bleeding after intercourse at some point during your first trimester. If your cervix—which is extremely sensitive at this stage of pregnancy—happens to get bumped by your partner's penis, a small amount of spotting may occur. Even though it can be alarming to see any type of bleeding coming from your vagina when you're pregnant, this type of bleeding doesn't pose any risk to the developing baby. Still, if it's going to cause you undue stress, it might be best to put the lovemaking on hold until you're into your second trimester and your cervix is a little less sensitive.

The concept of "safe sex" takes on an entirely different meaning when you're pregnant, by the way. While you'll still need to use a condom if you have unprotected intercourse with a new partner or if you have reason to suspect that your current partner may have a sexually transmitted infection, you also have to exercise caution if oral sex is part of your usual bedroom routine. It's okay to have oral sex (unless, of course, your doctor or midwife has forbidden any activity that could lead to orgasm), but it's not okay to allow your partner to blow air into your vagina. Believe it or not, this could cause an air embolism to travel to your brain, something that could result in stroke or even death. No sexual encounter is worth that kind of risk, so be careful.

While your doctor or midwife will probably talk to you about how the physical changes of pregnancy may affect your sex life—you're likely to find yourself with abundant vaginal secretions, super-sensitive breasts, and a belly that requires some manoeuvring to get around—what they might not discuss is how your feelings about sex may change over the course of your pregnancy. You may find that your interest goes through the roof, or that you couldn't care less if you ever have sex again. And you may find that your interest rises and falls as particular pregnancy-related complaints come and go. (Hint: Morning sickness isn't exactly an aphrodisiac.)

Here's what some of the women interviewed for this book had to say about their interest in sex during pregnancy:

- "In the beginning, exhaustion reigned supreme. In the second trimester, my sex drive was pretty much normal. In the third trimester, I don't know if it was hormones or my newly ballooned status, but I just couldn't get enough! Not every day, but some days it was on my mind all the time. My poor husband!"
- "My husband had heard stories of women who wanted sex all the time at certain points in their pregnancies. Boy, was he disappointed. We didn't lose our closeness, however. There was always lots of snuggling, et cetera, because we found the whole experience of sharing the pregnancies brought us closer together as a couple. But as for the rest—it just didn't happen."
- "Throughout my pregnancy I've had very little interest in sex. I just seem to have lost my drive. It's not that I don't feel attractive. My husband thinks I've never looked better and I feel great. Perhaps it's a hormonal thing. It's been a little hard on us, but we both realize that it's not that we don't love and aren't attracted to each other. I'm sure things will eventually get back to normal—maybe even better. Who knows—they say women reach their sexual peak at 30, and I'm still three years away!"
- "I always want more sex when I'm pregnant. I'm so scared of miscarriage though that we've only had sex once since we found out I was pregnant. It's hard, though, because I really, really want to! After the first trimester is over, I'm sure I'll feel more comfortable."
- "We only had sex a few times during the first trimester. After that, we completely stopped because my husband was worried that he was hurting the baby. We compensated with lots of affection, cuddling, hugging, and kissing."
- "With my first pregnancy, I was just as interested in sex as before pregnancy—maybe even more so!—and we had sex right up until the end of my pregnancy. With the subsequent two pregnancies, however, my sex drive went through the floor and there was not much action in the bedroom. When I went to bed, all I wanted to do was sleep."

Most couples find that it helps to keep your sense of humour and—if you can swing it—your sense of adventure, too. After all, you won't always have that watermelon–sized belly to manoeuvre around. Why not consider it a temporary challenge and make the most of it? See Table 8.4 for the lowdown on three positions that tend to work well during pregnancy.

8.4 **The Pregnant Kama Sutra: The Big Three**	
Wondering what positions work best while you've got a baby on board? Here's a sneak peek at what's going on inside the bedrooms of the nation.	
Position	**Why it's hot**
1. Woman on top ("female superior")	Allows you to control the depth and angle of penetration and keeps you from lying flat on your back (a position that may cause you to faint after your fifth month).
2. Side-by-side ("spoons")	Gets your tummy out front and out of the way and allows for lots of foreplay and cuddling.
3. Rear entry ("doggy style")	Gets your tummy out of the way, but allows for greater ease of movement than with the side-by-side position.

Your pregnancy sex questions answered

There's no need to spend the next nine months fumbling around in the dark, looking for answers to all your pregnancy-related sex questions. Not when you can find the answers right here . . .

My partner says I taste different during oral sex, what's that about? The hormonal changes of pregnancy can give your vaginal secretions a stronger taste and odour that can turn some people off.

Does an orgasm feel different when you're pregnant? It depends. For some women, it's business as usual; for others, it's a whole new world. While some women say that orgasms are more intense during pregnancy, others describe them as far less satisfying. And some women who've never had an orgasm in their lives report having them for the first time ever during pregnancy. So pretty much anything goes.

Is it normal to feel crampy after sex? Yes. That's your body's response to the oxytocin that is released while you're having an orgasm.

I can't believe how lubricated I become when I'm sexually aroused. Does this go along with being pregnant? Yes, you can blame—or thank—your body's increased estrogen levels for the extra lubrication.

Do I need to pack my sex toys away during pregnancy? According to Anne Semans and Cathy Winks, authors of *The Mother's Guide to Sex,* there's no need to pack your sex toys away because you're having a baby. Just keep them clean and well lubricated and be sure to adjust the angle and depth of insertion to avoid bruising your cervix.

My partner has been avoiding sex since the pregnancy test came back positive three weeks ago. He's totally freaking me out! Is this a typical guy reaction? Your partner's reaction is not at all unusual, believe it or not. Whether it's concern about hurting the baby or an irrational feeling that the baby could somehow be "watching" you that's motivating this bedroom boycott, try to be patient with his feelings. After all, he must be pretty concerned if he's voluntarily doing without sex!

Is there sex after baby? Eventually, yes. In the immediate short-run? Well, maybe. An often-cited study from south of the border found that only one in five couples managed to find the time and energy for sexual intercourse during the month following childbirth. And if you think that dodging that episiotomy site or Caesarean incision is the trickiest part of getting your sex life back on track, I've got news for you: the biggest obstacle between you and a night of passion is a tiny bundle of joy.

---

staying connected

Relationships tend to show up on the worry lists of most expectant parents at some point during pregnancy. If you and your partner have been sniping at one another a lot lately, you may wonder if coping with the needs of a newborn will end up driving the two of you even further apart. And if you're getting along famously, you may wonder if it really makes sense to jinx a terrific relationship by adding a baby to the mix.

The best thing you can do to alleviate this particular fear is to talk things over with your partner and to brainstorm some ways to stay connected through birth and beyond. Partners with solid communication skills and a strong attachment to one another are most likely to weather the transition to parenthood.

The Last Hurrah

The countdown to motherhood is officially on. At some point during the next few weeks, you will finally get to meet your new baby. While you might be tempted to fast-forward through the rest of your pregnancy in your eagerness to meet the pint-sized passenger who has been hitching a ride in your belly, these final weeks of pregnancy are actually a time to be savoured and enjoyed. They are, after all, your last chance to take advantage of the perks of the pre-baby lifestyle—in other words, your last hurrah!

As any veteran mother can tell you, having a baby changes your life forever. While some of the changes are temporary—you won't be pacing the floor at 3 a.m. with a fussy newborn forever!—some are practically permanent. (Your chances of maintaining Martha Stewart–like housekeeping standards after baby arrives are, at best, slim to none.) Here are nine experiences you'll definitely want to squeeze in before baby makes his or her grand entrance.

1. **Spontaneous sex.** I don't want to scare you by giving you the impression that the term *parenthood* is just a fancy euphemism for forced celibacy, but, during the early weeks of your baby's life at least, your odds of enjoying some good, old-fashioned spur-of-the-moment sex are pretty much non-existent. You see, newborns are equipped with a highly sophisticated radar device that tells them when things are about to get hot and heavy between their parents. They're programmed to let out a hearty cry whenever the sparks start to fly in the bedroom. Bottom line? If you only manage to accomplish one of the items on the to-do list this month, make sure this is the one.

2. **Time alone with your partner.** The other thing that quickly disappears when you're struggling to keep up with the demands of a newborn is time alone as a couple. This only makes sense: after all, you're going from two to three! That's why it's important to take advantage of the opportunity to spend some time alone together this month. Make breakfast together or flop out on the couch and watch all your favourite Saturday morning home renovation shows. Believe it or not, it won't be long until you're waxing nostalgic about these everyday aspects of couplehood. (It's a rare newborn, after all, who's willing to let his parents tune in to an entire morning of home reno shows without kicking up a bit of a fuss!)

3. **A meal at a fancy restaurant.** Even if you're not particularly into dining out at the types of restaurants that feature white linen and subdued music, make sure you enjoy a dinner out at such an establishment one last time. It won't be long before you start looking for places that feature plenty of noisy background music (to drown out the sounds of a fussy baby) and that have a more baby-friendly decor (strained peas do bad things to white linen, after all!), so be sure to seize the moment.

4. **A night at the movies.** You probably take trips to the movie theatres for granted, don't you? Believe it or not, it could be a while before you manage to enjoy date night at one of these establishments again. You see, babies and movie theatres don't make a particularly good mix—except during mom-and-baby movie matinees, when everyone has a babe in arms.

5. **An evening out with your girlfriends.** While babies have an almost magnet-like drawing power when it comes to attracting female visitors, friends without children tend to drift away after the initial novelty of seeing you in mommy mode wears off. You have to make an effort to stay connected with the friends who matter most to you. And even if you manage to get your girlfriends to show up on your doorstep for a late-night tête-à-tête, you'll probably find yourself dozing off each time there's a lull in the conversation. (Believe it or not, the need for sleep can beat out even the juiciest bit of gossip hands down.)

6. **The chance to strut your pregnant stuff.** You should definitely plan to pose for the camera at least once during the final home stretch of pregnancy. It won't be long before your huge belly is but a memory. Make sure you have some photos that capture this magical time in your life.

7. **The chance to sleep in.** Sleep: it's what new parents can only dream about. Don't miss the opportunity to sleep in as often and as late as possible during these last few weeks of pregnancy. The sandman is about to pack his bags and leave town.

8. **A nice warm (but not too warm) bubble bath.** It may not seem like a big deal now, but you'll thank me later on for encouraging you to squeeze in one last bubble bath. In just a few short weeks, it'll be darned near impossible for you to find an hour or two to bury yourself in the bubbles, trashy novel in hand.

9. **Time to write a love letter.** Take a moment to write a very special type of love letter—a love letter to your baby-to-be. Let your baby know about all your hopes and dreams for him. Better yet, make your letter the first entry in a journal chronicling the amazing journey you're about to make—the journey into motherhood. And while you're at it, dash off a second letter to your partner. Let your partner know that the rules of the game may be about to change, but you'll always be on the same team.

Have belly, will travel

Planning a pre-baby trip? Here are some tips on staying comfortable whether you're travelling by plane, train, or automobile.

Before you leave home, discuss your travel plans with your doctor or midwife. If you're experiencing a high-risk pregnancy or your due date is fast approaching, your caregiver may want you to stay relatively close to home (within a three-hour drive, for example) in case some complications arise or your baby decides to make an unscheduled early arrival. Even if your caregiver gives you the go-ahead to venture a little farther afield, she may want you to take a copy of your prenatal record with you. That way, if you unexpectedly run into complications while you're travelling, the doctor on call at whatever hospital or clinic you end up visiting will have the lowdown on your medical and obstetrical history.

Make sure that your health coverage is adequate if you will be travelling out of province. Most health insurance policies for travellers do not apply to women who are more than seven months pregnant, so be sure to let your travel agent know about your pregnancy when you're purchasing such coverage.

Dress in layers of comfortable, loose-fitting clothing. As your prenatal instructor no doubt told you, the hormonal changes of pregnancy cause your body temperature to shoot up. If you make the mistake of hopping on board an airplane wearing a long-sleeved wool dress, you won't have the option of removing a layer or two if you become overheated (unless, of course, you intend to carry your entire maternity wardrobe in your carry-on luggage).

Pack some healthy snacks to enjoy while you're on the road. Rather than having to rely on French fries and other fast foods while you're travelling— not exactly the most stomach-friendly cuisine if your world is being rocked by morning sickness!—you may prefer to eat fresh fruit, granola bars, and healthier (and less nauseating) foods instead. And don't forget to take advantage of every offer of a drink of water when the beverage cart goes by, if you're going to be travelling by plane: you'll want to counter the dehydrating effects of air travel.

Bring a small pillow or rolled-up towel with you. Placing it in the small of your back will help to reduce the amount of back discomfort you experience as a result of sitting in one position for prolonged periods of time.

If you're travelling by car

- Set a realistic travel itinerary for yourself. Your days of whizzing down the highway for hours at a time with not so much as a single bathroom break are a thing of the past—at least for now. In fact, if you're like most pregnant women, you're likely to find yourself mapping out your route based on washroom availability—the ultimate roadside attraction at this stage in your life.

- If your car has airbags, you'll want to make sure that there is at least a 25-centimetre (10-inch) gap between your belly and the dash. (You may have to move your seat back a little if you're mega-pregnant.) And while we're talking positioning, here's something important to keep in mind if you're the driver: you should tilt the steering wheel downward so that it's as far from your belly as possible to minimize the risk of injury to your baby in the event of a car accident.

- Wear your seatbelt. Your seatbelt should be fastened across your hips and underneath your belly (as opposed to across your belly). This will help to reduce the risk of injury to you and your baby in the event of an automobile accident. The shoulder belt should be positioned between your breasts. (If the shoulder belt is chafing your neck, try moving your seat back a little. That usually does the trick.

If you're travelling by plane

- Make sure you're clear about airline policies concerning pregnant travellers before you book your flight. Policies vary from airline to airline, but most carriers require some sort of doctor's certificate from any pregnant woman who is travelling during the mid- to late third trimester.

- If you're heading to exotic locales, make sure that any immunizations that are required can be safely administered during pregnancy. It's best to avoid live vaccines and certain other types of vaccines.

- Get out of your seat and move around whenever the opportunity presents itself. This will help to minimize leg cramps and ankle swelling. (Don't worry about setting the alarm on your watch to remind yourself to do this: your bladder will encourage you to make washroom treks on a regular basis!) If you end up being confined to your seat for a prolonged period of time, do calf stretches or rotate your ankles—whatever you can reasonably do to stretch your legs while you're stuck in one spot.

- If you're prone to varicose veins, you might want to pick up a pair of support hose (vascular tightening stockings) from your local medical supply store before you hop on board the plane. Flying increases your risk of developing varicose veins.

DOs and DON'Ts at the spa

FIRST TRIMESTER

✔ DO remember to spill the beans about your pregnancy the moment you call to book your day at the spa. That way, the staff will be able to help you steer clear of any treatments that aren't recommended for mothers-to-be—basically any treatment that involves high temperatures (whirlpools, saunas, steam rooms, heat wraps, etc.) or the use of any herbal or botanical products that could potentially be harmful to the developing baby. Note: If you're unsure whether or not it's safe to expose your baby to a particular product during pregnancy, call the Motherisk Clinic at the Hospital for Sick Children in Toronto: 1–416–813–6780.

✗ DON'T forget to let the therapist or esthetician who is treating you know if you're battling morning sickness. Once the person administering your treatment is aware of the problem, she can take steps to ensure that the treatment room is well ventilated and she can avoid using any strongly scented spa products that might inadvertently trigger your nausea.

SECOND TRIMESTER

✔ DO indulge yourself with a mid-pregnancy facial. Facial treatments designed to unplug oily pores can help to minimize the severity of the hormonally driven acne breakouts that are a pregnancy rite of passage for many moms-to-be.

✗ DON'T go near the tanning bed. Not only is the heat from the tanning bed potentially harmful to your developing baby, the man-made suntan you acquire will only serve to accentuate the butterfly-shaped area of pigmentation (chloasma) that can occur on the cheeks and forehead—the so-called "mask of pregnancy."

THIRD TRIMESTER

✔ DO treat those tired tootsies to an ultra-soothing foot massage and pedicure. Trying to apply nail polish to your own toenails is pretty much impossible at this stage of the game, so let someone else give you the ultimate pre-labour send-off: some fire-engine-red toenails to flash while you're giving birth. (Oh, baby!)

✗ DON'T overlook your belly. Treat it to a moisturizing body scrub. This particular spa treatment will help you to get rid of the buildup of dead skin cells that can otherwise lead to an itchy belly—a perennial source of annoyance for moms-to-be. At the same time, it will help replenish some of the moisture that's being lost as a result of hormone-induced skin dehydration.

MOTHER MASSAGE

Pregnancy massage could be just what the doctor—or midwife—ordered: a way to manage some of the more common pregnancy discomforts and to pamper yourself at the same time. It can help to reduce stress, improve your mood, decrease pain, lower the rate of obstetrical complications, and improve the health of your developing baby. A registered massage therapist can design a massage therapy program that's safe and effective for you and your baby.

Your increased sensitivity to touch may mean that you prefer a different amount of pressure than usual while you're being massaged. If you find the amount of pressure that your massage therapist is using too light or too heavy, let the therapist know so that she can adjust the amount of pressure accordingly.

Oh yeah: don't expect your massage to be business as usual once the pregnancy test comes back positive. Some minor modifications to your massage routine may be necessary for both comfort and safety reasons.

Early on in pregnancy, you'll want to avoid putting a lot of weight on those oh-so-tender breasts. Then, as your pregnancy progresses you'll need to work around your growing belly. After the fifth month, you'll need to avoid lying flat on your back because that position can lead to extreme dizziness, even fainting. While the side-lying position is a perennial favourite with moms-to-be, it's not the only position that works. Simply toss a few wedge-shaped pillows on the massage table and see where your body takes you!

Deep massage work—particularly on the legs—is a definite no-no for pregnant women. Pregnant women are highly prone to varicose veins, and vigorous leg massage could cause a blood clot in the leg to become dislodged, potentially leading to death or disability. Fortunately, massage doesn't have to be vigorous to be effective: your RMT's less vigorous massage strokes will still help you to do battle with leg cramps, headaches, fluid retention, swollen ankles, and other pregnancy-related aches and pains.

Oops, we did it again . . .

As excited as you may be about being pregnant with your second or subsequent child, it's only natural to worry about the disruption that may result from adding another baby to your family (the all-too-common ruining your first child's life worry). What if your happy, well-adjusted older child resents rather than welcomes the new arrival? What if she ends up talking to her therapist about this defining point in her childhood for the rest of her life?

Lori, a 29-year-old mother of four, remembers being haunted by these types of thoughts: "When I became pregnant with my second child, I began to worry that maybe it was too soon to have another baby. My son was 13 months old and so I wondered if I'd had enough time with him before bringing another child into the family. I thought it might be unfair to him, that he wouldn't get as much attention and that perhaps he'd feel as if we loved him less when the new baby was born."

After nine months of worrying, Lori found that the problem resolved itself. "By the time the new baby was born, my first child was six weeks away from turning two, and he had matured a great deal over the course of my pregnancy. He'd gained some independence and actually wanted to do more on his own." What's more, Lori discovered that "the new baby slept a lot and I still had a lot of time to do things with my son—something that helped to make the transition more gradual for him."

So relax! If this particular worry has made it onto your list, there's plenty you can do both during your pregnancy and after the birth to help make the transition as smooth as possible for baby number one. Here are a few tips:

- Tap into your child's natural curiosity about babies. Even very young children are fascinated by them. Look at picture books together and talk about what's going on inside your body right now and what the baby will be like after birth.
- Find ways to involve your child in your pregnancy. Have him accompany you to prenatal checkups so that he can listen to the baby's heartbeat or help the doctor or midwife measure your growing belly.
- Give your child a sneak preview of what babies are really like by visiting other families who have newborns. (Hint: If you don't know anyone who's had a baby recently, drop by your local family resource centre. There are always tons of moms with new babies hanging out there!) Visit the website of The Canadian Association of Family Resource Programs—www.frp.ca—for help in finding the closest centre. You might also find out whether the hospital in your community offers sibling preparation classes.
- Encourage your child to help you pick out clothes and other items for the baby. Your child will enjoy seeing the new baby wear the sleeper she picked out for him.
- Buy your child an inexpensive gift from the new baby. That way, when friends and relatives show up bearing gifts for the new arrival, your older child is less likely to feel left out.
- Don't oversell the new baby. Your child needs to know that it'll be at least a couple of years before the new arrival is able to play ball or go for a ride on a tricycle. Some young children are very disappointed when their new brother or sister who was supposedly going to be such a great playmate is actually kind of boring to have around.
- Arrange for a friend or relative to give your child some extra time and

attention after the baby arrives. A trip to the zoo or the playground with Grandma and Grandpa may be all that's required to let her know that she's still as special as always.

- Don't try to enforce a totally "hands off " policy. While you obviously don't want to allow your toddler to carry the new baby around the room, you can teach him to hold the baby's hand gently or to carefully pat the baby's tummy. Babies are just as irresistible to toddlers as they are to adults. Imagine how frustrated you'd feel if no one let you touch the new baby.
- Don't forget to take photos of your older child when you're snapping shots of the new baby. Otherwise, she may feel very left out when all the photos feature the new star attraction. Besides, this is the perfect time to capture those moments that melt a parent's heart: the first time the newborn stares at your older child's face, and your older child's big grin when she sees the baby's eyes open wide for the very first time.
- Don't panic if sibling love doesn't blossom overnight. It takes time for relationships to develop. Odds are that special sibling bond will begin to emerge over time.

The stuff of which pregnancy nightmares are made

It's easy to let your imagination run wild—to play out all kinds of crazy scenarios in your head. You might imagine yourself going grocery shopping with your baby only to accidentally leave her in the cart, or failing to detect the signs of some life-threatening illness that could have been prevented if only you'd been a little more on the ball.

These types of fears are very common in late pregnancy. If they don't catch up with you by day, they're likely to make cameo appearances in your nightmares. In many ways, these worries are a dress rehearsal for the awesome and exciting role you're about to take on. Despite what you might think, they're by no means an indication that you're woefully under-qualified for the job of parenting. In fact, by playing out these scenarios in your subconscious, your mind is making sure that you'll be über-prepared.

Don't fall into the trap, by the way, of assuming that everyone else in your prenatal class is far better equipped to care for a newborn than you are. No matter how many hours of babysitting they clocked as a teenager, or how many books they've read and courses they've taken on the ins and outs of baby care, nothing can fully prepare anyone for the challenges of parenthood. Despite what that obnoxiously overconfident couple in your class may believe, there's no way to cram for this particular final exam.

Prepare yourself for the fact that you're likely to experience a few moments of panic during the early weeks. You'll probably end up checking on the baby an inordinate number of times, just to be sure that she's breathing, and you'll likely end up making at least one unnecessary trip to the emergency ward because you're convinced she's developed some life-threatening disease when she's actually just come down with a case of baby acne. It's all part of the early-parenting turf! But before you know it, you'll be an old pro. You'll wake up one day and realize that you've mastered the art of detecting a fever by placing your hand on your baby's forehead, and that you've learned to distinguish between run-of-the-mill diaper explosions and bona fide diarrhea. All you need is a little practice—and, as we both know, that opportunity is fast approaching.

. . . And the stuff of pregnancy dreams

Pregnancy is a time made for dreaming. You probably catch yourself doing it all the time: imagining yourself at some point in the not-so-distant future with a baby in your arms. And why not? The nine and a half months of pregnancy are the perfect time to think about the type of parent you want to be and the family you hope to create after your baby is born. Here are eight key questions you may wish to consider as you make the transition from pregnancy to parenthood.

1. What are your basic beliefs about being a parent?
2. Where will you turn for parenting information and support?
3. How will you manage the stress that goes along with being a parent?
4. When others describe your family, what do you want them to say?
5. How will the family you are creating be different from (and similar to) the family you grew up in?
6. Are there lifestyle changes you would like to make now that you are becoming a parent? If so, where can you find support in making these changes?
7. Does your current neighbourhood meet your family's needs? Do you see yourself continuing to live in this neighbourhood as your child grows? Why or why not?
8. What are your hopes and dreams for your child? What kind of life-long relationship do you hope to establish with the baby you are cradling inside you right now?

CHAPTER 9

When Pregnancy Isn't Perfect

"Not everyone has a textbook pregnancy and delivery and ends up with a smiling chubby newborn who is breastfeeding with ease. A problem pregnancy, a preterm delivery, and a failed breastfeeding attempt do not make you less of a person. Having a baby is not a contest."

—SUSAN, 35, MOTHER OF TWO CHILDREN
WHO WERE BORN PREMATURELY

While some women enjoy the luxury of breezing through pregnancy with nothing more to worry about than whether the designer stroller will arrive on time, others have considerably more to feel anxious about—like how their pregnancy will be going a day, a week, or a month from now.

This chapter is all about the challenges of coping with a high-risk pregnancy, why your pregnancy might be classified as high risk, and what you can do to stay sane while you count down the days to delivery. We'll start off by talking about prenatal testing: which tests are likely to be offered to you at what stage in your pregnancy, and what you need to know about these tests in order to make informed decisions (so you won't have reason to second-guess those decisions after the fact, regardless of what you decide). Then we'll be zeroing in on multiple pregnancy and certain types of complications that can result in your pregnancy being designated as high risk. Next up? Preterm birth: what every pregnant woman needs to know about the risk factors and the warning signs. The chapter wraps up by touching on a subject you probably don't even want to think about—the possibility that your pregnancy could result in a less-than-happy ending. (It's up to you whether you read that part of the chapter, but at least it's there if you ever need it.)

To Test or Not to Test?

It's an issue that every pregnant woman will have to grapple with at some point in her pregnancy: whether or not to opt for prenatal genetic testing.

There's no right or wrong answer when it comes to prenatal genetic testing. There's simply the decision that's best for you. You may feel strongly about arming yourself with as many facts as possible about the well-being of your future child so that you can consider a variety of options, including pregnancy termination, or you may prefer to avoid the resulting stress and anxiety by skipping the testing altogether and letting nature take its course.

In order to make the best possible decision, you should ensure that you are being given the facts you need to exercise informed consent. For informed consent to apply

- You must be able to make decisions for yourself.
- Your health-care provider must have equipped you with the information you need to make the decision about the test, treatment, or procedures. In this case, the information might include the reason for doing the test, a description of the testing procedures, alternatives (if you decline this test, what other tests could be done in its place?), potential consequences of not having the test, and the risks and benefits of consenting to the test. (If some of this information is not known or not available, you should be told that, too.) You'll also want to find out how long you have to make up your mind. Sometimes time is not on your side (a particular test, if it is to be performed, may need to be carried out at a particular stage of pregnancy, for example), but, in most cases, your health-care provider should be able to give you a while to think through your options before you have to make your final decision.
- You must understand the information that has been provided. This means that you must be given the opportunity to ask questions about what you've just learned. Sometimes the best questions don't occur to you until after you've left your doctor or midwife's office, so be sure to find out how you can obtain answers to these after-the-fact queries.
- You must voluntarily grant your consent to the procedure without anyone pressuring you to do so.

What prenatal testing can—and can't—tell you

While every parent-to-be dreams of a storybook happy ending—of bringing home a healthy baby who's perfect from head to toe—not everyone's dream comes true. According to the Society of Obstetricians and Gynaecologists of Canada (SOGC), approximately 2 to 3 per cent of newborns are affected by major structural malformations and, contrary to popular belief, the majority of these babies are born to parents with no family history of congenital problems (problems that are present at birth).

While some of these infants adjust well to life outside their mothers' bodies, not all fare so well. A number of babies born with serious congenital abnormalities end up experiencing serious health problems or dying during their first year of life. In fact, according to the SOGC, 20 to 25 per cent of deaths occurring during the first 28 days of life (the perinatal period) are the result of congenital problems. You can find a list of the most common types of congenital problems in Table 9.1.

While medical science has made tremendous progress in figuring out what causes some babies to be born with congenital problems, there's still much we don't know about the causes of these types of problems. Less than half of congenital problems can be attributed to any known causes (such as a chromosomal problem, a genetic problem, an environmental factor such as maternal disease during pregnancy, or a combined factor).

While prenatal genetic testing can help you find out in advance whether your baby is affected by certain types of congenital problems, it's by no means the crystal ball that some expectant couples think it is. Even the most sophisticated diagnostic tests have a small margin of error, and what's more, not all problems can be detected through genetic testing. Even if a genetic test does indicate that your child has a particular abnormality, the test can't tell you to what degree your child may be affected, and what kind of quality of life your child will enjoy.

All that said, prenatal genetic tests can still be a source of valuable information. If they reveal that your baby is affected by a particular problem, this information can allow you to

- arrange for medical treatment in utero (a fetal bladder obstruction, for example, can be corrected prior to birth);
- make appropriate choices for the delivery (such as scheduling a Caesarean if you know in advance that you'll be giving birth to a medically fragile infant who might sustain injuries during a vaginal delivery);
- prepare to give birth to an infant with special needs in an appropriate setting (such as a hospital with state-of-the-art neonatal facilities, and

9.1 The Most Common Types of Congenital Problems

Approximately three out of every hundred live-born babies are born with congenital abnormalities (birth defects) that affect the way they look, develop, and function—either over the short term or for the rest of their lives. While there are literally thousands of different congenital abnormalities and syndromes identified in medical literature, the vast majority of these conditions are extremely rare—small solace, however, if your baby happens to be born with one of these abnormalities. This table lists the most common types of congenital problems.

Condition	How It Affects the Baby	What You Need to Know
Chromosomal abnormalities	How the baby is affected is determined by the particular chromosomal abnormality. In some cases, the baby survives until birth but does not survive the early weeks of life. For example, babies with an extra copy of chromosome 18 or chromosome 13 (called trisomy 18 or trisomy 13) have multiple birth defects and generally die in the first weeks or months of life. Babies with less severe chromosomal abnormalities, such as Down syndrome (trisomy 21), often survive, although with intellectual disabilities and often heart defects and other health problems.	In most cases, pregnancies with chromosomal abnormalities end in miscarriage.
Anencephaly	Most of the brain and skull are missing. Affected babies may be stillborn (the fetus dies before birth) or die in the first days of life.	A woman who has previously had a baby with anencephaly, or a related birth defect called spina bifida, should consult her health-care provider before getting pregnant again to find out how much folic acid to take, both prior to conceiving and during the pregnancy. Generally, a higher-than-normal dose is recommended (usually 4 milligrams).
Spina bifida	The spinal column fails to close properly during the early weeks of embryonic development. The newborn may initially appear to be normal other than for a small sac protruding from the spine.	Surgery must be performed to remove the sac and close the opening to the spine. Most babies with spina bifida develop such related physical problems as hydrocephalus (excessive increase in the fluid that cushions the brain—something that can result in a brain injury), muscle weakness or paralysis, and bowel and bladder problems. Spina bifida is the most common type of physically disabling congenital abnormality, occurring in 1 in 1,000 births.

		A woman who has previously had a baby with spina bifida, or a related birth defect called anencephaly, should consult her health-care provider before getting pregnant again to find out how much folic acid to take, both prior to conceiving and during the pregnancy. Generally, a higher-than-normal dose is recommended (usually 4 milligrams).
Hydrocephalus ("water on the brain")	Babies with hydrocephalus have a buildup of cerebrospinal fluid in the skull. If too much fluid builds up on the brain, developmental delays may result.	Hydrocephalus can be treated by inserting a shunt in the child's brain to drain off extra fluid. Children who are successfully treated with shunts have the potential to function at the standard level of intelligence.
Clubfoot (talipes)	The baby is born with the sole of one or both feet facing either down and inward or up and outward.	Clubfoot is treated by manipulating the baby's foot over a period of several months and bracing or splinting it into the correct position. If surgery is required, it can be performed when an infant is as young as 3 to 4 months old. Clubfoot is twice as common in boys as it is in girls.
Dislocated hip	The ball at the head of the thigh bone doesn't fit snugly in its socket in the hip bone, something that results in a dislocated hip.	Treatments such as manipulation and splinting can resolve most problems, but surgery may be required in the most severe cases. This problem is far more common in girls than in boys, and is also more likely to occur in breech births and in pregnancies in which there was an abnormally small amount of amniotic fluid. Approximately four out of every thousand babies are born with a dislocated hip.
Epispadias and hypospadias (penile abnormalities)	A baby with epispadias has a urethral opening on the upper surface of the penis rather than on the tip, and his penis may curve upward. A baby with hypospadias has a urethral opening on the underside of the glans of the penis, and his penis may curve downward. In rare cases, baby boys are born with a urethral opening in between the genitals and the anus, something that may give the genitals a female appearance.	Surgery during early childhood can correct these problems. None of these abnormalities causes infertility or otherwise affects sexual functioning. Approximately three out of every thousand babies are born with some sort of abnormality in the position of the urethral opening on the penis. Note: Circumcision is not an option for babies with penile abnormalities. The foreskin needs to be maintained so that it can be used for penile reconstruction when the child is older.
Congenital heart defects	About 1 in 125 babies is born with some type of congenital heart problem. Most affected babies survive and do well. Your baby's prognosis is very much determined by the disease. The most common type of problem is a hole in the ventricular septum (the dividing wall between the right and left pumping chambers of the heart).	Babies can be born with a number of different types of congenital heart problems. Some types of heart problems repair themselves over time, others can be repaired with surgery, and still others are untreatable and/or may prove fatal. Heart defects are the most common birth defect–related causes of death during the first year of life. Heart defects are responsible for about 25 per cent of infant deaths.

continued

9.1   The Most Common Types of Congenital Problems (continued)

Condition	How It Affects the Baby	What You Need to Know
Lung defects	A baby may be born with a malformed or underdeveloped lung or lungs.	In most cases, lung defects are the result of birth defects, or occur because pregnancy complications interfered with lung development.
Cleft lip and cleft palate	If the parts of a baby's face are not properly fused together, the baby may end up with a cleft lip (a separation of the upper lip that can extend into the nose) or a cleft palate (when the roof of the mouth is incomplete). Babies with a cleft of the lip or the soft palate only are most likely to be able to breastfeed. Babies with a cleft of the lip as well as the soft and hard palate are generally unable to breastfeed. Use of a football hold position while breastfeeding or offering expressed breast milk in a squeeze bottle designed for babies with feeding difficulties may make feeding easier.	A cleft lip can be repaired shortly after birth, but surgery on a cleft palate is typically delayed until a baby is 6 to 9 months of age or older. Children with cleft palate problems may face speech delays and have other associated problems with their hearing and their teeth.
Pyloric stenosis	Pyloric stenosis refers to a thickening in the muscle leading to a narrowing in the pylorus (the passage that leads from the stomach into the small intestine). The baby's stomach contracts violently in an attempt to force a buildup of food through the narrow passageway, which results in powerful projectile vomiting. The baby may also experience constipation and dehydration.	Pyloric stenosis is more common in boys than in girls, with symptoms typically presenting themselves at some point during the second to fourth weeks of life. The condition can be corrected with surgery.
Imperforate anus (sealed anus)	Some babies are born with an anus that is sealed, either because there is a thin membrane of skin over the opening to the anus, or because the anal canal failed to develop properly.	Surgery must be conducted as soon as the problem is detected (typically during the newborn exam).

where it will be possible to make contact with other parents who have been through the experience of giving birth to a baby with special needs and who are willing to share their wisdom and offer their support);

- begin to prepare yourself emotionally for the fact that you may be carrying a baby who could be stillborn or have life-threatening health problems; or

- make the heart-wrenching decision to terminate the pregnancy.

Is prenatal genetic testing the right choice for you?

While no one can help you to decide what to do about prenatal genetic testing, it can be useful to find out who is—and isn't—generally considered to be a good candidate for the tests.

Health-care professionals tend to recommend prenatal testing to

- couples who have a family history of genetic disease or who know they are carriers of a particular disease;

- pregnant women who have been exposed to a serious infection such as rubella, parvovirus 19, or toxoplasmosis during pregnancy, or who have been exposed to a substance known to cause birth defects;

- couples who've had three or more miscarriages or who've previously given birth to a baby with a diagnosable birth defect;

- couples who are anxious to find out whether or not their baby has any sort of detectable birth defect or other anomaly.

On the other hand, prenatal genetic testing is generally not recommended for couples

- who have concerns about the accuracy of certain types of prenatal tests;

- who feel that taking this sort of test will add to (rather than alleviate) their stress;

- who have already decided they wouldn't consider terminating their pregnancy under any circumstances;

- who are afraid to undergo certain types of prenatal tests (such as amniocentesis) because the procedure may be painful or may cause miscarriage or otherwise harm a healthy baby.

While health-care providers used to recommend prenatal testing to all women based on age (with 35 being the magic number), they are no longer taking that one-size-fits-all approach to prenatal testing. Caregivers are now taking into account the unique circumstances of each pregnant woman and making a recommendation on that basis. In fact, the Society of Obstetricians and Gynaecologists of Canada states that maternal age screening is inferior to newer screening approaches which combine a number of screening methods to assess risk and then proceed to more specific diagnostic testing, if warranted and if a woman chooses.

In 2007, the SOGC published guidelines entitled *Prenatal Screening for Fetal Aneuploidy*, which note that screening practices vary across Canada and are constantly changing, and that screening programs "should show respect for the needs and quality of life of persons with disabilities. Counselling should be nondirective and should respect a woman's choice to accept or to refuse any or all of the testing or options offered at any point in the process."

looking beyond your age	Despite the fact that older women face an increased risk of giving birth to a baby with a chromosomal abnormality, the vast majority of babies with Down syndrome are born to women age 35 or younger. This is simply because there are many more babies born to women under age 35 than over age 35. It is another reason why it doesn't make sense to recommend prenatal testing to every woman on the basis of age alone. It is a lot more reasonable to consider a woman's feelings, her entire medical history, and the family medical histories for herself and her partner when weighing the pros and cons of prenatal testing.

Screening tests vs. diagnostic tests

There are two major categories of prenatal tests: screening tests and diagnostic tests.

Screening tests are designed to screen a large number of pregnant women in order to identify those who have a greater-than-average chance of giving birth to a baby with a serious or life-threatening birth defect. They aren't designed to determine whether there *is* a problem, but rather to alert a pregnant woman and her caregiver that there *could be* a problem. The first trimester or integrated screening blood test (its exact name may vary depending on where you live) is an example of a prenatal screening test. Ultrasound can also be used for screening purposes, although it's frequently used as a diagnostic tool as well. (See Table 9.2.)

Diagnostic tests are designed to pick up where screening tests leave off: they get down to the real nitty-gritty, providing a much clearer answer about what is—or isn't—going on with your baby. Unfortunately, there's no single diagnostic test capable of screening for every possible problem, and there are still a significant number of serious health problems that can't be detected prior to birth.

Amniocentesis and chorionic villus sampling are examples of prenatal diagnostic tests. (See Table 9.2.)

Many pregnant women mistakenly expect screening tests to perform like diagnostic tests. For example, they may become angry if they receive a false positive on the first-trimester blood test (the test says their baby may have a problem, when in fact the baby is perfectly healthy). What they're forgetting is that in order to ensure that as many problems are detected as possible, screening tests inevitably end up generating a certain percentage of so-called false positives. The alternative would be to make the testing criteria so rigid that the test would ignore any results that were less than clear-cut, which would dramatically increase the number of false negatives (situations in which the test says the baby is perfectly healthy, when in fact there is a problem).

It's also important to keep in mind that an all-clear test result doesn't offer any guarantee that the baby that you're carrying will be perfect. Some conditions can be tested for and others cannot. Furthermore, certain conditions may arise as the pregnancy progresses and therefore cannot be predicted ahead of time. And a test can't tell you the extent to which your baby will be affected by a particular condition. The test answers the question, "Is my baby affected? Yes or No?" It doesn't answer the questions "How severely is my baby affected?" or "What will my baby's life be like?

gestational diabetes

If your doctor or midwife feels that you are at risk of developing gestational diabetes, you may be screened for the condition toward the end of the second trimester or the beginning of the third. The one-hour glucose-screening test is designed to indicate whether you're at increased risk of having this condition, not to state definitively whether you actually do. In fact, if you test positive there's an 85 per cent chance that you *don't* actually have gestational diabetes.

Some health-care providers send anyone who tests positive on the one-hour glucose-screening test for a glucose tolerance test, which involves fasting for at least eight hours, consuming a beverage with a very high concentration of glucose (which makes some pregnant women feel quite nauseous), and having your blood sugar levels measured both prior to and at regular intervals after drinking the sugary beverage. Only when your result is positive on this test will you be diagnosed with gestational diabetes.

Other caregivers prefer to do fasting and post-meal blood sugar tests rather than relying on the glucose tolerance test. If your blood sugar readings are high on this test, you will be instructed to start monitoring your blood glucose levels at home and will be given some tips on modifying your diet. If your blood sugars continue to climb, you may have to start taking insulin.

What to Do if the Test Brings Bad News

It's something that every couple going for prenatal testing needs to think about up front: what they'll do if the test reveals a serious or even life-threatening birth defect. While some couples will opt to carry the pregnancy to term, others will make the difficult and painful decision to terminate the pregnancy as soon as possible.

If you find yourself faced with heartbreaking news and you're trying to decide whether to carry your pregnancy to term, you'll want to weigh the following factors carefully:

- whether you're prepared to raise a child born with a severe disability or give birth to a baby who may either be stillborn or die shortly after birth;
- how much your child would suffer physically and emotionally if he or she were to survive past birth;
- whether the baby's disabilities are treatable and, if so, the odds of treatment being successful;
- whether new methods of treating your baby's disabilities are likely to be developed in the near future;
- whether your baby would be able to live at home or whether he or she would need to be cared for in the hospital or a long-term-care setting for an indefinite period of time, perhaps forever;
- whether your relationship with your partner is strong enough to survive the emotional and financial stresses of caring for a severely disabled child;
- whether you and your partner are opposed to abortion under all circumstances or just under certain circumstances;
- whether you'd prefer to cherish the remaining time you have left with your baby by carrying your pregnancy to term or whether you'd find it excruciatingly painful to continue your pregnancy, knowing that your baby would likely die prior to or shortly after birth;
- whether you would prefer to have a funeral for your baby, a private memorial service, or to grieve in a less public way;
- whether you're concerned that your child may be subjected to painful medical interventions if he or she were to survive beyond birth.

There are no easy answers to these questions, so be sure to seek counselling to help you make the decision. You'll likely find yourself second-guessing whatever decision you make, so it's important to remind yourself in the weeks and months to come that the decisions you made for your baby, however heart-wrenching and difficult, were made out of love. As Deborah Davis, Ph.D., notes in *Empty Cradle, Broken Heart,* you did the best you could, given the options you had: "You had to make an impossible choice between 'terrible' and 'horrible.'"

Whether your baby dies prior to or after birth, or is born with a severe disability, you'll need to take time to grieve the loss of "the perfect baby" you'd hoped for from the moment you first found out you were pregnant. Please visit the book's website (www.having-a-baby.com) for suggestions on where to turn for information and support.

> *boutique ultrasounds*
>
> The first ultrasound baby boutique in Canada opened its doors in 2003. Today, you can expect to pay about $300 for a 30-minute ultrasound featuring such frills as live broadcasting of your session to the web, a web page for your baby, and gender prediction. You'll also receive video and prenatal baby pictures to take home with you—this despite the fact that the Society of Obstetricians and Gynaecologists is firmly opposed to the operation of such clinics in Canada. The SOGC has been calling for a complete ban on the non-medical use of fetal ultrasound since the publication of its April 2007 policy statement entitled "Non-Medical Use of Fetal Ultrasound." It has three key concerns: boutique ultrasounds can provide a false sense of reassurance if there are abnormalities present but not detected by an ultrasound operator who is taking baby pictures, not conducting a diagnostic test; unsafe levels of abdominal pressure may be applied in an effort to obtain high-quality pictures; and the appropriate safeguards (operator expertise and fetal energy exposure, for example) are simply not in place in a non-medical environment.

What Does the Term "High-Risk Pregnancy" Really Mean?

While it can be pretty scary to have your pregnancy labelled "high risk," it's important to keep in mind that the term tends to be applied quite liberally. Doctors and midwives will consider your pregnancy high risk if you face a higher-than-average chance of experiencing complications during pregnancy or birth, or of delivering a baby who's in less-than-ideal health. The label is by no means a self-fulfilling prophecy: the vast majority of women to whom it's applied end up giving birth to healthy babies after all. That high-risk label is simply your health-care provider's method of flagging your pregnancy as one that needs to be monitored a little differently than a low-risk pregnancy.

In general, you can expect your pregnancy to be labelled high risk if

9.2 Prenatal Genetic Tests

Serum integrated prenatal screen (first-trimester blood test with ultrasound)

When It's Performed	Between the 11th and 14th weeks of pregnancy.
How It's Performed	The first-trimester blood test (quadruple screen) screens for alpha-fetoprotein, unconjugated estriol, human chorionic gonadotropin, and dimeric inhibin. The test is combined with an ultrasound screen for nuchal translucency.
What It Can Tell You and How Long It Takes to Get the Results	Can tell you whether you face a higher-than-average risk of giving birth to a baby affected by Down syndrome, a neural tube defect, placental dysfunction, and trisomy 18. You'll generally have your test results within a week.
Accuracy	The detection rate for Down syndrome is 75 to 80 per cent, and the false positive rate is 3 to 5 per cent. A follow-up blood test at 16 weeks has been shown to reduce the false positive rate and improve the ability to detect problems with the developing baby.
Risks	No direct risks to the fetus, but a false positive on the test may lead to other, more invasive tests that may carry a risk of miscarriage. It can also massively increase your stress level. Moreover, false negatives tend to be falsely reassuring. The test can't tell you for certain that your baby is not affected by the types of birth defects that are tested for. It can only tell you that the odds of the baby being affected are very slim.

Ultrasound

When It's Performed	The Society of Obstetricians and Gynaecologists of Canada recommends that all Canadian women be offered a screening ultrasound at 18 to 20 weeks' gestation. Most major fetal anatomic abnormalities can be detected by such a screen. Other data picked up by the screen can be used to modify the assessed risk for certain types of chromosomal abnormalities. Early ultrasound is done as part of the first-trimester screen (see above). The ultrasound's primary focus is to ensure fetal well-being and to measure the nuchal (back of the baby's neck) thickness. Can be used for screening or diagnostic purposes at any point during pregnancy.
How It's Performed	High-frequency sound waves are bounced off the fetus and used to create a corresponding image on a computer screen. The test can be performed by rubbing a transducer across the woman's abdomen or by inserting an ultrasonic probe into her vagina (more common early on in pregnancy when it's more difficult to detect a fetal heartbeat via the abdomen).

What It Can Tell You and How Long It Takes to Get the Results	Early in pregnancy, it can be used to detect a fetal heartbeat or to rule out an ectopic pregnancy (by detecting the presence of an amniotic sac in the uterus). Later on, it can be used to confirm your due date; check for the presence of multiples; monitor the growth and development of your baby; detect certain types of fetal anomalies; locate the fetus, the umbilical cord, and the placenta during amniocentesis and chorionic villus sampling; measure the quantity of amniotic fluid; determine the cause of any abnormal bleeding; assess the condition and position of the placenta; determine the condition of the cervix; check for evidence of miscarriage, an ectopic pregnancy, a molar pregnancy, or fetal demise; determine the baby's sex; assess whether a Caesarean might be required; determine the baby's position and size; and so on. If your doctor is performing the ultrasound, you'll have the results immediately. If a technician is performing the test, you may have to wait to see your doctor in order to receive the results.
Accuracy	Accuracy depends on the type of problem being screened for, with detection rates for various disorders ranging from 25 to 71 per cent, according to the Society of Obstetricians and Gynaecologists of Canada. In most cases, ultrasound is generally considered to be quite accurate when performed by a skilled technician. Note: The most accurate time to date a pregnancy is during the first trimester. The most accurate time to screen for fetal anomalies is at 18 to 20 weeks of pregnancy. The Society of Obstetricians and Gynaecologists of Canada recommends that all pregnant women be offered a late-second-trimester ultrasound.
Risks	While no specific risk factors have been identified, ultrasound is still a relatively new technology and consequently should not be used indiscriminately. The Society of Obstetricians and Gynaecologists of Canada's April 2007 publication entitled the "Non-Medical Use of Fetal Ultrasound" states that "the fetus should not be exposed to ultrasound for commercial and entertainment purposes" and that it "strongly opposes the non-medical use of ultrasound to view or photograph the fetus for the sole purpose of determining the fetal sex when there is no medical indication to scan."

Amniocentesis

When It's Performed	Typically performed after 15 weeks' gestation. Results can generally be obtained prior to 20 weeks.
How It's Performed	A fine needle is inserted through the abdomen and into the amniotic sac. A small amount of amniotic fluid (under 30 millilitres, or less than an ounce) is withdrawn for analysis. Note: The procedure can be done with or without local anaesthetic.

continued

9.2 Prenatal Genetic Tests (continued)

Amniocentesis (continued)

What It Can Tell You and How Long It Takes to Get the Results	Can be used to detect chromosomal defects, neural tube defects, certain genetic and skeletal diseases, fetal infections, central nervous system diseases, blood diseases, and chemical problems or deficiencies. It can also be used to determine the sex of the baby (important if a couple is known to be a carrier for a disease such as hemophilia that is only a problem for babies of a particular sex), assess the baby's lung maturity (important if the mother is experiencing premature labour or pregnancy-related complications that may necessitate a premature delivery), and measure the bilirubin count of the amniotic fluid (which can help the doctor determine whether a baby with Rh disease may need a blood transfusion prior to birth). It generally takes one to three weeks to obtain the results of your amniocentesis if the purpose of the procedure is to screen for chromosomal abnormalities. Results for amniocentesis that has been performed to assess fetal lung maturity, however, can usually be obtained within 24 hours.
Accuracy	Generally considered to be highly accurate, although specific accuracy figures vary according to the specific type of test. Note: Sex determination tests are 100 per cent accurate if the result is male and 99 per cent accurate if the result is female, because there is a slim chance that maternal cells may have affected the test result.
Risks	Approximately one out of 100 to 600 women who undergo amniocentesis will miscarry or go into premature labour as a result of the procedure. Note: If you experience an increased vaginal discharge after amniocentesis, notify your caregiver immediately. You may be experiencing an amniotic fluid leak. Your caregiver will likely recommend that you rest and wait to see if the problem will resolve itself. Other potential complications include bleeding and uterine irritability.

Chorionic villus sampling (CVS)

When It's Performed	Between 10 and 12 weeks' gestation (12 to 14 weeks of pregnancy).
How It's Performed	A catheter is passed through the cervix or a needle is inserted through the abdomen to obtain a sample of chorionic villus tissue (the tissue that will eventually become the placenta).
What It Can Tell You and How Long It Takes to Get the Results	Can be used to detect Down syndrome, sickle-cell disease, thalassemia, cystic fibrosis, hemophilia, Huntington's disease, or muscular dystrophy. Unlike amniocentesis, however, it cannot be used to measure alpha-fetoprotein (AFP) levels to detect spina bifida. Note: It can take anywhere from a few days to a few weeks to obtain the results.

Accuracy

Less accurate than amniocentesis, due to the risk that the sample may become contaminated with maternal cells.

Risks

The miscarriage rate is approximately 0.5 to 1 per cent, which is higher than the miscarriage rate for amniocentesis. Chance of successful sampling: 99 per cent. Approximately 10 to 20 per cent of women who undergo transcervical CVS will experience some sort of bleeding. The transabdominal method is associated with increased uterine discomfort and cramping. Note: Some early research that linked CVS to limb reduction abnormalities has since been disproven. Infection has not been identified as a significant concern. (This is more of a concern with amniocentesis.)

Note: In most Canadian centres, RAD (rapid aneuploidy detection) (primarily FISH) is only available to select high-risk cases to provide more rapid results to women faced with time-sensitive decisions about pregnancy termination. Fluorescence in Situ Hybridization (FISH) is undertaken as an add-on test for selected pregnancies deemed to be at very high risk for chromosome abnormalities, or in cases of advanced gestational age, in order to provide results as soon as possible to couples faced with time-sensitive decisions about pregnancy termination.

Prenatal tests are constantly evolving. What's more, the types of tests that are offered to pregnant women tend to vary slightly, depending on where in Canada you live. The best places to find out about what prenatal tests are recommended in your jurisdiction are the websites of your provincial or territorial ministry of health and your local health unit.

- you're expecting multiples;
- you have a chronic medical condition that may affect your pregnancy (see Chapter 2 for a discussion of the effects of various medical conditions on pregnancy);
- you have a history of pregnancy-related complications (see Table 9.3) or appear to be developing one of these in your current pregnancy;
- you are an older mother (which can be 35 or 40, depending on the criteria that your health-care provider uses);
- you are obese;
- you had a Caesarean section less than two years ago;
- you have a history of miscarriage (usually meaning three consecutive first-trimester miscarriages);
- you have experienced stillbirth;
- you've had a baby who died shortly after birth or who was diagnosed with a genetic disorder;
- you're a carrier for a genetic disorder;
- your membranes have ruptured and you're not yet 36 weeks pregnant;
- you have a history of gynecological problems, such as large, symptomatic fibroids (non-cancerous growths in the uterus);
- you have a sexually transmitted infection that could be passed on to your child during pregnancy or birth (such as herpes, HIV, or hepatitis B or C);
- you conceived using high-tech fertility methods (which may increase your odds of experiencing a multiple birth, and which may increase your risk of other complications. Babies conceived through high-tech fertility procedures—either as a singleton or a multiple birth—have an increased likelihood of low birth weight, fetal growth restriction, perinatal mortality, and being born preterm. It is not known whether the fertility treatment procedures themselves or the underlying fertility problems are responsible for the increased risk);
- your mother took an anti-miscarriage drug called diethylstilbestrol (DES) when she was pregnant with you.

If your pregnancy is diagnosed as high risk, you may find yourself feeling angry and resentful that every other pregnant woman you know seems to be enjoying a blissfully uneventful pregnancy while you have to worry about every little symptom and complaint. Or perhaps you feel worried and upset about what the pregnancy may mean for you and your baby. You may even experience some guilt feelings if you believe (rightly or wrongly) that you may have done something to put your pregnancy at risk. It's important to talk about how

9.3 Conditions That Can Arise During Pregnancy

Type of Condition	Risks	Treatment
Amniotic Fluid Problems		
Chorioamnionitis (infection of the amniotic fluid and fetal membranes)	Chorioamnionitis increases your risk of premature rupturing of the membranes (PROM) or of premature labour. It can also occur after your membranes have ruptured.	Your doctor will either treat the problem with antibiotics or decide to deliver your baby early.
Oligohydramnios (too little amniotic fluid)	Oligohydramnios can indicate that you're carrying a baby who has missing or malfunctioning kidneys, that you may be leaking amniotic fluid due to premature rupture of the membranes, or that the placenta is not functioning properly. Olidohydramnios may lead to umbilical cord compression and fetal distress during labour, or premature rupture of membranes (PROM).	This condition is generally treated by delivering the baby as soon as possible.
Polyhydramnios (too much amniotic fluid)	Polyhydramnios can indicate that you're carrying a baby with Rh-incompatibility problems, a gastrointestinal anomaly, or diabetes, or that you're carrying more than one baby.	If your baby is believed to be at risk as a result of a high amniotic fluid level, excess fluid may be removed through amniocentesis. Your doctor will want to pinpoint the cause of the problem, if possible, in case treatment may improve your baby's outcome. Unfortunately, in almost 50 per cent of cases it's impossible to determine the cause of the problem. The good news about polyhydramnios is that in 40 to 50 per cent of cases, the problem resolves itself spontaneously and the baby does well.
Fetal Health Problems		
Intrauterine growth restriction (your baby is consistently measuring small for its gestational age)	Intrauterine growth restriction is an issue in 5 to 10 per cent of all pregnancies and up to 30 per cent of multiple pregnancies. Placental insufficiency is the leading cause of intrauterine growth restriction, responsible for 60 per cent of cases. Intrauterine growth restriction can lead to stillbirth or the growth of a low birth weight baby with a range of health problems.	If your doctor believes the baby would do better outside the womb, labour may be induced or your baby may be delivered by Caesarean section.

continued

9.3 Conditions That Can Arise During Pregnancy *(continued)*

Type of Condition	Risks	Treatment
Fetal Health Problems *(continued)*		
	Note: Intrauterine growth restriction is more likely to occur in women with chronic health problems, who have an unhealthy lifestyle, who have high blood pressure, who are carrying multiples, who are on their first or fifth (or subsequent) pregnancy, or who are carrying a fetus with chromosomal abnormalities.	
Maternal Health Problems		
Gestational diabetes (a form of diabetes that can develop during pregnancy)	Gestational diabetes puts you at increased risk of giving birth to an excessively large baby who may have difficulty adjusting to life outside the womb, of giving birth to a stillborn baby, and of having your diabetes recur later in life. Your baby may also be at increased risk of developing diabetes in adulthood. Note: Women who are overweight, who have high blood pressure, who have recurrent yeast infections, who have a history of polycystic ovarian syndrome (PCOS), who have experienced gestational diabetes in a previous pregnancy, who have a family history of diabetes, who have previously given birth to a baby weighing more than nine pounds (4.1 kilograms), or who have experienced an unexplained stillbirth face an increased risk of developing gestational diabetes. Gestational diabetes occurs in 3.7 per cent of pregnancies in the non-Aboriginal population in Canada and 8 to 18 per cent of the Aboriginal population. Women who develop gestational diabetes during pregnancy face a 20 to 50 per cent chance of developing diabetes in the future, and their children are at increased risk of obesity and diabetes during childhood and adolescence as compared to other children.	The condition is controlled through diet, exercise, and—if necessary—insulin injections.

Condition	Description	Treatment
Intrahepatic cholestasis (impairment of bile secretions in the liver characterized by severe itching and mild jaundice)	Intrahepatic cholestasis increases your risk of experiencing either a premature delivery or a stillbirth.	Your pregnancy will be monitored carefully and your baby may be delivered prematurely if it's believed that the baby would do better outside the womb.
Pre-eclampsia (a serious health condition characterized by very high blood pressure)	Pre-eclampsia can develop into eclampsia, a potentially life-threatening condition for both mother and baby. Note: The warning symptoms of pre-eclampsia include swelling of the hands and feet, sudden weight gain, high blood pressure (140/90 or higher, or a marked increase over your baseline blood pressure reading), increased protein in the urine, headaches, and nausea, vomiting, and abdominal pain during the second or third trimesters. The condition is more likely to occur in first-time mothers (and in women who are giving birth to their first baby with a new partner), women who are carrying multiples, women who are over 40 or under 18, and women with chronic high blood pressure, diabetes, kidney disease, or a family history of pre-eclampsia. If seizures are present, the condition is known as eclampsia. Note: A study published in the November 2009 edition of *BMJ* reported that women who develop pre-eclampsia during pregnancy may be at increased risk of experiencing reduced thyroid function during the final weeks of their pregnancy and again later on in life (20 years after giving birth). Reduced thyroid function (hypothyroidism) can lead to overall weakness and fatigue, and also increases the risk of cardiovascular disease. Pre-eclampsia occurs in 3 to 5 per cent of pregnancies.	Your doctor may recommend bedrest (in cases of mild pre-eclampsia) or an immediate delivery (in situations where both your life and the baby's life are at risk). Your doctor may also treat you with medication in order to safeguard your own health and to try to buy your baby some more time in the uterus. If you develop serious complications such as seizures, or liver or kidney complications, your doctor will have no choice but to deliver your baby as soon as possible.
Pregnancy-induced hypertension (PIH) (high blood pressure that occurs during pregnancy)	Severe high blood pressure can be dangerous—even fatal—to both mother and baby.	Your doctor will prescribe blood pressure medication to try to bring your blood pressure down. It may also be necessary to deliver your baby prematurely.

continued

9.3 Conditions That Can Arise During Pregnancy (*continued*)

Type of Condition	Risks	Treatment
Placental Problems		
Placental abruption (premature separation of the placenta from the uterine wall)	A placental abruption can result in stillbirth or the birth of a disabled baby and can lead to severe hemorrhaging and even death in the mother. Note: The warning symptoms of a placental abruption include heavy vaginal bleeding, premature labour contractions, uterine tenderness, and lower back pain. Placental abruptions are more common in mothers who've had two or more children, who have pregnancy-induced or chronic high blood pressure, who have experienced a previous placental abruption, who smoke, who use cocaine, or whose membranes have ruptured prematurely.	Treatment may include careful monitoring and bedrest (if the placental abruption is only partial) or an emergency Caesarean (if it appears that a full abruption is inevitable—something that could put both your life and the baby's life at risk). Note: If your baby has already died as a result of the abruption, your doctor will induce labour rather than performing a Caesarean section, because of the risk of hemorrhage.
Placental insufficiency (your baby is not receiving adequate nutrition from the placenta)	Placental insufficiency can be caused by restricted blood flow due to a clot, a partial abruption, a placenta that's too small or underdeveloped, a postdate pregnancy, high blood pressure, cigarette smoking, lupus or lupus antibodies, or maternal diabetes. It can lead to stillbirth or the birth of a small-for-date baby who may have some serious health problems.	Treatment may include careful monitoring and bedrest, or a premature delivery (if it's believed that your baby would be better off being delivered early). You will likely receive two injections of steroids to help mature your baby's lungs if a premature delivery is anticipated. You may also be prescribed baby aspirin to decrease clotting in the placenta.
Placenta previa (the placenta is blocking all or part of the cervix—the exit from the uterus)	Placenta previa may prevent you from giving birth vaginally. In most cases, a low-lying placenta that's diagnosed early in pregnancy will correct itself before you go into labour. In the meantime, your health-care provider will monitor it to see how close it gets to the cervix, which will determine intervention. Note: The warning symptoms of placenta previa include bleeding (usually painless) whenever you cough, strain, or have sexual intercourse. The condition is more common in women who've had several children, who have closely spaced pregnancies, who have a history of abortion (multiple D&Cs) and/or Caesarean section, or who have endometrial scarring from a previous episode of placenta previa. Placenta previa is a problem in 2.8 of every 1,000 singleton pregnancies and 3.9 of every 1,000 twin pregnancies.	Treatment may include bedrest, careful monitoring, hospitalization, and/or delivery via Caesarean section. Placenta previa can cause life-threatening hemorrhaging and, in up to 10 per cent of cases of complete placenta previa, a hysterectomy may be required to control the bleeding. Note: If placenta previa is diagnosed during the second trimester and the placenta is barely touching the cervix at that point, there is generally less cause for concern. As the uterus grows, the area of placental contact will move upward, away from the cervix.

Placenta accreta (a serious obstetric complication that occurs when the placenta implants itself too deeply in the uterine wall)	Placenta accreta results in a potentially life-threatening hemorrhage and an average blood loss of 6.5 to 10.5 pints (3 to 5 litres) of blood at delivery. Placenta accreta has been on the rise along with the increase in Caesarean deliveries. It is now estimated at one per one thousand deliveries. Note: Placenta increta occurs when the placenta works its way into the uterine muscle. Placenta percreta occurs when the placenta forces its way through the uterine wall and attaches itself to another organ, such as the bladder. Placenta increta and placenta percreta are far less common than placenta accreta.	A hysterectomy may be required to save your life.

Other Problems

Hyperemesis gravidarum (severe morning sickness)	Hyperemesis gravidarum can lead to dehydration, malnutrition, intrauterine growth restriction, and/or premature labour. Note: Hyperemesis gravidarum is more common in first-time mothers, mothers carrying multiples, and mothers who have experienced this condition in a previous pregnancy.	Anti-nausea medication (Diclectin) may be prescribed. In very severe cases, you may require intravenous feeding (TPN). You may be hospitalized so that intravenous drugs and fluids can be administered.
Premature labour	Your baby may be born with some medical challenges and possibly some chronic health conditions. If your baby is born too prematurely, he or she may not survive. You face a higher-than-average risk of going into premature labour if you smoke, you are younger than 16 or older than 35, your mother took DES when she was pregnant, you've been diagnosed with placenta previa or polyhydramnios, you haven't gained an adequate amount of weight during your pregnancy, you've been experiencing some unexplained vaginal bleeding, you've had abdominal surgery or have developed a high fever or kidney infection during your pregnancy, you have high blood pressure, you have an abnormal uterine structure, you have fibroids, or you are experiencing a great deal of physical or emotional stress. Note: Uterine irritability, a result of poor hydration, can seem like premature labour, and can also lead to premature labour if not treated. It can be treated with proper hydration.	If your baby is very premature, your treatment plan may be designed to hold off labour for as long as possible. Unfortunately, bedrest, intravenous fluids, and/or drugs tend to be ineffective at delaying or stopping labour if your cervix has dilated by more than 3 centimetres or has already begun to thin out (efface). In this situation, your doctor will simply be hoping that these forms of treatment will buy your baby an extra couple of days before birth—just long enough for the steroid shots to help mature your baby's lungs.

continued

9.3 Conditions That Can Arise During Pregnancy *(continued)*

Type of Condition	Risks	Treatment
Other Problems *(continued)*		
Premature rupture of membranes (PROM) or preterm premature rupture of membranes (PPROM)	Premature rupture of membranes is the term used when a pregnant woman is at least 37 weeks pregnant and her membranes rupture before the onset of labour. Preterm premature rupture of membranes is the term used when a pregnant woman is not yet 37 weeks pregnant and her membranes rupture before the onset of labour. PPROM is associated with 30 to 40 per cent of cases of preterm delivery and is the leading identifiable cause of preterm birth. It occurs in approximately 3 per cent of all pregnancies. Low body mass index, tobacco use, preterm labour history, urinary tract infection, vaginal bleeding at any time in pregnancy, cerclage (a procedure in which a stitch is inserted into and around the cervix early in the pregnancy, usually between weeks 12 to 14, and then removed toward the end of pregnancy when the risk of miscarriage has passed), and amniocentesis are all associated with PPROM. PROM is less common during the second trimester (0.4 per cent of pregnancies), but when it occurs, it can pose major risks to mother (infection, placental abruption, sepsis) and baby (fetal death occurs 30 per cent of the time).	If you think you could be leaking amniotic fluid, get it checked out. Sometimes it can be difficult to tell because your vaginal secretions increase during pregnancy, and you could be leaking urine, too. To find out whether or not your membranes are leaking, your caregiver will conduct a vaginal exam using a speculum (to check for amniotic fluid leaking from the cervix and/or pooling in the vagina) and test the composition of a fluid sample to see if it is amniotic fluid. If your membranes rupture at term, you will generally go into labour within 24 hours. The risk of infection increases the longer your membranes have been ruptured, so your health-care provider may recommend labour induction if you do not go into labour on your own after this time. Get in touch with your health-care provider immediately if you think your membranes may have ruptured. If your membranes rupture before term, efforts will be made to postpone labour and to prevent infection. You may be given a shot of corticosteroids to encourage your baby's lungs to mature rapidly. It is generally not possible to hold off labour for more than three to four weeks. Spontaneous resealing of the membranes occurs in less than 10 per cent of cases (usually when the leak was related to amniocentesis).

breast cancer

Breast cancer is the most common cancer in pregnant women, occurring in one to three out of every 10,000 pregnancies. That said, there is no evidence that pregnancy triggers or contributes to the progression of cancer. It's probably more an issue of demography. Breast cancer occurs in a certain percentage of women of childbearing age—and a certain number of those women get pregnant. Because it is difficult to detect abnormalities in breast tissue while you are breastfeeding (your breasts become lumpier), a thorough breast exam at your first prenatal checkup is recommended. You should continue to examine your breasts throughout pregnancy and while you're breastfeeding: 90 per cent of breast cancers are detected this way. A woman knows her own breasts best. If a lump is detected, a mammogram will be scheduled.

Your risk of developing breast cancer increases slightly during the three to four years after you have a baby, but your lifetime risk is lower than that of women who never have children. And if you breastfeed your baby or babies for an extended period of time (you breastfeed for at least 24 months of your life), you enjoy some added protection against breast cancer. Breastfeeding at a younger age also works to your advantage.

you're feeling with your midwife, doctor, or a counsellor, or with other women who are currently experiencing or who have been through a high-risk pregnancy in the past.

Hey baby, what's happening?

The Society of Obstetricians and Gynaecologists of Canada recommends daily monitoring of fetal movements starting at 26 to 32 weeks in all high-risk pregnancies. Its September 2007 publication "Fetal Health Surveillance: antepartum and intrapartum consensus guideline" also states that "Healthy pregnant women *without* risk factors for adverse perinatal outcomes should be made aware of the significance of fetal movements in the third trimester and asked to perform a fetal movement count if they perceive decreased movements."

What you do is start counting fetal movements at one point during your day over a period of two hours. (Ideally, you should do this in the early evening when you are lying down, semi-reclined, or you have your feet up and you're relaxed.) As soon as you reach six fetal movements, your work is done for that day. You don't have to continue counting fetal movements for the entire two-hour period. If you don't detect six fetal movements over a two-hour period, you should contact your health-care provider or go to the hospital as soon as possible—but don't panic. In most cases, everything is fine, but it's best to err on the side of caution by seeking medical help. That way, additional tests can be done to check on the well-being of your baby.

Wondering why a two-hour period was picked? Sleep cycles in healthy babies tend to last for 20 to 40 minutes and they almost never last longer than 90 minutes in utero. A baby with six or more movements in a two-hour interval is almost always healthy. (Note: It's important to distinguish between contractions and fetal movements.) Babies who are less active are more likely to have health problems. Diagnosing these problems early may make it possible for an affected baby to receive treatment prior to birth or as soon as possible after birth, depending on the nature of the problem.

Bedrest?

The medical profession is rethinking its approach to bedrest during pregnancy after a research review found that bedrest is not effective in preventing preterm birth or reducing the incidence of perinatal death. (In fact, the review found that rather than preventing harm, bedrest can actually cause harm by stressing out moms-to-be.) That's not to say that bedrest will never be recommended under any circumstance: what's changed is that bedrest has lost its status as the catch-all treatment for any woman experiencing a high-risk pregnancy.

The Unique Challenges of a Multiple Pregnancy

Approximately 3 per cent of Canadian births are multiple births, with about 95 per cent of these multiple births resulting in the birth of twins. Approximately 35 per cent of all Canadian multiple births are the result of infertility treatments (both fertility drugs and assisted reproductive technologies). However, it is estimated that over 80 per cent of higher-order multiples (triplets and more) result from these treatments.

The incidence of multiples conceived naturally (*without* the assistance of infertility treatments) is about 1 in 90 births for twins, 1 in 8,100 births for triplets, 1 in 729,000 births for quadruplets, and 1 in 65,610,000 births for quintuplets. (Source: Multiple Births Canada.)

There are few things as exciting or overwhelming as discovering that there's more than one baby on the way. You may feel special because you've been blessed with more than one, but you may also feel a bit nervous about the challenges you could face both prior to and after your babies' birth.

You or your caregiver will begin to suspect that you're pregnant with multiples if fraternal twins tend to run in your family, you were taking fertility drugs when you became pregnant, you're experiencing excessive vomiting and nausea, your uterus is larger than what would normally be expected for someone at your stage of pregnancy, or you're experiencing a lot of fetal movement. These suspicions will be confirmed if your caregiver is able to pick up more than one fetal heartbeat on the Doppler or ultrasound screen.

If you're carrying multiples, you can expect to face some special challenges during your pregnancy:

- The day-to-day aches and pains of pregnancy tend to be magnified if you're carrying more than one baby. You can expect to experience heightened early-pregnancy symptoms such as morning sickness, breast tenderness, and fatigue due to the high level of pregnancy hormones in your body. As your pregnancy progresses, you can expect to experience symptoms caused by the pressure of your heavy, stretched uterus on your surrounding organs (including shortness of breath, heartburn, constipation, pelvic discomfort, urinary leakage, back pain, and hemorrhoids).
- You will gain more weight than a woman who's pregnant with a single baby. (See Chapter 5 for details.)
- You face an increased risk of experiencing certain types of pregnancy complications. You're more likely to become anemic, develop pre-eclampsia or gestational diabetes, or experience pregnancy-induced hypertension (high blood pressure) than women who are carrying a single baby. What's more, your babies are at risk of experiencing such complications as growth discordance (when one baby develops more quickly or slowly than the others) and intrauterine growth restriction (due to limited space in the uterus and competition for nutrients). They're also at risk of twin-to-twin transfusion syndrome (a condition that occurs when there's an unequal sharing of nutrients in an identical twin pregnancy with a single placenta, causing one twin to get more than his or her share of nutrients and blood flow).
- You face an increased likelihood of delivering via Caesarean section. Caesarean section is required for over 50 per cent of twin pregnancies and almost all higher-order multiples.
- Women with a pre-pregnancy Body Mass Index (BMI) of 30 or greater are at a significantly increased risk of conceiving dizygotic multiples.
- You face a higher-than-average risk of going into labour prematurely. A mother carrying twins can expect to deliver her babies about four weeks earlier than a mother carrying a single baby. What's more, moms carrying triplets tend to deliver about seven weeks early, while moms carrying quads

tend to deliver about 10 weeks early. It's important to remember, of course, that these figures are averages. Some women deliver sooner or later than this.

- You're more likely to require a Caesarean delivery because of presentation problems (problems with the position the babies assume at the time of birth) and because, as the uterus begins to collapse down with the delivery of one of the babies, the risk of a placental abruption increases.

- You face a higher-than-average risk of giving birth to a low birth weight baby. Although multiples represent only one in 34 births, they account for one in five preterm births, one in four low birth weight births and one in three and a half very low birth weight births. While a typical singleton weighs about 7 pounds (3.2 kilograms) at birth, multiples are considerably lighter, with twins weighing in at 5 pounds, 5 ounces (2.4 kilograms) on average, and triplets and quadruplets at 3 pounds, 12 ounces (1.7 kilograms).

- You face a higher-than-average risk of giving birth to a baby with a birth defect. Birth defects are twice as common in multiple pregnancies, and are far more common in identical twins (twins that develop from the splitting of a single egg) than fraternal twins (twins that develop from two separate eggs).

- You face an increased risk of pregnancy loss. Studies have shown that women carrying twins are twice as likely (and women carrying triplets are four to six times as likely) to experience a stillbirth as women who are carrying singletons. The risks tend to be particularly high if you're carrying monoamniotic twins (twins that share the same amniotic sac): there's a 50 per cent mortality rate with such twins, due to the high risk that the babies will be born conjoined (Siamese twins) or that they'll become tangled up in one another's umbilical cords, cutting off the supply of oxygen.

- You face a higher-than-average risk of having a baby die shortly after birth. Twins are three to five times more likely than singletons to die during the first 28 days of life, largely due to health problems associated with prematurity. Furthermore, the risk of sudden infant death syndrome (SIDS) is twice as high in twins as it is in singletons. This is because many of the risk factors for SIDS are commonly associated with multiples: low birth weight, premature birth, and bed sharing.

- You face a higher-than-average risk of experiencing a postpartum hemorrhage. Because the uterus has been severely stretched during pregnancy, it may have more difficulty contracting after the delivery.

- You may be faced with the difficult issue of fetal reduction if you discover that you're carrying four or more babies. (Note: Since the outcomes of twin and triplet pregnancies are relatively similar, fetal reduction is not routinely recommended during triplet pregnancies.) This can be a heart-breaking decision for couples, particularly since there's a 10 to 13 per cent risk that all the fetuses will be miscarried as a result of the procedure.

That's not to say that all women who are pregnant with multiples experience complications. Many end up giving birth to two or more healthy term or near-term babies. You can increase your odds of enjoying a healthy pregnancy by listening to your body (eat, drink, and rest when you feel the need), tapping into your support network both before and after the birth, and communicating with your health-care provider about any and all concerns.

If you'd like to learn more about what having multiples may mean for you before, during, or after the birth, get in touch with Multiple Births Canada (www.multiplebirthscanada.org). They can connect you with other parents who have given birth to twins and higher-order multiples, and can provide you with practical advice on coping with the physical, emotional, and financial challenges of raising multiples.

fertility treatments and multiples

In an effort to reduce the number of babies being born preterm (more than 50 per cent of twins and 90 per cent of triplets are born preterm), the Society of Obstetricians and Gynaecologists of Canada and the Canadian Fertility and Andrology Society issued joint guidelines entitled "Guidelines for the Number of Embryos to Transfer Following In Vitro Fertilization" in September 2006. The guidelines note, "Decisions on the number of embryos to transfer should be based upon prognosis determined by variables including the woman's age, prior outcomes, and the number and quality of embryos available for transfer, and should be made to minimize the risk of multifetal gestation while maintaining a high probability of healthy live birth." The guidelines also recommend public funding for IVF-ET (in vitro fertilization embryo transfer) treatment: "A strategy for public funding of IVF-ET must be developed for the effective implementation of guidelines limiting the number of embryos transferred. In the context of this strategy, total health care costs would be lower as a result of reductions in the incidence of multifetal pregnancies and births."

The SOGC is also concerned about the number of multiples being conceived through the use of ovulatory drugs. "At present, there are no limitations on the ability of medical practitioners to prescribe these medications and there are no mechanisms to ensure appropriate prescribing other than through extensive professional and consumer education," says the SOGC.

Preterm Labour

Approximately 1 in 13 Canadian babies decide to make their grand entrance before the 37th completed week of pregnancy. In 25 to 30 per cent of these cases there's no apparent reason for the early arrival, while in the remaining 65 to 70 per cent the premature birth is triggered by conditions affecting the mother, the baby, or the placenta.

9.4   The Warning Signs of Preterm Labour

Every pregnant woman needs to know the warning signs of preterm labour, whether or not she is specifically at risk of a preterm birth. You should get in touch with your health-care provider right away if you suspect that you are experiencing preterm labour. Getting help sooner rather than later can make a big difference for your baby.

Warning signs to be watching for are

- menstrual-like cramps or stomach pains that don't go away;
- cramps with or without diarrhea;
- bleeding and/or a trickle or gush of fluid (clear, pink, or brownish) from your vagina;
- lower back pain or pressure, or a low, dull backache;
- a feeling that the baby is pushing down;
- pelvic pressure;
- contractions (especially a change in the strength or number of contractions: preterm labour contractions may feel more regular, they do not go away if you move around or lie down, and they may or may not be painful);*
- an increase in the amount of vaginal discharge;
- your gut instinct says that something isn't right. If you feel unwell and your body is telling you that something's wrong, it's possible that you're experiencing preterm labour. Always err on the side of caution.

---

* Note: While it's normal to experience some uterine tightening when you're exercising, you should be concerned if these contractions continue after you stop exercising, and if they don't go away when you drink a large glass of water or juice, empty your bladder, and lie down on your side.

Possible health problems

Babies who are born prematurely face a higher-than-average risk of experiencing such complications as respiratory distress syndrome (breathing problems in the newborn), bleeding of the fragile blood vessels in the brain (a stroke-like experience that can lead to developmental delays, cerebral palsy, learning disabilities, and/or behavioural problems such as attention deficit hyperactivity disorder), and infection.

If your baby is born prematurely, she may develop a condition known as respiratory distress syndrome (RDS). This is usually caused by a lack of surfactant (the dish detergent–like liquid that prevents the hollow sacs in the lungs from collapsing and sticking together each time the baby exhales) and can lead to such serious complications as pneumonia (which is particularly common if the baby has contracted an infection prior to or during birth, or if the baby is on a ventilator for an extended period of time), persistent pulmonary hypertension/persistent fetal circulation (a condition that occurs if the pressure in the blood vessels of the lungs fails to drop after birth, thereby reducing the amount of blood that's able to flow through them), bronchopulmonary dysplasia (the abnormal development of the lungs and the bronchial tubes—a condition that's common in babies who've been on ventilators for an extended period of time), and intraventricular hemorrhage (bleeding in the brain).

Risk factors

The age at which a mother becomes pregnant affects the odds of her giving birth to a baby who is preterm or small for gestational age (SGA) (another measure of fetal well-being). Babies who are born to younger mothers (teenagers) or women over the age of 35 are more likely to be preterm or SGA. According to the Canadian Institute for Health Information, in 2006–2007, mothers age 35 and older had a preterm birth rate of nearly 10 per cent, as compared to 8 per cent for those age 20 to 34.

Studies have shown that certain risk factors are associated with premature birth. You are more likely to give birth to your baby prematurely if

- you're a first-time mother or a mother with three or more other children;
- you've had a cone biopsy performed on your cervix at some point in the past (a cone biopsy involves removing a cone-shaped portion of tissue from the cervix);
- you're pregnant with multiples (multiples are nearly 17 times as likely to be born preterm as singletons);
- the baby you're carrying has severe congenital anomalies;
- you've experienced premature rupture of the membranes (PROM), placenta previa, or a placental abruption;
- you've been diagnosed with an incompetent cervix, fibroids, uterine abnormalities, or polyhydramnios (excess amniotic fluid);
- your mother took diethylstilbestrol (DES) when she was pregnant with you;
- you have a urinary tract infection or other type of infection (with or without a fever);

- your lifestyle is not as healthy as it should be (for example, if you smoke, use illicit drugs, or are under extreme stress);
- you have pre-existing health problems that put you at risk of experiencing a premature birth (such as diabetes, hypertension, kidney disease, or cardiovascular disease. Mothers who are diagnosed with diabetes or hypertension are six times more likely to deliver preterm than mothers without these conditions);
- you've previously given birth to a premature baby;
- your mother gave birth to you prematurely.

Seventy per cent of preterm births occur spontaneously. The other 30 per cent are medically indicated. These are situations in which preterm delivery by Caesarean section is necessary because continuing the pregnancy poses a serious risk to mother, baby, or both. Complications such as hypertensive disorders, maternal bleeding, intrauterine growth restriction, and fetal distress are among the most common reasons for medically indicated preterm deliveries.

Four major categories of triggers for spontaneous preterm birth have been identified: maternal and fetal stress (specific types of stress trigger a series of events that can lead to the onset of labour), inflammation, hemorrhage or abruption, and an overly distended (stretched) uterus.

Babies born even just a few weeks prematurely—between 34 and 36 weeks' gestation or 36 and 38 weeks of pregnancy—can still face a number of long-term health problems. They are more than three times as likely as full-term babies to have cerebral palsy, and they also face an increased risk of developmental delays. These babies tend to feed more slowly and may need to be fed more often than full-term babies.

Prevention

While researchers have yet to come up with a way to prevent all premature births, there are certain things you can do to reduce your risk of giving birth prematurely:

- Avoid sexually transmitted organisms that are known to or suspected of triggering premature labour (such as bacterial vaginosis—a vaginal infection characterized by a thin, milky discharge with a fishy odour).
- Promptly seek treatment for any urinary tract infections and don't allow your temperature to climb too high before seeking medical treatment for a fever (a high temperature can cause your uterus to start contracting).

- Call your doctor if you're unsure about any fluid that is leaking from your vagina.
- Avoid accidents and injuries that could trigger premature labour.
- Don't smoke or take illicit drugs, and lead a generally healthy lifestyle during pregnancy.

If you've experienced a premature birth in the past, your doctor will monitor any future pregnancies closely. You can expect to be tested for bacterial vaginosis (a vaginal condition characterized by the overgrowth of normal bacteria in the vagina, which can either be symptomless or accompanied by a greyish discharge with a foul odour) and fetal fibronectin (fFN) (a type of biological glue which can be detected in vaginal discharge approximately one to two weeks before you go into labour), and to have your cervical length measured via ultrasound.

If it appears that you may be going into preterm labour, the condition of your cervix will be assessed. If there are no changes or only minor changes to your cervix, you will probably be sent home with instructions to follow up with your doctor or midwife.

If your cervix has already started to open or to shorten and there is concern that you will give birth in the near future, you will be admitted to hospital for treatment. You will be injected with corticosteroids to help your baby's lungs to mature quickly. You will also receive a medication to try to delay or stop your labour (necessary to give the corticosteroids a chance to work). In some cases a stitch (a cerclage) can be inserted into the cervix to keep it from opening further.

Welcoming a premature baby or a baby with special needs

If your baby is born prematurely or has a lot of health problems, she'll likely spend her first weeks or months in the hospital. This can be very upsetting to you and your partner. After all, your dreams of the perfect birth didn't include watching your baby be whisked away to the neonatal intensive care unit or you checking out of the hospital without your baby.

Here are some tips on surviving your baby's hospitalization:

- Spend time getting to know your baby. "It's difficult to bond with your baby when your baby's in an Isolette hooked up to a bunch of machines, but it is possible," says Rita, 35, whose son was born prematurely. "Touch your baby, caress your baby, talk to your baby. I didn't think touching the baby did much good until my friend noticed that my son's heartbeat would change when I was with him and he would breathe more relaxed."

- Try to master the neonatal intensive care unit (NICU) lingo. Ask a nurse or another parent to explain the terminology so that you won't feel quite so confused and overwhelmed.
- If your baby is seriously ill, find out as much as you can about his or her medical condition, either by talking to the hospital staff and visiting the library, or by asking a friend or family member to do some research on your behalf. "Be realistic about your expectations, however," warns Bonnie, whose second child died at nine months. "Denial is your worst enemy."
- Play as active a role as you can in your baby's care, but don't put superhuman demands on yourself. No one expects you to hang out at the hospital 24 hours a day, nor should you expect this of yourself. If you don't like the idea of leaving your baby alone, see if another family member will stay at the hospital for a couple of hours so that you can enjoy a guilt-free break, suggests Monique, a 28-year-old mother of two, whose daughter, Maddy, was hospitalized for 11 weeks as a result of heart problems associated with her Down syndrome. "I arranged for my mother to spend time with Maddy a couple of times when I needed a break. That helped to ease my guilt a little, knowing that my mom would be there."
- Ask if you can practise kangaroo care. Researchers who have studied the benefits of kangaroo care (skin-to-skin contact between parent and baby) have found that it can stabilize the baby's heart rate, regularize the baby's breathing pattern, improve oxygen delivery to the baby's organs and tissues, help Baby sleep better, improve weight gain, decrease crying, encourage breastfeeding, and result in earlier discharge from hospital. Kangaroo care also delivers significant benefits to the parents by increasing the mother's breast milk supply, encouraging bonding and increasing confidence in their ability to care for their baby, reassuring them that their babies are being well cared for, and giving them back some control in a situation in which they often feel like they have none.
- Don't let the fact that your baby is premature discourage you from breastfeeding. Your baby might initially have to drink breast milk via a tube, but you can plan to gradually switch him over to the breast as he gets stronger and bigger.
- Bring a support person along with you when you're speaking to the medical staff. Not only can this person help you remember all the important details about what the doctor or nurse has to say about your

baby's progress, he or she can also help to spread the news to other friends and family members on your behalf. This can really help to alleviate your stress, notes Susan, a 35-year-old mother of two (both born prematurely). "You don't need to be telling the same story over and over again, particularly if the news is not good."

- Start preparing for the day when you'll be able to bring your baby home. The more you participate in your baby's day-to-day care while she's in the hospital, the less intimidated you'll feel when it's time to leave. And before you check your baby out of the hospital, line up as much support as you can on the home front: some insurance companies cover the services of a visiting nurse, particularly if you've given birth to multiples.

post-traumatic stress disorder

Post-traumatic stress disorder (PTSD) is relatively common among parents whose newborns spent time in the NICU. And there's no link between the severity of the trauma and the extent of the symptoms experienced by the parent, according to Richard Shaw, MD, a child psychiatrist and an associate professor at the Stanford University School of Medicine, who has studied the phenomenon. "Some individuals seem to be quite resilient and less likely to develop symptoms of PTSD. Others, especially those with prior history of trauma exposure, or those with poor coping abilities, are more vulnerable."

Shaw found that mothers and fathers followed different patterns in dealing with the trauma: "We were surprised to find that fathers had a delayed reaction in terms of their trauma response. By four months, maternal trauma symptoms had diminished, but fathers' symptoms had increased, and in fact exceeded those of the mothers. It appeared that fathers tend to keep their emotional reactions in check for the first few months, perhaps to allow full support to be given to the mothers. However, by four months, when the mothers are recovering, the fathers go through a very difficult period. Awareness of this phenomenon is essential to ensure that the fathers' needs are not overlooked or neglected."

Parents need to be informed about the types of symptoms they might experience and to be offered appropriate supports, including access to parent-to-parent support groups. Parents benefit greatly from advice from other parents who have gone through similar NICU experiences, according to Shaw.

When a Baby Dies

There are few experiences in life that can compare to the grief of losing a child. Whether that baby is miscarried, stillborn, or dies during or after birth, the loss can be devastating to both you and your partner. As Deborah Davis, Ph.D., notes in her book *Empty Cradle, Broken Heart*: "While the death of a parent or friend represents a loss of your past, when your baby dies you lose a part of your future. You grieve not only for your baby, but for your parenthood. Times you had looked forward to—maternity leave, family gatherings, and holidays—can seem worthless or trivial without your baby."

Pandora, 45, whose second child died of SIDS, feels that expectant parents are ill-prepared for anything other than a storybook happy ending to their pregnancies: "Western society fills us with 'great expectations'—that's literally the name of a magazine on the subject!—and we have no preparations for the empty crib, the unused baby clothes and diaper coupons, and the calls from baby photographers for months afterwards."

> "I loved being pregnant . . . watching my tummy get bigger and feeling tiny movements inside of me late at night. I loved wearing maternity clothes and looking at tiny cotton dresses and miniature denim overalls at Baby Gap. I loved reading *Little House in the Big Woods* aloud at night, hoping the baby would hear. I loved the excitement in my mother's voice when I called her, and the big smile on my father-in-law's face every time he saw me. I started noticing pregnant women everywhere. I felt like I had finally joined this sort of sacred sisterhood, this exclusive club I had longed to be a part of for so long. And then, as another bereaved mother ruefully put it to me, 'I got kicked out of the club.'"
>
> —LORI, 39, WHOSE DAUGHTER WAS STILLBORN AT 26 WEEKS

What can go wrong

While you might feel as if you're the only person to experience the death of a baby, miscarriage, stillbirth, and infant death are far more common than most people realize:

- Between 20 and 25 per cent of pregnancies end in miscarriage, ectopic pregnancy (a pregnancy that occurs outside the uterus), molar pregnancy (a pregnancy that results in the growth of abnormal cells rather than the development of a healthy placenta and embryo), or stillbirth.
- Miscarriages (the death of a baby before the 20th week of pregnancy) are the most common type of loss, occurring in 10 to 15 per cent of confirmed pregnancies. (According to the March of Dimes, as many as 40 per cent of pregnancies may end in miscarriage, with the majority of losses occurring before a woman even realizes she is pregnant.)
- Ectopic pregnancies occur in 1 to 2 per cent of pregnancies.

- Stillbirth occurs in approximately 1 in 160 pregnancies. When a baby dies during labour, the death is classified as an intrapartum death.
- Molar pregnancies occur in 1 out of every 1,000 to 2,000 pregnancies.

Here's what you need to know about each of these types of losses.

Miscarriage

Miscarriage is the term used to describe the spontaneous death of an embryo or fetus prior to the 20th week of pregnancy. (Medically, miscarriages are referred to as "spontaneous abortions"—a term that many couples who've lost a baby find upsetting and insensitive.) Some hospitals also use the term "miscarriage" to describe the deaths of babies who weigh less than 1 pound, 2 ounces (500 grams) at birth—something that can apply to babies whose mothers are as much as 23 or 24 weeks into their pregnancies.

While many women who are having a miscarriage report heavy bleeding and other symptoms (see list below), other women who've had a "missed abortion" have no idea that they've had a miscarriage until many weeks after the fact (see Table 9.5). Their miscarriage is diagnosed when their caregiver is unable to detect a fetal heartbeat using a Doppler or ultrasound. Note: An ultrasound can detect the fetal heartbeat as early as six weeks after the first day of your last menstrual period, while a Doppler can detect the fetal heartbeat about 12 to 14 weeks into your pregnancy—although it may take a little longer than that if you are overweight.

You should seek medical attention if you're experiencing one or more of these symptoms:

- spotting or light bleeding with or without menstrual-like cramping
- heavy or persistent bleeding (with or without clots) accompanied by abdominal pain, cramping, or pain in the lower back
- a gush of fluid from the vagina (an indication that your membranes may have ruptured)
- the sudden disappearance of all pregnancy symptoms (such as morning sickness or breast tenderness)

What treatment is required if you're experiencing a miscarriage?

In most cases, your body does not require any special treatment. If you are miscarrying, you body will do so naturally. If you are more than a few weeks along, you will experience severe cramping (painful enough that you will need to use

9.5   How Miscarriages Are Classified

Your caregiver may use one or more of the following terms when describing your miscarriage.
Note: "Abortion" is the medical term for "miscarriage."

Term	What It Means
Threatened abortion	You appear to be miscarrying (you're likely experiencing some vaginal bleeding and possibly some pain as well), but the miscarriage is not yet inevitable. Up to 50 per cent of these pregnancies continue successfully.
Inevitable abortion	Your cervix has begun to dilate and a miscarriage is in progress.
Incomplete abortion	You have experienced a partial miscarriage. Some of the so-called products of conception (the gestational sac, the fetus, the umbilical cord, and the placenta) remain in the uterus. Generally, a dilation and curettage (D&C) or suction curettage are performed to remove the remaining material.
Complete abortion	You have miscarried and all the products of conception have been expelled from your uterus.
Missed abortion	Your baby has died, but neither the baby nor the placenta have been expelled from the uterus. You may not realize there's a problem with your pregnancy until your caregiver is unable to detect the fetal heartbeat.
Early miscarriage	The term "early miscarriage" is used to describe a miscarriage that occurs prior to the 12th week of gestation.
Late miscarriage	The term "late miscarriage" describes a miscarriage that occurs between 13 and 19 weeks' gestation. (Sometimes miscarriages that occur at this stage of pregnancy are referred to as second-trimester miscarriages or fetal deaths.) Late miscarriage is much less common than early miscarriage, occurring in 1 to 5 per cent of pregnancies between weeks 13 and 19.
Blighted ovum	A pregnancy sac that doesn't contain a fetus. Either the embryo didn't form or it stopped developing very early on in pregnancy. A blighted ovum can be the result of chromosomal abnormalities. With a blighted ovum, you may notice that your pregnancy symptoms have disappeared. You may also experience some dark brown vaginal bleeding. An ultrasound will reveal an empty sac. Miscarriage will eventually occur, but it may not occur for weeks.

coping strategies to deal with the pain) and a lot of bleeding. Don't expect to be able to just go on with your day, in other words. If there are concerns that you may be retaining tissue (your bleeding is heavy and prolonged), your health-care provider may suggest a dilation and curettage (D&C). Some caregivers offer the option of using medication (misoprostol) to help pass the remaining tissue (an option that is effective in about 84 per cent of cases).

If you have been diagnosed with a blighted ovum or a missed miscarriage, your health-care provider may give you the option of waiting for a miscarriage to occur naturally, having a D&C, or using medication (misoprostol). If your miscarriage is really intense (your bleeding is really heavy, you are in a lot of pain) or you are concerned that you might be experiencing some of the symptoms of an ectopic pregnancy or a molar pregnancy, seek medical treatment right away.

The causes of miscarriage

While there's still much that medical science doesn't know about the causes and treatment of miscarriage, scientists have identified some of the major causes of these early pregnancy losses:

Chromosomal abnormalities. Chromosomes are the tiny, thread-like structures in each of our cells that carry our genetic material. We have 23 sets of chromosomes—46 chromosomes in total—with one chromosome in each pair coming from our mother and the other from our father. Chromosomal abnormalities are thought to be responsible for approximately 60 per cent of miscarriages. These randomly occurring genetic errors happen either prior to conception (if there's a defective egg or sperm cell) or during the earliest stages of cell division. Researchers estimate that the incidence of congenital anomalies in newborns would jump from 2 or 3 per cent to 12 per cent if miscarriages did not occur.

Maternal disease. Certain types of health problems in the mother increase her risk of experiencing a miscarriage. These conditions include immune system disorders such as lupus, congenital heart disease, severe kidney disease, uncontrolled diabetes, thyroid disease, and intrauterine infection.

Hormonal imbalances. Hormonal imbalances can also cause a woman to miscarry. If, for example, she has a luteal phase defect (her body doesn't secrete enough progesterone to sustain the pregnancy), she may end up miscarrying. (Think of progesterone as pro-gestation: a hormone needed to promote and sustain pregnancy.)

Rhesus (Rh) disease. Rh incompatibility occurs when the mother's blood is Rh-negative and the father's is Rh-positive. If the baby has Rh-positive blood too, this can pose problems during the pregnancy. The mother may become Rh-sensitized if some of the baby's blood cells get into her bloodstream, which can cause her to develop antibodies that may attack the baby's red blood cells, leading to anemia and possibly even the death of the baby. Rh-negative women with Rh-positive partners can generally avoid Rh-sensitivity problems if they receive a shot of Rh immune globulin (RhoGAM) whenever there's any sign of bleeding or suspected bleeding during pregnancy (such as following amniocentesis or in cases of placenta previa), during the 28th week of each pregnancy, and following each birth or miscarriage. Note: Fetal deaths caused by Rh disease are most likely to occur during the second trimester of pregnancy.

Immune system disorders. Immune system disorders are believed to be the cause of 5 to 10 per cent of recurrent miscarriages. They occur when a pregnant woman's immune system mistakenly concludes that her baby is an "intruder" and starts attacking the baby. Some recent research suggests that immune system responses inhibit the rise in progesterone levels, resulting in eventual miscarriage.

Allogeneic factors. If you develop antibodies to your partner's leukocytes (white blood cells), your baby may be miscarried. Sometimes this condition can be treated by immunizing you with either your partner's or a third party's leukocytes—a technique believed to trick your body into producing the blocking antibodies that prevent you from rejecting the developing baby.

Anatomical problems of the uterus and cervix. Congenital abnormalities of the uterus and the cervix, uterine adhesions and fibroids, complications arising from an elective abortion (such as infection or cervical trauma), and an incompetent cervix (a grossly insensitive term that simply means your cervix opens prematurely) are just a few of the problems that can lead to miscarriage or stillbirth. Some of these problems can be treated with surgery.

Viral and bacterial infections. Viral and bacterial infections have been proven to play a role in miscarriage. Some of them are unlikely to recur during a subsequent pregnancy (such as chicken pox) while others are more likely to be a problem again (group B strep). Note: Group B strep is more likely to be a problem during late pregnancy or during labour itself.

Recreational drug and alcohol use. Women who use recreational drugs or consume large quantities of alcohol during pregnancy face a higher-than-average risk of miscarriage.

Exposure to harmful substances. Exposure to high-dose radiation, certain types of chemicals, chemotherapeutic drugs, cigarette smoke, and moderate to heavy doses of caffeine may result in an increased risk of miscarriage. (A recent study found that women who consume about 200 milligrams (one 12-ounce cup of coffee) or more of caffeine every day are twice as likely as women who consume no caffeine to experience a miscarriage.)

Maternal age. A woman's chances of experiencing a miscarriage increase as she ages. While women in their 20s have just a 10 per cent risk of miscarrying during any given pregnancy, the risk for women in their 40s is believed to be approximately 50 per cent.

> *Fifth disease*
>
> If you have been exposed to or develop symptoms of parvovirus B19 (fifth disease), you should be assessed to find out if you are immune to the virus or if you have been infected. If you are immune (as is the case for 50 to 65 per cent of women of reproductive age), you don't have to worry about becoming infected or having parvovirus B19 affect your pregnancy. If you are not immune and you have not yet developed the virus, you may wish to minimize further exposure. (This can be a bit tricky if you work in a school or daycare because parvovirus tends to get transmitted in these environments, particularly in springtime, and yet taking leave from the workplace to avoid exposure is not routinely recommended.) If it appears that you have developed the infection, referral to an obstetrician or a maternal-fetal medicine specialist may be suggested so that you can be advised on the likelihood that this virus has been transmitted to your baby (the maternal-fetal transmission rate is 17 to 33 per cent), the odds of fetal loss (14.8 per cent before 20 weeks of pregnancy; 2.3 per cent after 20 weeks of pregnancy), and what would happen if your baby was affected. (In most cases, your baby will be fine, but there is a small risk that your baby could develop a serious condition known as fetal hydrops in which the baby accumulates a lot of fluid.)

Will it happen again?

Miscarriage is a one-time event for most women, but 1 per cent will go on to experience recurrent miscarriages. While doctors used to wait until you had experienced three or more consecutive miscarriages before launching an investigation into their cause, many caregivers are now willing to start looking into the problem after your second consecutive loss, particularly if you're over age 35. Your doctor may recommend blood tests (to detect any hormonal or immune system problems that could be causing you to miscarry), genetic tests (to determine if you or your partner are carriers of any genetic disorder that could be causing you to miscarry), a genital tract culture (to look for the presence of any sort of infection that could be causing you to miscarry), an endometrial biopsy (to assess whether your uterine lining is sufficiently thick to allow for implantation), a hysterosalpingography (an X-ray of the uterus and Fallopian tubes), or a hysteroscopy (an examination of the inside of the uterus using a telescope-like instrument inserted through the vagina and the cervix) to look for blockages and other problems, or an ultrasound or sonohysterography (to look for any structural problems and/or fibroids or adhesions that could be causing you to miscarry).

Depending on what your doctor is able to uncover during this investigation, he or she may recommend one or more of the following treatments:

- surgery to remove large (for example, grapefruit-sized) or problematic fibroids, or to correct any uterine abnormalities that may be causing you to miscarry;
- the insertion of a stitch in your cervix (cerclage) at the beginning of the second trimester to help stop the cervix from opening prematurely during your next pregnancy;
- a course of antibiotics to cure any infections that may be causing you to miscarry repeatedly;
- the improved management of chronic diseases such as diabetes or lupus that may be causing you to miscarry;
- hormone therapy to correct any hormonal imbalances that may be causing you to miscarry;
- treatment for immune system problems;
- treatment for allogeneic problems.

Less important than how many miscarriages you've had is whether or not you've been able to give birth to at least one living baby. Women who've had two or more miscarriages and who've never given birth to a living baby have a 40 to 45 per cent chance of miscarrying the next time around, whereas women who've given birth to a living baby but who've experienced as many as four miscarriages in the past have just a 25 to 30 per cent chance of miscarrying the next time around. (It's worth bearing in mind, when you're pondering this statistic, that 15 to 20 percent of all confirmed pregnancies end in miscarriage.)

Here's some good news to hold on to while you're trying to figure out what's behind your miscarriages: even without treatment, about 60 to 70 per cent of women who have experienced repeated miscarriages in the past have a successful next pregnancy.

Ectopic pregnancy

Ectopic pregnancies occur in 1 in every 40 to 1 in every 100 pregnancies. An ectopic pregnancy occurs when the fertilized egg implants somewhere other than in the uterus. In 95 per cent of ectopic pregnancies, the fertilized egg implants in one of the Fallopian tubes, and in the remaining 5 per cent of cases, it implants in the abdominal cavity, the ovaries, or the cervix. The ectopic pregnancy rate in Canada was 11.9 per 1,000 reported pregnancies in 2004–2005. The rate has been declining for the past ten years after rising steeply from the early 1970s through the early 1990s.

An ectopic pregnancy can pose a significant threat to a woman's health. If the Fallopian tube ruptures and results in massive internal bleeding, it may put her life at risk. That's why it's so important to be aware of the warning signs of an ectopic pregnancy (see Table 9.6) and to seek treatment before a rupture occurs. An ectopic pregnancy is classified as unruptured or subacute if it's detected before a tubal rupture occurs, and ruptured or acute if it isn't detected until after the tube has burst, causing pain, internal bleeding, and shock.

9.6 The Warning Signs of an Ectopic Pregnancy

You should seek medical treatment immediately if you experience one or more of the signs of an ectopic pregnancy:

- abnormal vaginal bleeding (especially bleeding that's either lighter or heavier than what you'd experience during a normal menstrual period)
- abdominal pain (either sudden and acute or sharp and aching), especially pain that's felt more on one side of the body than the other
- shoulder pain (caused by the pooling of blood in the abdomen)
- weakness, dizziness, fainting, and/or a weak but rapid pulse (caused by substantial blood loss)
- and you have reason to suspect that you could be pregnant (for example, you are experiencing early pregnancy symptoms like breast pain and/or nausea.)

Familiarize yourself with the risk factors for an ectopic pregnancy so that you'll know whether you face a higher-than-average risk of experiencing this type of problem:

- scarring of the Fallopian tubes caused by a past ectopic pregnancy, a prior infection of the Fallopian tubes, or surgery to the Fallopian tubes;
- a history of tubal infections caused by pelvic inflammatory disease, sexually transmitted infections, postpartum endometritis, or post-abortion infections (all of which can damage the mucus surface of the Fallopian tubes and make it more difficult for the fertilized egg to pass through the tube and into the uterus);

- a history of tubal or pelvic surgery such as surgery to deal with endometriosis or a ruptured appendix (which can lead to tubal adhesions);
- a structural abnormality of the Fallopian tubes;
- a hormonal imbalance (for example, insufficient progesterone—the hormone that causes the Fallopian tube to contract and propel the egg toward the uterus);
- conceiving while you're using Depo-Provera or another progesterone contraceptive (your Fallopian tube's ability to contract and propel the fertilized egg toward the uterus is affected);
- conceiving through in vitro fertilization (there's a possibility that you could have both a uterine and ectopic pregnancy simultaneously).
- smoking (nicotine is thought to interfere with the Fallopian tube's ability to contract and propel the fertilized egg);
- douching;
- becoming pregnant with an IUD in place or after a tubal ligation (sterilization) or a tubal ligation reversal procedure;
- a past history of ectopic pregnancy (you're 12 times as likely to experience an ectopic pregnancy if you've already experienced one in the past).

Ectopic pregnancies cannot continue to term. The developing pregnancy poses a threat to the mother's life. In fact, ectopic pregnancy is the leading cause of maternal mortality during the first trimester of pregnancy. If you are concerned that you might be experiencing some of the symptoms of an ectopic pregnancy, seek emergency medical attention immediately. If the pregnancy is still small and the tube has not yet ruptured, the ectopic pregnancy may be treated with methotrexate (a drug given by injection) that stops the pregnancy from developing and saves the Fallopian tube. (Your body gradually absorbs the pregnancy.) If the pregnancy is detected when it is slightly larger, but before the Fallopian tube ruptures, the embryo may be removed via a tiny incision in the Fallopian tube, thereby preserving the tube. If the ectopic pregnancy is diagnosed after the Fallopian tube has begun to stretch or after it has ruptured, it will be necessary to remove part or all of the Fallopian tube.

Fifty to 80 per cent of women who have had an ectopic pregnancy experience healthy pregnancies in the future. The odds of conceiving and carrying a baby to term after an ectopic pregnancy depend on such factors as the woman's age, whether or not she already has children, and the cause of the initial ectopic pregnancy. The success rates are about the same for women who have been treated with methotrexate and women who have had surgery. Any woman who has experienced an ectopic pregnancy in the past faces about a 10 per cent chance of experiencing another ectopic pregnancy in future, so all future pregnancies will need to be monitored carefully.

Molar pregnancy

The terms molar pregnancy, hydatidiform mole, and gestational trophoblastic disease are used to describe a pregnancy that results in the growth of abnormal tissue rather than a healthy placenta and embryo. Researchers believe that molar pregnancies result from a genetic error at the very beginning of pregnancy. Early on in pregnancy, the placenta develops into an abnormal mass of cysts known as a hydatidiform mole that resembles a bunch of white grapes.

There are two types of molar pregnancies: complete molar pregnancies and partial ones. In a complete molar pregnancy, thousands of fluid-filled cysts develop instead of a fetus. All of the fertilized egg's chromosomes come from the father. (The chromosomes that come from the mother are either lost or inactivated, and the chromosomes that come from the father are duplicated.)

In most partial molar pregnancies, the mother's 23 chromosomes remain, but there are two sets of chromosomes from the father (so the embryo has 69 chromosomes instead of the normal 46). This can occur if the fathers' chromosomes are duplicated or if two sperm manage to fertilize a single egg. In a partial molar pregnancy, there's an abnormal fetus as well as thousands of these fluid-filled cysts. In very rare situations—approximately 1 in every 22,000 to 100,000 births—a normal twin is also present and will be born very prematurely.

In most cases, a molar pregnancy is miscarried spontaneously. In some cases, however, it's diagnosed only when a woman begins to experience its symptoms: vaginal bleeding (usually dark brown in colour) during the first trimester, a uterus that grows too quickly (due to the increasing number of cysts), enlarged ovaries (caused by cysts on the ovaries), extremely high levels of hCG, and severe nausea, vomiting, and high blood pressure (possibly even pre-eclampsia) caused by unusually high hormone levels. Once a diagnosis has been made (via ultrasound and by measuring hormone levels), the pregnancy is terminated and the uterus is carefully emptied to ensure that no abnormal tissue is left behind.

In rare cases, a molar pregnancy will become cancerous. After the uterus is emptied, about 20 per cent of complete moles and less than 5 per cent of partial moles persist. The remaining abnormal tissue may continue to grow. If this occurs, the condition is known as persistent gestational trophoblastic disease (GTD). The key way of detecting this condition is by measuring the level of human chorionic gonadotropin (hCG) in your blood during the months following your delivery.

You won't be able to become pregnant during this time because it would be impossible for your doctor to determine whether your hCG levels were rising because of the choriocarcinoma (the cancerous form of GTD) or because of your new pregnancy. If your hCG levels are normal for six months to one year after your molar pregnancy, your doctor will likely give you the go-ahead to try again. If persistent GTD is detected, treatment with one or more cancer drugs will be recommended. This form of treatment cures persistent GTD nearly 100 per cent of the time. Rarely, choriocarcinoma develops and spreads to other organs. Use of multiple cancer drugs usually is successful at treating this cancer.

According to the Society of Obstetricians and Gynaecologists of Canada, women should avoid conceiving again after a molar pregnancy until hCG levels have been normal for six months following removal of the molar pregnancy, and for one year following chemotherapy for a gestational trophoblastic tumour (GTT). Note: It is safe to take the combined oral contraceptive pill if you are being treated for a GTT.

Certain women are more likely to experience a molar pregnancy than others:

- women of Southeast Asian descent;
- women with a family history of molar pregnancy;
- women who have previously experienced a molar pregnancy (there's a 1.3 to 2.9 per cent chance of recurrence).

Stillbirth

Stillbirth is the name given to losses that occur after the 20th week of gestation. Stillbirth occurs in approximately 1 out of 160 pregnancies and is more common in women under the age of 15 and over the age of 35, in pregnancies that last for longer than 42 weeks, in multiple pregnancies, and in pregnancies involving a male fetus.

> "I have talked, once or twice, to other parents who have lost babies at birth. Once unleashed, their grief is like a flood. I recognize the sandbags that they keep stacked between it and the rest of life. It does not recede, this flood. It is on the other side, always and forever. It is a peculiar grief, a pregnancy that never ends."
>
> —BETH POWNING, *SHADOW CHILD: AN APPRENTICESHIP IN LOVE AND LOSS*

While approximately 60 per cent of stillbirths are unexplained, researchers have been able to come up with a few clues about the causes of the other 40 per cent. Here's what is known about the most common causes.

- **Birth defects.** About 15 to 20 per cent of stillborn babies have one or more birth defects.
- **Chromosomal abnormalities.** While just 2 to 3 per cent of live-born infants have chromosomal problems, 6 to 13 per cent of stillborn babies have chromosomal problems.
- **Maternal health problems.** Certain types of maternal health conditions increase the risk of stillbirth, including diabetes, epilepsy, high blood pressure, heart disease, kidney disease, liver disease, lung disease, parathyroid disease, sickle-cell disease, systemic lupus erythematosus, and pre-eclampsia.
- **Maternal obesity.** Because obesity may increase a woman's risk of stillbirth, women who are obese may wish to consider losing weight before attempting to conceive.
- **Fetal growth problems.** Babies who are growing too slowly face an increased risk of stillbirth. About 40 per cent of stillborn babies exhibit signs of poor growth.
- **Infection during pregnancy.** Some types of infections are able to cross the placenta and harm the developing baby. In severe cases, they may result in stillbirth or cause labour to begin before the baby is capable of surviving outside the womb. These infections include group B streptococcus (the leading cause of fatal infection in newborns), cytomegalovirus (CMV), human parvovirus B19 (fifth disease), listeriosis, rubella (German measles), chicken pox, toxoplasmosis, and certain types of sexually transmitted infections.
- **Problems with the placenta.** The placenta is the baby's life-support system prior to birth. If serious problems arise, the baby may not be able to survive. There are three major types of problems that can arise with the placenta: placental insufficiency and placental failure (when the placenta is unable to meet the baby's need for nutrients and oxygen), placental abruption (when the placenta begins to separate prematurely from the uterine wall), and placenta previa (when the placenta blocks all or part of the exit to the womb). Problems with the placenta are responsible for about 25 per cent of stillbirths.
- **Problems with the uterus.** You are at increased risk of experiencing a stillbirth if you've been diagnosed with cervical insufficiency (a cervix that opens prematurely, resulting in miscarriage or premature birth; potential causes may include damage to the cervix during surgery, injury during a previous birth, and exposure to certain drugs), fibroids (non-cancerous

growths of tissue that occur in the wall of the uterus), or uterine abnormalities (such as a bicornate uterus or septate uterus). Note: Neonatal survival rates may be as high as 93 per cent after a cerclage (a procedure in which the cervix is stitched closed to prevent it from opening prematurely) as compared to 27 per cent before the cerclage.

- **Umbilical cord accidents.** Accidents involving the umbilical cord are responsible for about 2 to 4 per cent of stillbirths. The umbilical cord is the baby's lifeline prior to birth, carrying oxygen and nutrients to the baby and carrying away waste products. A problem with the umbilical cord can result in the death of the baby.
- **Umbilical cord problems.** These may include excessively long or short cords (cords that are shorter than 30 to 32 centimetres, or 12 to 12.5 inches, are associated with an increased risk of asphyxia at birth while cords that are longer than 75 to 100 centimetres, or 29.5 to 39 inches, are more likely to develop knots, to twist, or to prolapse), two-vessel cords (a normal umbilical cord has three vessels: when an umbilical cord only has one artery—as is the case with 0.55 per cent to 1 per cent of newborns—there is an increased risk of cardiovascular, gastrointestinal, and genitourinary anomalies), straight umbilical cords (which are more likely to tangle than telephone-cord-like umbilical cords), umbilical cords that are abnormally inserted into the placenta (for example, a velamentous insertion, which occurs with 1–2 per cent of placentas: the cord is inserted into the membranes so that the vessels run between the amnion and chorion before entering the placenta, potentially leading to rupture, fetal hemorrhage, or fetal death), prolapsed cords (umbilical cords that slip into the vagina ahead of the baby during labour), umbilical cord knots, umbilical cords that get wrapped around the baby's neck (generally a problem only if the cord has been wrapped around the neck a number of times), torsion of the umbilical cord (twisting that cuts off the supply of oxygen), cord strictures (a cord with insufficient amounts of Wharton's jelly—the thick substance that prevents the cord from becoming constricted), and amniotic band syndrome (a condition that can prevent oxygen from reaching the baby if the amniotic bands happen to be located on the umbilical cord).
- **Complications resulting from a multiple pregnancy.** As we noted earlier in this chapter, women who are carrying multiples face an increased risk of experiencing the death of one or more of their babies prior to birth.

- **Other causes.** Other causes of stillbirth include car accidents, postdate pregnancy (a pregnancy that lasts longer than 42 weeks), and Rh disease (when the mother's blood and the baby's blood are incompatible). All of these causes are rare.

What happens once a stillbirth has been confirmed?

Labour generally begins naturally within two weeks of a baby's death in utero. Some parents prefer to allow labour to begin on its own; others prefer to be induced as soon as possible. In some cases, continuing the pregnancy simply isn't an option. (Your health-care provider will recommend inducing labour as soon as possible if it appears that the baby has been dead for more than two weeks. There is a small risk of developing blood clots—something that could be very dangerous to you—after this amount of time.)

To induce labour, your health-care provider may start out by trying to encourage your cervix to dilate. She may use a synthetic form of prostaglandins and laminaria (seaweed sticks that swell, manually dilating the cervix). You will also be offered medication to reduce your anxiety level and help you sleep during this initial phase of labour. With any luck, you'll wake up in the early stages of active labour.

When you're planning for the delivery, talk to your caregiver about what pain relief methods you wish to use. (While you might want to be completely out of it so that you can block out the grief and the pain, it's healthier for your long-term healing if you can give birth to, spend some time with, and say goodbye to your baby.)

Think about whom you would like to have with you—to offer you support and encouragement during what will still be a labour of love (you love your baby so much), but what will be a journey toward an end rather than a beginning.

Intrapartum death

Most stillborn babies die before labour begins, but a few die during labour itself. This is more likely to occur in a labour that is prolonged, in which there are excessively frequent contractions, in which there are problems with the placenta or the umbilical cord, or in which the baby is in a medically fragile condition (perhaps due to a congenital anomaly).

If you experience an intrapartum death, you will be in shock and you will be traumatized. That's a given. Call in your support team—friends, family, the hospital social worker (who can help you to connect to other support services in your community), and others who can help you through this devastating time—right away. There is no need to suffer alone.

Neonatal and infant death

Despite all the amazing advances in neonatal medicine we've witnessed over the past few decades, there are still a number of problems that medical science is unable to treat or prevent. As a result, approximately 1 in every 196 babies dies during the first year of life.

Approximately two-thirds of infant deaths occur during the first month of life—during the so-called neonatal period. The two leading causes of neonatal death are conditions originating in the perinatal period (these include respiratory distress syndrome; problems associated with prematurity and/or low birth weight; maternal complications of pregnancy, such as gestational diabetes or pre-eclampsia; problems with the placenta, umbilical cord, and amniotic sac; complications of labour and delivery; slow fetal growth and fetal malnutrition; birth trauma; intrauterine hypoxia and birth hypoxia—when the baby is deprived of oxygen prior to or during birth; hemorrhage; and perinatal jaundice) and congenital anomalies (for example, neural tube defects such as anencephaly, spina bifida, and hydrocephalus; heart and other circulatory system defects; problems with the respiratory, digestive, genitourinary, and musculoskeletal systems; and chromosomal anomalies such as Down syndrome). The two leading causes of post-neonatal death (deaths occurring between one month and one year of age) are sudden infant death syndrome (SIDS) and congenital anomalies.

Some parents know ahead of time that their babies are going to be born with medical conditions that are incompatible with life. If you find out in advance that your baby has a serious health problem that will not allow her to survive for very long after birth, you'll want to decide in advance how you'd like to spend your baby's few short days or hours of life. Here are some questions you'll need to consider:

- Would you prefer to spend that time alone with your baby and your partner?
- Would you prefer to have your baby's siblings or your baby's grandparents there as well?
- Would you prefer for your baby to receive pain relief if she seems to be experiencing a lot of discomfort or pain?
- Would you prefer to be holding your baby as she passes away?

- Would you prefer to spend some time alone with your baby after her death?
- Do you intend to donate your baby's organs?

> "The fullness of motherhood was compressed into that day. A mother's deep love for her son, her tender concern, her exquisite pain of separation, her comforting touch for a lifetime of scraped knees, her worry for a lifetime's danger, her peace in their inseparable bond, all came together in that rich moment as she gazed upon her precious little boy."
>
> —PEDIATRICIAN ALAN GREENE, RECALLING THE EXPERIENCE OF A PATIENT WHO LOST A BABY TO TRISOMY 13 SHORTLY AFTER BIRTH

Sudden infant death syndrome

The term sudden infant death syndrome (SIDS) is used to describe the death of an infant that remains unexplained after a thorough investigation has been completed.

While there's still much we don't know about SIDS, researchers have identified some risk factors involved and have recommended some strategies for minimizing the number of SIDS-related deaths. Here's what we know so far.

Some babies face a greater risk of dying as a result of SIDS than others. The key risk factors for SIDS include prematurity (especially babies with birth weights of less than 4.4 pounds, or 2 kilograms), being a multiple as opposed to a singleton, abnormal or irregular breathing in the newborn (particularly if the baby periodically stops breathing), a minor respiratory infection in the newborn (one-third of infants who die of SIDS had a runny nose or slight cough in the two to three days prior to their deaths), being formula fed, maternal smoking or illicit drug use during pregnancy, sex (male babies are more likely to die from SIDS than female babies), ethnicity (African-American and Aboriginal babies face a greater SIDS risk), age (the peak risk period for SIDS deaths is between two and four months), the time of year (SIDS deaths are more common during the winter months than at other times of the year), and placental problems during pregnancy.

While there's nothing you can do to guarantee that your baby won't die from SIDS, there's plenty you can do to reduce the risk:

Place your baby to sleep on his back. The risk of SIDS is much higher when your baby sleeps on his front or side than on his back. The SIDS risk skyrockets if a baby who usually sleeps on his back is placed to sleep on his stomach. Note: Sleep positioners and rolled-up blankets pose a suffocation risk to babies. Your baby will get used to sleeping on his back with practice. (If he protests consistently, consult your physician. A baby who *really* hates sleeping on his back may be suffering from gastroesophageal reflux disease or GERD.) One more thing; You don't have to get up in the middle of the night to check your baby's position or to roll him back over on to his back. If he rolls himself over (a skill he'll start to master at around 5 months of age), he can stay on his tummy or side.

Create a safe sleeping environment for your baby. Make sure the mattress is firm but not soft and that the crib, bassinet, or bed where your baby will be sleeping is free of pillows and other soft bedding that could increase the risk of suffocation or cause large quantities of carbon dioxide to pool around your baby's head. (A lack of oxygen or an excess of carbon dioxide is thought to be responsible for some SIDS deaths.) Do not allow your baby to sleep on a waterbed.

Room-share with your baby during the first six months. Health Canada recommends having your baby sleep in a crib next to your bed.

Don't smoke—or allow anyone to smoke around you when you're pregnant, and don't allow anyone to smoke around your baby after the birth. Second-hand smoke doubles a baby's chances of dying from SIDS, while babies whose mothers smoked during pregnancy are three times as likely to succumb to SIDS.

Don't allow your baby to become overheated. Some studies have shown that infants who are overdressed or bundled in too many blankets may face a greater risk of SIDS.

Breastfeed your baby. Some research has found that breastfeeding may help to reduce the risk of losing a baby to SIDS.

Two excellent sources of information and support to grieving parents are the Canadian Foundation for the Study of Infant Deaths (www.sidscanada.org) and the Canadian Infant Safe Sleep Project (@CdnInfSafeSleep on Twitter).

Grieving the Loss of Your Baby

Grief is painful. As you begin to come to terms with the fact that your pregnancy has ended and your baby has died, you may find yourself experiencing some of the following physical and emotional symptoms of grief: thoughts of the baby you lost, irritability, restlessness, anxiety, fear, yearning, hopelessness, confusion, shortness of breath, tightness in the throat, fatigue, crying spells, an empty feeling in your abdomen, sleeplessness, a change in appetite, heart palpitations, and other physical symptoms of anxiety. Some bereaved parents experience some additional symptoms: empty, aching arms and having illusions about seeing, hearing, or feeling the presence of the baby.

You may feel shocked that this has happened, and overwhelmed by the extent of your grief. You may feel as though you're going through the motions of everyday living even though your mind is preoccupied with the task of making sense of something that makes no sense at all. You may also find yourself denying that your baby has died or wishing desperately that he hadn't, blaming yourself or others for his death, and coping with feelings of depression and despair.

Some parents who have lost a baby are afraid to work through their grief, believing that doing so will enable them to move on and cause them to forget about the baby they lost. Here are some reassuring words from Deborah Davis, Ph.D., author of *Empty Cradle, Broken Heart*: "You will never forget your baby. Many people mistakenly believe that resolution means you stop grieving, forget about the baby, and meekly abandon your baby to death. To the contrary, grief does not end. You will always feel some sadness and wish that things could have turned out better. But, with time, the denial, failure, guilt and anger fade; the sadness becomes manageable . . . The peaceful feelings that come with resolution are a blessed change from the ravages of grief."

Here are some suggestions on surviving the first few weeks and months after the death of your baby:

- Be prepared to make some difficult decisions. If you are experiencing a miscarriage, you may be asked to decide whether you prefer to miscarry naturally at home or go to the hospital for a D&C. If your baby is stillborn or dies shortly after birth, you'll have to decide whether to have an autopsy performed and what to do about a baptism, burial, memorial service, and so on. If you're worried that you won't be able to afford to bury your child properly, talk to your doctor or midwife about burial options for families in your situation. You may find that a local funeral home offers a significant discount or waives its fees entirely for families who have lost a child.

- Plan to spend some time with your baby after the death. In addition to holding and dressing your baby, you might want to take some photographs of her in your arms, in your partner's arms, with other special people in your life (such as her grandparents or her siblings), and, in the case of a twin pregnancy, with her surviving twin. These photos may become some of your most treasured mementos of the time you spent with your baby.

- Find ways to collect other memories of your pregnancy or your baby's short life. You might want to start a scrapbook and include cards you received when you found out you were pregnant, pictures of yourself when you were pregnant, and so on. Or you may decide to write a letter to your baby, reflecting on the joys of your pregnancy and letting your baby know how much she is missed.

- Recognize that there's no one "right" way to grieve. You may spend a lot of time crying or you may find that you feel numb and frozen. Your grief may come in waves or it may be with you 24 hours a day. There's no such thing as "normal" when it comes to grief. "Keep one thing that belonged to your baby or that you bought for your baby, suggests Liz, a 36-year-old mother of four who has experienced four miscarriages. "If you can, take a picture of your baby so that when you're grieving . . . you'll have something tangible to hold on to and cry with."

- Accept the fact that your partner may grieve differently from you. Don't automatically assume that he's less affected by the loss just because he's less willing to express his emotions. Many bereaved fathers feel tremendous pressure to "hold it together" when their partners are falling apart. Because fathers tend to be less verbal about their grief, their grief has been underestimated in grief research. A 2002 study conducted by researchers at the University of Queensland in Australia found that grief in fathers tends to peak around 30 months after the death of a baby, whether that baby is stillborn or whether that baby dies shortly after birth. And understand that sex may either bring comfort to one or both of you right now, or act as a painful reminder of your loss. It's important to keep communicating as you work through the potential minefield of emotions surrounding your loss. Shutting out your partner will only add to the loneliness of grief.

- Find ways of involving your living children in the grieving process. They may wish to help pick out flowers for the funeral bouquet or to draw a picture for the baby who died. It's important to explain what's happening to even very young children. They will pick up on your emotions and sense that something has gone wrong. They need to know that they are safe and that you and the family will be okay: you're just sad about the baby who died. The way you handle this loss with them will begin to set the stage for the way future losses are handled within your family.

- Understand that some children avoid expressing their feelings of grief openly, for fear of upsetting their parents. Others become very clingy, reacting out of fear that something could happen to you. Some will respond with attention-seeking behaviours, sensing (quite rightly) that your attention is elsewhere right now. Girls aged 7 to 12 who had strongly identified with their mother's pregnancy are especially likely to want to "fix" their mother's grief. They may feel the loss of the baby particularly acutely or may fear for their own death. Children who may have expressed feelings that they may regret now (such as negative feelings toward the pregnancy or the baby) need to be given an opportunity to work through any feelings of guilt they may be harbouring. Children who have lost a baby sibling suffer in other ways as well. At the very time they need their parents most, their grieving parents may be emotionally treading water themselves.

breast symptoms after a loss

If your baby is stillborn or dies shortly after birth or after breastfeeding has already been established, you'll have to cope with breast engorgement (overly full and uncomfortable breasts). Having milk leaking from your breasts after your baby has died can be both physically and emotionally stressful. You may feel as though your entire body is mourning the loss of your baby—which, in fact, it is. The period of engorgement tends to last for about 48 hours, but it could last for up to a week. You can relieve your breast tenderness in the meantime by expressing a small amount of milk. (Don't express too much or your body will start producing more milk.) Binding your breasts tightly, applying ice packs or cabbage leaves to your breasts, and wearing a snug bra at all times can also help to reduce your discomfort. Note: If you notice red, warm, hard, or tender areas in your breasts; develop a fever of more than 37.8°C (100°F), notice that the lymph nodes under your arms are becoming uncomfortable, or feel generally ill, it could be because you're developing a breast infection. Contact your doctor or midwife to talk about treatment options.

- Don't forget that grandparents grieve, too. They grieve the death of their grandchild and they hurt because their children are hurting. Sometimes a bereaved grandmother will try to "shut down" her daughter's grief—an indication of her own feelings about the power of grief and the fact that women are vulnerable to suffer losses like stillbirth.

- Let family and friends know how they can be helpful to you. Tell them that their phone calls and visits are important to you: grief is lonely. Let them know what you would appreciate most right now: personal visits, daily phone calls, someone to run errands for you (or with you), someone to help you with chores at home. And thank them for their patience and support.

- Families need some time to grieve in privacy—some time and space to process their loss without a constant stampede of visitors. This needs to be balanced with the need for care and support from the community.

- If you still have questions about what happened, set up an appointment with your doctor or midwife to go over your medical records so that you can find out as much as possible about what went wrong. Include your partner in this follow-up appointment so that he/she can also benefit from this sharing of information and express his/her feelings of loss.

- Take care of your physical needs as well as your emotional ones. Get the sleep you need, exercise regularly, and make a point of eating nutritious, well-balanced meals. Don't forget that you'll also need time to recover from the delivery if your baby was miscarried or stillborn, or died shortly after birth. If you had a miscarriage, you'll need about six weeks to physically recover from the experience. If your baby was stillborn or died shortly after birth, you can expect to experience all the usual postpartum discomforts associated with a vaginal or Caesarean delivery on top of trying to cope with your grief.

- Resist the temptation to bury your grief by turning to alcohol or prescription drugs or by throwing yourself into your work and refusing to face your feelings. You can't avoid working through your grief—you can only postpone it. Grief is patient; it will wait for you.

- Find ways to honour your baby's memory. You might wish to make a donation to a charity in your baby's name, light a candle on special days and holidays, plant a tree or small garden, create a piece of art, or invite friends to come together to help you to remember your baby in a way that is meaningful to you.

- Reach out for support from other women who have experienced the loss

"I had known women who had suffered miscarriages, but I never knew how painful it was until I went through it. It took months to 'get over' it. I cried so much and was so desperately sad. It was horrible. I asked my midwife to collect all the medical records from the ER and OR and I made an appointment at the hospital records department to read through my chart to see what the doctors and nurses had found. To see what might have caused the miscarriage or to see exactly what was wrong. I spoke with the obstetrician who did the D&C and with my midwife and no one could tell me anything. It was just 'one of those things.' I think the worst part was not knowing how it happened or why."

—LORI, 29, MOTHER OF FOUR

of a baby. Lori, a 29-year-old mother of four who's also been through a miscarriage, feels that support groups have a lot to offer: "There are so many shoulders to cry on—so many people to listen to. And it helps tremendously when you can help another person," she explains.

- Be prepared for insensitive comments from people who fail to understand the extent of your grief. "Don't let anyone tell you you'll 'get over it,'" insists Lori, whose daughter was stillborn at 26 weeks due to intrauterine growth restriction. "You never get over it. You just learn—gradually—to live with your loss. In time, it does get easier to cope with day-to-day life, but you never, ever forget."

- Don't be afraid to reach out for professional help if you find your feelings of grief overwhelming, if you are becoming depressed or extremely anxious, or if you are experiencing some of the symptoms of post-traumatic stress disorder in the wake of your baby's death. Researchers in the Netherlands found that the prevalence of PTSD in women experiencing pregnancy loss was 25 per cent one month after their loss and 7 per cent four months after their loss.

- Understand that there is no statute of limitations on grief. Your grief doesn't magically disappear after a certain period of time. "Childbearing losses may affect women and their families for a lifetime. The effects of childbearing losses may occur well after the childbearing years have ended," notes the Wisconsin Association for Perinatal Care. But, over time, your grief ceases to be crippling. You learn to live with grief. It becomes part of your life story.

- Remind yourself that you have the strength to get through this—that as painful as it is to have to say goodbye to a baby you desperately wanted, you can survive this heartbreak. As hard as it may be for you to believe right now, you will find joy in your life again. Researchers at Millersville University in Pennsylvania found that the majority of bereaved parents describe their child's death as precipitating a crisis in meaning that resulted in stronger connections with other people, desire to engage in activities that would give their child's life and death meaning, enriched beliefs and values, personal growth, and feelings of connection with the child who had died.

Preparing for Another Pregnancy

It takes courage to start trying again when your previous pregnancy has ended in heartbreak. As you know only too well, there are no guarantees when it comes to conception, pregnancy, and birth.

Your doctor or midwife will likely suggest that you give yourself time to heal before you embark on another pregnancy. If you had a miscarriage or an uncomplicated vaginal delivery, you'll likely be advised to wait until you've had at least one normal menstrual cycle before you start trying to conceive. This will help to reduce your chances of experiencing a miscarriage since, if you conceive right away, your uterine lining may not have had the chance to build back up to healthy levels again. If you had a Caesarean section, on the other hand, you'll be advised to wait for six months before you start trying to conceive again. It takes a couple of months for your uterine scar to heal, and becoming pregnant too quickly could increase your odds of experiencing a uterine rupture or other complications during your subsequent pregnancy. And if your baby died as the result of a birth defect, you may want to consider consulting with a genetic counsellor before you start trying to conceive again.

You can't base your decision about whether or not to start trying again on physical factors alone, however. You also need to assess your emotional readiness for another pregnancy. That means considering whether you've had the opportunity to work through some of your grief, whether you'd be able to cope if you were to have trouble conceiving or experience another loss, whether you're ready to cope with the stress of a subsequent pregnancy (a major consideration if your next pregnancy is likely to be classified as high risk), whether you actually want another baby—or whether what you really want is the baby who died, and how your partner feels about trying again.

You may be eager to start trying again right away, or you may decide that it's important for you to let certain key milestones pass before you become pregnant again—the due date of the baby you lost, the anniversary of your baby's death, and so on. You'll find a detailed discussion of these issues in my book (with John R. Sussman, MD) *Trying Again: A Guide to Pregnancy After Miscarriage, Stillbirth, and Infant Loss.*

Getting pregnant again won't make all your worries go away. In fact, it'll make a whole bunch of new worries appear on the horizon! Here are some tips on weathering the emotional highs and lows of pregnancy after a loss:

- Be prepared to experience a range of emotions—everything from joy at being pregnant again, to fear that something could go wrong this time too, to guilt at "betraying" the baby you lost by moving on with your life. You may also have strong feelings about conceiving a baby of a particular sex—feelings that may be difficult to admit even to yourself.

- Surround yourself with people who are prepared to support you during your subsequent pregnancy. You might wish to join a pregnancy-after-loss support group (if there's one available in your community) or an on-line support group. At the very least, you should arrange for a friend or family member to accompany you to your prenatal appointments and/or ultrasound appointments in case you need some additional support.

- Make sure you've got a supportive caregiver. You need a doctor or midwife who will understand that you'll likely need extra reassurance—and perhaps even extra prenatal visits—this time around. If you're not getting that kind of care and support from your current caregiver, it's time to consider making a change.

- Find out as much as you can about the cause of your previous loss and what, if anything, can be done to prevent the problem from recurring this time around. The more knowledge you have about the medical aspects of your pregnancy, the more in control you'll feel.

- Accept the fact that this pregnancy will be different. Some parents who have been through a loss are more guarded in sharing their news with other people the next time around. Some prefer not to have a baby shower until after their baby has arrived safely—and others are afraid to shop for Baby, set up the baby's room, or choose a name for Baby until the very end of pregnancy, fearing that not waiting might somehow jinx the pregnancy. If you have other children, they may also avoid growing attached to the new baby for fear that the family will be devastated by another loss—and they may feel guilty for feeling this way.

- Fathers who have had babies that died prior to birth tend to experience an overwhelming sense of relief once they have had a chance to hold their healthy newborn. For them, the period of anxious waiting is over. Mothers, on the other hand, tend to continue to crave reassurance that the baby is really okay and to feel anxious about anything else that could harm their newborn. This period of heightened anxiety can continue through the peak risk period for SIDS (2 to 4 months of age) and, for some mothers, it becomes part of their approach to parenting: hypervigilance.

• Nearly all mothers report that the birth of the new baby helped them with their feelings of grief, and nearly all couples who welcomed a new baby after a loss report increased closeness and less conflict following the birth.

• Take things day by day—hour by hour, if you have to. Rather than dwelling on the fact that there are 40 weeks of pregnancy ahead of you, focus on achieving the next milestone—making it to the end of the first trimester, passing the point at which you lost your previous baby, and so on. Cyndie, a 35-year-old mother of two, found that taking this approach was the only thing that kept her sane when she became pregnant again after experiencing three consecutive losses: "It was like holding your breath for nine months, afraid to breathe, afraid to let your guard down," she recalls. "Every waking moment was lived literally from moment to moment. Every internal twinge or sensation signalled a rush of adrenaline as a surge of panic raced through my bloodstream. How I lived through nine months' worth of seconds like this I still have no idea. I guess because I never allowed myself to live in the future. Every day, every hour, even every minute, was only that and nothing more."

• Expect certain milestones to be particularly tough: the anniversary of your previous baby's due date or death, the week of pregnancy when you lost your previous baby, and so on. You might want to

hand-held Dopplers

Thinking about renting or buying a hand-held Doppler so you can hear your baby's heartbeat whenever you need some added reassurance? Some health-care providers have started to advise against their use, citing a report published in the *British Medical Journal* in 2009 in which a mother-to-be postponed seeking medical care after using such a device, with tragic consequences for her baby. (It is much easier to pick up the mother's heartbeat or blood flow through the placenta than it is to detect the baby's heart rate.)

schedule your prenatal visit around this time so that you'll have the reassurance you crave when you need it most.

- Rather than focusing on all the scary things that could go wrong, try to remain positive. The majority of couples who have experienced miscarriage, stillbirth, or infant death go on to give birth to healthy babies the next time around.

"When Renée was born—five and a half years after the birth of my first child, and following three losses—she brought me completion. She gave me pure satisfaction and joy. I smile inside every day. She alone numbs the pain of my losses and makes three and a half years of hell worth every step. I'd do it all again if I knew she'd be the reward. Now I take nothing for granted and I enjoy every moment with my children. They are my priority, my happiness, my life."

—CYNDIE, 35, MOTHER OF TWO

CHAPTER 10

Labour Day

"I think that nine months is the perfect length for pregnancy. By the end, you want to be able to move around easily again and you're so excited and eager to hold your baby."

—CHRIS, 36, MOTHER OF THREE

Starting to feel as though you're going to be pregnant forever? Convinced that you're destined to spend the rest of your days coping with insomnia, back pain, and the other third-trimester discomforts? The good news is you're in the home stretch now. At some point over the next few weeks, your baby will get tired of using your bladder as a trampoline and will decide it's time to be born.

In this chapter we're going to talk about the things you're likely to be most concerned about at this stage of the game: the physical changes you can expect to experience as your body prepares for labour, what to bring to the hospital (if that's where you'll be giving birth), the decisions you'll have to make that will affect the type of birth you have, why you might want to use the services of a doula (a professional labour support person), what a birth plan can—and can't—do for you, what you can do to reduce the odds that you'll experience perineal tearing, what types of comfort measures and pain relief options you may wish to draw upon during labour, how to tell if you're in labour (and the answers to other questions that may be worrying you), how to stay sane if you go overdue, what to expect if your labour is induced, what to expect from a vaginal delivery and a Caesarean delivery, the facts about vaginal birth after Caesarean (VBAC), and what those first moments after the birth may be like.

Eight Months and Counting

While you might feel as though you're in a bit of a holding pattern, waiting for your baby to make his or her grand entrance, there's actually a lot going on inside your body. Here are just a few of the physical changes and sensations you might notice as your baby's birthday approaches:

- Your baby may be doing fewer somersaults than she was a few weeks ago. While a reduction in the number of fetal movements can indicate a possible problem, don't be too concerned if the movements simply become a bit less vigorous and more like rolling than kicking. That's pretty standard at this stage of the game. If you're worried, however, check in with your caregiver. That's why you've got her number programmed into your cellphone, after all.
- You may be experiencing a lot of pain underneath your ribs. Since she can no longer amuse herself by doing somersaults, your baby's doing some heavy-duty stretching instead. Unfortunately, once she moves into the head-down position (the position that 97 per cent of babies assume before labour), what she likes pushing against most with her feet is the area just underneath your ribs. Fun for her: not so fun for you.
- You may feel some sudden, darting movements. Your baby may be vigorously rooting around, trying to get her thumb back in her mouth (yes, that thumb-sucking habit often starts before birth), or she may have gulped back enough amniotic fluid to give herself the hiccups.
- You may feel as though your pelvic floor muscles are supporting a cantaloupe. And, frankly, that's not far off the mark. Once your baby descends into your pelvis (which can happen a few weeks ahead of time or right as labour begins), her head begins pressing against your perineum, which can make walking and even sitting rather uncomfortable. You may also notice an odd buzzing sensation—like either a mild electric shock or a tickle. This occurs as your baby raises and lowers her head against your pelvic floor muscles, and can be more than a little disconcerting.
- You may feel increased pressure in your pelvis and rectum during the last month of pregnancy. This can result in abdominal cramping, groin

pain, and persistent lower backache. Note: You're more likely to experience this particular symptom if this is your second or subsequent baby.

- You may find that your breathlessness decreases, but that annoying urge to urinate every hour on the hour returns. You may also find yourself experiencing a variety of other pregnancy complaints: sciatica, varicose veins, hemorrhoids, and stretch marks. (See Chapter 7 for the lowdown on these common late-pregnancy symptoms.)

- Your Braxton Hicks contractions may become increasingly uncomfortable—and perhaps even painful. These practice contractions, which can feel like a gigantic blood pressure cuff around your belly, are busy preparing your body for the hard work that awaits it when "labour day" arrives. Note: Some childbirth instructors no longer talk about Braxton Hicks contractions, arguing that every type of contraction that occurs prior to the onset of actual labour is a practice contraction, and that it doesn't make sense to differentiate between Braxton Hicks contractions and the pre-labour contractions that occur in late pregnancy. Frankly, it's an argument that makes a lot of sense. I've left the term Braxton Hicks in this edition of the book, but it may disappear in future revisions.

- Your eating habits may change. You may find you need smaller, more frequent meals rather than several large meals each day. Crowded conditions inside your body prevent your stomach from holding a lot of food at one time.

- You may feel more—or less—energetic. Some women get a burst of energy as labour approaches (that much-talked-about nesting instinct). Others are reluctant to do anything more ambitious than lifting their head off the couch. Both reactions are perfectly normal, so don't assume you're never going to go into labour just because you've got absolutely no urge to clean out all your closets.

- You may lose weight. Even though your baby is still packing on the pounds, your weight may drop by a pound or two during the last month of your pregnancy. This is because the total amount of amniotic fluid in your body is decreasing—a change triggered by the hormonal fluctuations of late pregnancy—and because crowded conditions around your stomach may make it difficult for you to eat as much as you usually do.

You may also notice that your emotional state changes. Even if you've been thoroughly enjoying your pregnancy, you may find yourself becoming irritable and impatient: eager to get on with the show. This whole business of being pregnant has long since lost its novelty, and you're ready to meet your baby.

And then there's the business of the impending labour—something that can have you tossing and turning at 3:00 a.m., wondering what on earth you were thinking when you decided to get pregnant eight months ago.

As your baby's birthday approaches, you may find that you become increasingly introspective, more tuned in to what's going on with your baby and less interested in the world around you. Be sure to treasure this special time before the birth, says Lori, a 29-year-old mother of four. "Enjoy every minute you have your baby to yourself because once the baby enters the world, life becomes a little chaotic and time flies by. When your baby is still being held inside your womb, you can sit back, relax, and appreciate the bond you already have with your child."

Pre-labour symptoms

Despite what the movies would have you believe, labour seldom kicks off with gut-wrenching contractions at two-minute intervals. Most of us experience at least a bit of pre-labour pain to warn us that labour day isn't far off. Unfortunately, this pre-labour can hurt as much as the early stages of the real thing, and—to add insult to injury—it doesn't even guarantee labour any time soon. Does Mother Nature have a twisted sense of humour or what?

That said, you still need to be aware of the classic symptoms of pre-labour. They may not guarantee you'll have your baby today, but they sure as heck indicate that the big day is fast approaching. Here's what to look out for:

- Your baby drops. At some point during the last few weeks of pregnancy, you may notice that instead of being pressed against your lungs, your baby is now sitting on your bladder. If you check out your profile in the mirror, you'll see that the change can be quite dramatic. While a first-time mother's baby typically drops sometime during the two weeks leading up to delivery, many women giving birth for the second or subsequent time find their babies don't drop until labour actually starts. (This is because the mother's pelvic muscles have already been stretched during a previous pregnancy, so there's not the same need for a pre-game workout.) Just a quick footnote on terminology before we move on: the terms "dropping," "lightening," and "engagement" are used pretty much interchangeably. So if your doctor or midwife happens to say that your baby's head is engaged, it means your baby has dropped.
- Your pre-labour contractions (sometimes called Braxton Hicks

contractions) become stronger. Instead of feeling like a mild tightening sensation, they're starting to resemble menstrual cramps. While they aren't as strong as the contractions you'll feel during labour, they're effective nonetheless. Their job is to thin out (or efface) your cervix, changing it from a thick-walled cone to a thin-walled cup so that it'll be ready to start dilating (opening up) when you actually go into labour. In women who are giving birth for the second or subsequent time, effacement and dilatation occur simultaneously.

- You may have a lower backache that you can't relieve by changing position.
- You'll experience some diarrhea and possibly some nausea. As your body prepares for labour, your hormones trigger abdominal cramps that cause loose, frequent bowel movements—nature's way of emptying your intestines before labour begins. Unfortunately, these hormones can leave you feeling a bit nauseated. In fact, you might (wrongly) conclude that you're coming down with a touch of the stomach flu.
- Your vaginal discharge thickens. You may notice more egg white or pink-tinged vaginal discharge as labour day approaches. This is caused by hormonal changes rather than the cervical dilation that is responsible for the "bloody show."
- You may experience some "bloody show." This is the name given to the blood-streaked mucus that typically passes out of the vagina as the cervix begins to dilate. This mucus plug seals the cervix during pregnancy, protecting your baby from infection. The mucus becomes streaked with blood as some of the tiny blood vessels in your cervix break as your cervix thins. The mucus typically has a pink or brownish tinge. The passage of the mucus plug typically indicates that your labour will start within the next three days, but some women do manage to hang on for another week or two. Passing your bloody show isn't painful, despite what you might think, given its rather alarming name. In fact, if it passes gradually, you might not even notice that you've passed it at all. Note: If there seems to be a lot of blood and not much mucus you could be experiencing potentially serious complications and will need to notify your caregiver immediately.
- You may experience a premature rupture of membranes (the rupture of your bag of waters prior to the onset of labour). Approximately 10 per cent of women experience the rupturing of their membranes before they're actually in labour. If this happens to you, you can expect your labour to begin within the next few hours or at least within the next day. Due to

the risk of infection, your caregiver may want to induce you if your membranes have ruptured and you haven't gone into labour. Whether or not you'll be induced will depend on how much amniotic fluid has been lost and how close you are to your due date. Note: You should avoid baths and sexual intercourse once your membranes have ruptured.

By the time this period of pre-labour has ended you'll be approximately 1 to 2 centimetres dilated. You're ready for active labour to begin.

> "The most unusual thing I brought with me to the hospital was a Tupperware rolling pin. You can fill these with liquid, so I was able to put hot or cold water in it and have my coaches roll it over my back. I had a lot of lower back and hip pain, so it saved my coaches' hands and gave me the exact pressure I wanted over an entire section of my back at a time."
>
> —DOROTHY, 33, MOTHER OF TWO

Decision Time

Your coffee table is overflowing with pregnancy books and your fridge is plastered with pamphlets about various aspects of prenatal health. Sometimes you feel as though you've read enough to earn your Ph.D. in motherhood!

Well, believe it or not, you're not finished hitting the books yet. You've still got a few more important issues to read up on before Baby arrives, namely, types of births, doulas, birth plans, and pain relief during labour.

Pre-birth planning

A lot of people don't figure out the connection between birth and what comes afterward until a few months, even years, after the fact. It's only when they have the luxury of a good night's sleep and a spare moment for retrospection that they start to see the links between what happened during labour and birth and how the first few days, weeks, and months played out for them as a family.

It only makes sense. If you embark on motherhood exhausted, in pain, and with a newborn who is having a difficult time figuring out how to breastfeed, you may find the early days of parenthood a lot more challenging than another mother who is more euphoric than tired after she gives birth, who is achy and sore rather than in pain, and whose baby takes to the breast like she's been watching breastfeeding videos in utero.

Some of what happens after the birth comes down to luck, good or bad.

(You can't order a baby of a particular temperament or control everything that happens during labour and birth.) But some decisions that come up while you are in labour will be within your control. What you won't realize, unless you do your homework ahead of time, is how much hinges on each of those decisions. Each time you say yes or no to a particular birth intervention or procedure, you're making a choice that could have implications for the type of labour and birth you experience, and how the postpartum period plays out for your family. It's an important point to keep in mind as you make your way through this section and the remainder of this chapter.

Choices that affect the type of birth you will have

Where you give birth. The types of birthing policies that are in place and the types of medical technology that are available vary from one setting to another (hospital, birth centre, home). Choose a birth setting that supports your philosophies about birth and where you will feel comfortable and relaxed giving birth. For some women, that will be at home. For others, that will be in a birth centre (where birth centres are available) or in a hospital.

Note: If you are planning to give birth at home or at a birth centre, but unanticipated complications arise, you will need to give birth in hospital. According to the Society of Obstetricians and Gynaecologists of Canada (SOGC), the most common reasons for maternal transport during labour include preterm labour, preterm rupture of membranes, severe gestational hypertension, hemorrhage, multiple birth, intrauterine growth restriction, fetal abnormalities, inadequate progress during labour, malpresentation, and maternal trauma.

---

planned home birth

Planned home birth is safe for women who are at low risk of complications and who are in the care of licensed midwives with access to a nearby hospital. That was the conclusion of a major Canadian study of home birth published on the *Canadian Medical Association Journal* website on August 31, 2009.

The study compared the outcomes of 2,889 planned home births attended by registered midwives in British Columbia during the years 2000 to 2004 to the outcomes of midwife-attended and physician-attended hospital births occurring over the same time period.

Here are the key findings of the study:

- 78.8 per cent of the women in the group who were intending to give birth at home had a planned home birth, and 96.9 per cent of the women in the group who were intending to give birth in the hospital with a midwife in attendance had a planned hospital birth.

- There were no significant differences between the planned home-birth group and either comparison group in terms of the health of the baby after birth. Factors tracked included a diagnosis of asphyxia at birth, Apgar scores of less than 7 during the five minutes after the birth, seizures, or the need for assisted ventilation beyond the first 24 hours of life.

- Women in the planned home-birth group were significantly less likely than those who planned a midwife-attended hospital birth to receive obstetric interventions or to experience maternal complications such as a third- or fourth-degree perineal tear or a postpartum hemorrhage. The findings were similar when the planned home-birth group was compared to physician-assisted hospital births.

- Newborns in the home-birth group were less likely than those in the midwife-attended hospital-birth group to require resuscitation at birth or oxygen therapy beyond 24 hours. The findings were similar as compared to newborns in the physician-delivered hospital births.

- The rate of perinatal death per 1,000 births was lower for the planned home-birth group (0.35 for the planned home-birth group as compared to 0.57 for hospital births attended by a midwife and 0.64 for hospital births attended by a physician).

The researchers pointed out that further research is required before anyone can reach the definitive conclusion that a planned home birth is as safe as a hospital birth. They noted that women who opt for home birth versus hospital birth may have already assessed some of their obstetrical risk factors, something that would prevent women in the two groups from being totally comparable:

"We cannot exclude the possibility that differences in findings between the groups were attributable to unmeasured characteristics of the women who chose home birth. Although our study cohorts were closely matched on prognostic variables, we do not underestimate the degree of self-selection that takes place in a population of women choosing home birth. This self-selection may be an important component of risk management for home birth."

Only a randomized control study (where women are randomly assigned to the home-birth group or the hospital group) would produce two such groups. Still, in the absence of the perfect study, the researchers conclude that planned home birth is safe for women who are at low risk of complications and who are in the care of "appropriately qualified and licensed midwives with access to timely transfer to hospital if required."

Your labour and birth support team. Choose a health-care provider (doctor or midwife) who is in sync with your philosophies about childbirth, who anticipates and answers your questions, and who provides you with referrals to pregnancy, birth, breastfeeding, and motherhood-related services and supports in your local community. If you don't have the luxury of choice (and in some parts of Canada, it is a luxury), you may find yourself having to work with a caregiver you would not otherwise have chosen. If you're not on the same page when it comes to your ideas about pregnancy and birth, you may want to bring someone with you to your appointments to support you as you advocate for yourself. If it's more of a personality clash, remind yourself that you don't have to love this person (although it's a lot more pleasant if you and your caregiver "click"): you simply need to work together well, and to focus on the same shared goal: ensuring that you and your baby receive the best possible care. Once again, you may find it works well to bring someone else along to your appointments to help ease the tension between you and Dr. Not-Quite-Right.

Round out your labour and birth support team with a supportive labour partner and, if possible, a labour doula (see the following section) who will be able to help you to develop the skills to advocate for yourself and provide you with emotional support when the going gets tough. (Having continuous emotional and physical support during labour from a doula or other professional labour support person makes a huge difference for labouring women and their families. Receiving comfort and encouragement as well as information about what is happening during the birth increases the odds of a vaginal birth, decreases the likelihood that an epidural will be required or that a baby will need to be resuscitated after birth, and improves breastfeeding outcomes. Women who do not benefit from this type of support during labour are less likely to feel supported during labour, to feel prepared for parenthood, and to discuss postpartum concerns and problems with their caregivers.)

Your ability to trust your body. Fear is your greatest enemy as a labouring woman. If you can trust your body, you will have the confidence to ask your caregiver if certain procedures are medically necessary (or simply being ordered because the caregivers in that practice have gotten in the habit of ordering them for every pregnant woman). You will also feel much more satisfied about your birth experience if it turns out that your birth doesn't go exactly as you had hoped. (The more involved you are in making informed choices about each aspect of your care, the more in control you will feel about your birth experience, regardless of how things actually play out. It's when women feel that they surrendered control, or that they were poorly informed about the choices available to them, that are the least satisfied about their birth experience.) Here are a few examples of labour policies and medical interventions you may wish to discuss with your caregiver in advance, and why:

- **Labour induction:** In most cases, your body knows when your baby is ready to be born. If labour is induced artificially, your body and your baby may not be ready, and there is an increased risk that other interventions will be required (labour augmentation, for example). Of course, in some situations, labour induction is medically necessary because either the mother or the baby is at risk. That changes everything. What I'm talking about here is inducing labour because someone is becoming antsy about getting that baby delivered, even though there's no justifiable medical reason to induce labour now.

- **Diagnosis of dysfunctional labour:** Dystocia (ineffective or dysfunctional labour) is a word you don't want to see on your labour chart—particularly if it ends up being there for no good reason. If you end up being admitted to the hospital before you are 3 centimetres dilated, the odds are good that someone will decide at some point that your labour isn't progressing as fast as it should, or that it is otherwise dysfunctional. (Dystocia tends to be diagnosed during the latent phase of labour—when you're not yet into active labour—and up to 40 per cent of Caesareans for labour dystocia are performed at this time.) A better alternative is to do more of your labouring at home. That way, by the time you check into the birthing unit, you'll be well in active labour and no one will have time to worry about how functional your labour is. Things will be chugging right along.

- **Augmentation of labour:** Every labour is unique. It simply takes some babies a little longer to be born than others. Speeding up labour with

thinking about a midwife?

If you are planning to have a home birth, you should aim to make contact with a midwife as soon as you find out you are pregnant. There are far more women who hope to have midwife-attended home births than there are midwives available, and midwifery is not yet regulated in all Canadian provinces and territories. According to the Canadian Association of Midwives, "Midwifery is recognized as a legal and regulated profession in some Canadian provinces and territories while in others it is not yet regulated. Check with your provincial or territorial ministry of health to inquire about the current status of midwifery in your province or territory."

Pitocin (the synthetic form of oxytocin) increases the likelihood that you'll end up requiring additional labour interventions. If Pitocin is introduced too early in labour (dilation of less than 5 centimetres or when contractions are coming 3 to 5 minutes apart), there is a greater risk for Caesarean due to failure to progress.

- **Pain relief methods:** Choose pain relief methods that allow you to remain mobile during labour. You want gravity (the pressure of the baby's presenting part on your cervix) and biology (your pelvis opens up considerably when you are performing squats and lunges or sitting on a birthing ball) on your side. There are also other benefits to opting for non-pharmacologic pain relief methods, such as labouring in water, massage, cold and hot compresses, and focused breathing: both you and your baby will be awake and ready to make the most of the period of wakefulness that newborns enjoy shortly after the birth.

- **Fetal monitoring during labour:** Having your baby's heartbeat monitored intermittently (using a fetoscope or a hand-held Doppler) as opposed to continuously (by an electronic fetal monitor) will free you up so you can move around or take advantage of the pain-relief benefits of labouring in the shower or a birthing tub. What's more, routine continuous electronic fetal monitoring during low-risk labours increases the likelihood of an instrumental vaginal delivery or a Caesarean section being required, while failing to reduce rates of low Apgar scores (used to evaluate the health of your newborn), stillbirth and newborn death rates, admissions to special care nurseries, or the incidence of cerebral palsy. According to the SOGC, if emergency Caesarean sections were performed whenever a non-reassuring fetal heart rate reading was obtained from a low-risk mother, in 99 per cent of cases, the baby would be found to be doing just fine. This is because tests like continuous electronic fetal monitoring (EFM) have a very poor positive predictive value (ability to accurately detect actual problems without falsely flagging non-problems as potential emergencies) when they are used during low-risk labours. For this reason, the SOGC does not recommend the use of continuous EFM during low-risk labour. (On the other hand, women who are being induced, are experiencing high-risk labours, or have used pain medications should have continuous EFM. Some hospitals offer wireless telemetry, which provides continuous EFM but allows you to stay mobile and even go into the shower.)

- Touch base with your doctor or midwife to let her know what's happening. Ditto for your doula. (Your doula will want to know how you're coping and when you'd like her to come over to provide some in-person support.)
- Slip into comfortable, loose-fitting clothing. Clothing that is tight or too restrictive will add to your discomfort.
- Get as much rest as you can during early labour. Sure, you're excited, but rather than wearing yourself out too early on in this process, nap or relax while you can. When the contractions are coming fast and furious later on, you'll be grateful for any sleep you stockpiled during early labour.
- Keep your energy up in other ways. Graze on light snacks that are easy to digest, and keep yourself well hydrated, too.
- Focus on staying calm and centred. Keep the lights low and the noise level down, and let the phone screen your calls.
- As your contractions become more challenging, start experimenting with various types of pain relief methods (see "Pain relief during labour" later in this chapter). You may find that changing your position (a birthing ball or a V-shaped pillow can be useful to have around), having a warm shower or bath, or having your partner apply counter pressure to your back provide a great deal of relief.

- **Birthing positions:** Giving birth in any position other than on your back (or, worse, with your feet in stirrups) will make a huge difference in the effectiveness of your pushing contractions and your ability to work with—not against—gravity. If you adopt a sitting, squatting, standing, side-lying, or on-all-fours birthing position—try them all to find the one that works best for you—you'll find the pushing stage much easier. It's also important to be patient, to wait for the urge to push to kick in naturally (as opposed to allowing other people to coach you into pushing before you feel that urge, which is totally counterproductive). Otherwise, you may end up trying to push your baby through the pelvic bones. If you wait until the baby is through the pelvis, you only have to push a bit to get the baby through the vaginal opening. It all comes down to trusting your body and its ability to provide you with the cues you need to do what comes naturally. It's been doing that with all other biological functions all your life. Why would it fail you now?
- **Newborn policies:** Enjoying skin-to-skin contact with your baby right after the birth is good for you and your newborn. Your body helps to keep your baby warm and to regulate his heartbeat and breathing. And

the weight of your baby on your abdomen helps to stimulate uterine contractions (gentle ones, don't worry), something that helps with the process of involution (the shrinking down of the uterus) and the expulsion of the placenta. You'll also have the opportunity to gaze into your baby's eyes (and see him gaze back), respond to your baby's hard-wired feeding cues (he'll make his way to the breast on his own, if given enough time), and to get breastfeeding off to a good start. Let your health-care provider know that it's important to you that your baby remain with you as much as possible immediately after the birth. Many newborn checks and exams can be done while your baby is on your chest. Others can be delayed until after this initial period of mom-and-baby togetherness. Let your health-care provider know that you want your baby to be accompanied by your partner or another support person if he has to go to the special care nursery or another area of the hospital for tests or treatment after the birth.

- **Cord clamping:** The placenta continues to transfer oxygenated blood, nutrients, and stem cells for several minutes after the birth. A 2007 study published in the *Journal of the American Medical Association* found that waiting for three minutes to clamp the baby's umbilical cord as opposed to clamping the cord during the first minute following the birth may have health benefits for the newborn. The researchers, who conducted 15 trials involving 1,912 newborns, found that delayed cord clamping was associated with an 80 per cent reduction in the likelihood that the newborn would be anemic 24 to 48 hours after the birth, and a 50 per cent reduction in the likelihood that the baby would be anemic two to three months after the birth.

You don't have to be adversarial when you're discussing birth policies with your health-care provider. Your goal should be to have a respectful conversation in which you challenge your health-care provider to provide maternity care that is customized to your needs as a one-of-a-kind pregnant woman experiencing a one-of-a-kind pregnancy (as opposed to offering one-size-fits-none care that shortchanges pregnant and birthing women by treating each one as the same). You can move the conversation in this direction by asking such questions as, "Do you order that test for every pregnant woman?" "Why do you feel that it is medically necessary for me?" and "Are there any alternatives?"

The first step, of course, is to be informed about the many care options that you could potentially encounter and what the implications are for the health of you and your baby. You can learn about these options by reading books like this (and by checking out other resources recommended on the website for this book, www.having-a-baby.com). It is important to be informed. If you don't understand your options, you risk handing over the ability to make important decisions about your health and your baby's health to other people. Remaining in control of that decision-making process simply requires that you be pro-active: learn as much as you can ahead of time. That way, you can make the best possible choices each step of the way.

To find out more about policies that promote healthy birth, you may want to download a free copy of "Having a Baby? Ten Questions to Ask" from www.motherfriendly.org.

Why a doula is a mom's best friend

Looking for a way to decrease the length of your labour, reduce your need for pain medication, decrease your chances of needing a forceps delivery or a Caesarean, and leave you feeling satisfied about your birth experience? What you need is a doula—the birthing world's equivalent of a fairy godmother.

Think I'm exaggerating? Consider the evidence for yourself. There's a grow-ing body of research proving that doulas (experienced non-medical female com-panions who provide continuous labour support) can help to improve the birth and postpartum outcomes for both mother and baby. Klaus and Kennel found, for example, that when doulas are involved in labour and delivery, requests for epi-durals decrease by 60 per cent, the Caesarean rate decreases by 50 per cent, oxy-tocin use during labour decreases by 40 per cent, requests for pain medications decrease by 30 per cent, and labours are 25 per cent shorter. And a study at the University of Texas Medical School found that women who used the services of a doula were more nurturing toward their babies two months after the delivery.

Doulas typically charge $300 to $1,200 for supporting a birth. This fee includes one or more meetings prior to the birth to talk with you and your part-ner about your plans, helping you to draft a birth plan, making herself available by phone to address any concerns the two of you may have about the birth, provid-ing continuous support during labour, and providing support and breastfeeding help during the first few hours postpartum. Doulas do not, however, perform medical checks (such as monitoring your blood pressure or doing internal exam-inations as they are not clinicians, like midwives and doctors), nor are they licensed to deliver babies. Their role is to provide labour support (most doctors are too busy to do this and some birthing unit nurses simply do not have the time) and, if necessary, to help you communicate your decisions to the medical staff.

The best way to get a referral to a doula who's practising in your community is to contact your nearest midwifery practice. If there isn't a midwifery prac-tice in your community, you might want to contact Doulas of North America

(DONA) via their website (www.dona.org) or CAPPA Canada (1–866–CDN–BIRTH (236–2478) or www.cappacanada.ca) to ask for the names of certified doulas in your area.

Here are 10 great reasons why you may want to think about inviting a doula to your baby's birth:

1. A doula can help you to feel better about your birth experience. A group of researchers in California found that women who had the support of a doula during their babies' births were more likely to feel positive about their birth experiences (82.5 per cent) than women who did not have the benefit of such support (67.4 per cent).

2. A doula can leave your partner free to focus more fully on his key role during the birth: providing you with emotional support. Doulas have knowledge of birth that partners, who may have no prior experience with birth, simply may not have.

3. A doula can help to take some of the pressure off your partner. Having someone else on hand to support you can allow him to take a guilt-free dinner or bathroom break. (It's hard for your partner not to feel like the world's biggest heel if he or she has to take a bathroom break just when your contractions are starting to peak.)

4. A doula can help to reduce the likelihood that you will require an epidural. A study conducted at Case Western Reserve University in Cleveland, Ohio, found that 7.8 per cent of women using doulas requested an epidural as compared to 55.3 per cent of women labouring without a doula.

5. A doula can offer helpful suggestions on ways to cope with the labour when you've pretty much run through your own repertoire of coping strategies.

6. A doula can help breastfeeding get off to the best possible start. A study conducted in South Africa found that women who have support from doulas during labour are more likely to be breastfeeding exclusively when their babies are six weeks old than other moms.

7. A doula can help to answer your questions about the birthing process and provide on-the-spot reassurance when you need it—something that can be truly invaluable if you find yourself with a lot of questions and concerns.

8. A doula can help you advocate for yourself with the hospital staff and ensure that your voice is heard.

9. A doula can promise to be there, even if your partner can't. If there's a chance that your partner isn't going to be there at the birth (possibly because he or she is scheduled to work out of town around your due date) or if you're going to be giving birth without a partner, a doula can provide you with some much-needed support.

10. A doula can act as your cheering section. When you're trying to weather the storms of transition, sometimes you just need someone to tell you that you've got what it takes to get through this—and to say it with enough conviction that you actually believe her. (That's an important part of the doula job description, by the way.)

Writing a birth plan

Something else you need to think about at this stage is whether you and your partner would like to write a birth plan.

Contrary to popular belief, a birth plan doesn't have to be overly long or complicated. It's not a business plan, after all. Birth plans today tend to be much shorter and less formal than they were a decade ago. A birth plan can be as simple as a one-paragraph letter addressing a point of particular concern to you, or it could be a more detailed document addressing such issues as

- where you intend to give birth;
- your plans regarding the use of medication during labour;
- whom you'll be inviting to your baby's birth, and what each person's role will be;
- the atmosphere you hope to create while you're in labour (for example, dim lights and quiet music);
- where you're intending to do the bulk of your labouring (such as in a birthing tub or squatting on a birthing ball);
- what types of birthing equipment you intend to use (a birthing stool, a birthing bed, a birthing ball, a squatting bar, or a birthing tub, for example) and what comfort measures and/or pain relief options you plan to use;
- your desire to have your baby kept with you after you give birth so that you can spend time getting to know one another and initiate breast-feeding as soon as possible;
- whether you want your baby to be placed skin-to-skin on you after the birth, and if you want your baby's hands to remain unwashed until after you've initiated breastfeeding (the scent on her hands can help her

to recognize the scents associated with your breasts and breastfeeding as familiar);

- whether you want your baby to be placed skin-to-skin on your partner's chest if you're not able to hold her immediately after the birth.

Your birth plan should be developed based on your understanding of current policies that are in place at the hospital or birth centre where you intend to give birth (something your health-care provider, doula, or childbirth instructor can help to provide) and/or your midwife's practice guidelines, if you will be giving birth at home. It's important to take a hospital tour to see what equipment is available and what you're allowed to bring in. There's no point wasting time or energy worrying about antiquated policies that are no longer in place at the facility where you will be having your baby—or wasting money renting a birthing pool if you won't be allowed to BYOP (bring your own pool) to the high-risk pregnancy unit where you are scheduled to deliver.

It's important to remember, however, that a birth plan is just that—a plan. It's not a blueprint for labour. Sometimes the way your labour progresses requires you to rethink various aspects of that plan—something that Stephanie, 27, learned for herself when her daughter was born two and a half years ago. She explains: "I had hoped for a non-medicated birth with a midwife, but I found myself in a room with the midwives, an obstetrician, two nurses, and a pediatrician for my child." If you are able to make informed decisions whenever it becomes necessary to amend your original plans, you are less likely to experience after-the-fact regrets. It's when women lose control over the process of giving birth—they are no longer able to make decisions about what is happening because those choices are being made for them—that they tend to feel dissatisfied, even devastated, by the way things played out. Since you may be too busy to decide when the time comes, making sure your supporters are aware of your birth wishes and are prepared to assist you in communicating and clarifying them can help you maintain control of the situation.

Birth plans aren't necessarily for everyone. Marguerite and her husband found that writing one actually contributed to their sense of failure when their first birth didn't go as they had hoped. Consequently, when it came time to prepare for the birth of baby number two, they decided to pass on the plan. "We discussed the relevant issues with our midwife, but we didn't write a formal plan," the 36-year-old mother of two recalls.

There are, of course, some situations in which a birth plan can be very helpful. If, for example, you have a history of sexual abuse and you are worried you may have flashbacks or begin to dissociate yourself (psychologically distance yourself) from the birth as a means of protecting yourself from further trauma, you might want to let the birthing unit staff know what will help to reassure you. Similarly, if you've previously experienced the death of a baby either prior to or shortly after birth, you might want to let the birthing unit staff know whether or not you'd prefer to give birth in the same room as the last time around.

If you and your partner want to write a birth plan but aren't sure how to get started, you might want to consult the sample birth plan in Appendix B. You can either photocopy it and use it as is, or—if you'd like to go with the trend toward short-and-sweet birth plans—simply highlight the points of the birth plan that are most important to you in a letter to your doctor or midwife. If you'll be giving birth in a hospital or birth centre, include a copy of this letter with your pre-registration documents and tuck an extra copy in your labour bag.

What's up down there?

You know how squeamish guys get when someone starts talking about vasectomies? The closest thing to that we women will ever experience is reading up on episiotomies and perineal tears during labour.

Episiotomies

Women who have episiotomies (the medical term for the surgical cut that's sometimes made to the perineum, which is the area between the vagina and rectum) are more likely to experience such complications as blood loss, infection, pain during the postpartum period, the involuntary passage of gas or fecal matter after delivery, rectal tears, weaker pelvic floor muscles, pain during intercourse, and worse sexual functioning. Midline episiotomies (where the incision goes straight up and down) are associated with higher rates of anal incontinence (the involuntary passage of fecal material) and flatus incontinence (the involuntary release of gas from the bowel) following the delivery, while mediolateral episiotomies (where the incision veers slightly to the right or left) are more likely to result in painful intercourse.

All that said, they do have their place in the world of obstetrics: they can make it possible for a baby that is in distress to be delivered in a hurry, or for a mother to avoid a very bad tear in the event of an instrument-assisted (forceps or vacuum) delivery.

What women of previous generations were so eager to say goodbye to (and what has thankfully, for the most part, become a footnote in the obstetrical history books) is the routine episiotomy. It's no longer standard practice to perform an episiotomy during a vaginal delivery.

If you do require an episiotomy, your doctor or midwife will inject anaesthetic into the perineum during the height of a contraction (when pressure from the baby's head is helping to numb the area). (If you've had an epidural or your doctor has injected other anaesthetic into the area—such as a pudendal block—you won't need to have any additional anaesthetic injected at this point.) The incision will also be made during a contraction to take advantage of this natural form of pain relief. Most of the discomfort you experience will occur after the freezing wears off. You can minimize the pain by sitting on one of those doughnut-shaped cushions that work wonders for hemorrhoid sufferers, by squeezing your buttocks together before you sit down, and by pouring water across your perineum while you urinate to prevent the urine from burning. It can take a couple of weeks for your episiotomy to heal—sometimes even longer. Your doctor or midwife will check your episiotomy at your six-week checkup, but call before that if you suspect that your episiotomy site has become infected.

The Canadian episiotomy rate declined by 34 per cent between 1995–1996 and 2004–2005 from 31.1 to 20.4 episiotomies per 100 hospital vaginal deliveries (*Canadian Perinatal Health Report*, 2008). The reduction is likely the result of recommendations from organizations such as the World Health Organization, which now recommends against routine episiotomy. And the December 2008 *Joint Policy Statement on Normal Childbirth*, issued and approved by the Society of Obstetricians and Gynaecologists of Canada (SOGC), the Association of Women's Health, Obstetric and Neonatal Nurses of Canada (AWHONN Canada), the Canadian Association of Midwives (CAM), the College of Family Physicians of Canada (CFPC), and the Society of Rural Physicians of Canada (SRPC), states that "A normal birth does not include . . . routine episiotomy."

Avoiding perineal tears

But enough about episiotomies. Let's talk about what you can do to avoid a perineal tear. A number of studies have demonstrated quite conclusively that perineal massage can help women giving birth for the first time to avoid episiotomies and severe tearing.

The techniques involved are extremely low-tech. You simply gently massage and stretch the tissues at the opening of the vagina while you're soaking in the bathtub. Or, if you don't mind turning this particular activity into a team sport, your partner can help to massage and stretch your tissues when you're lying on a towel on the bed. You might want to use a small amount of olive oil or natural cocoa butter for lubrication if you're going to be doing the perineal massage on dry land. Regardless of where you decide to do your massage, however, you should plan to do it for about four minutes, three to four times per week from the 34th week of your pregnancy onward.

Just one small disclaimer: there are no guarantees. You could massage your little heart out during the weeks leading up to the birth and still end up with an episiotomy or a significant-sized tear. In certain situations an episiotomy may be unavoidable—if your baby is breech, in distress, or in fragile medical condition; in cases of operative vaginal delivery (forceps or vacuum); or your baby's shoulders are too wide to be delivered without an episiotomy (shoulder dystocia). As well, some caregivers will perform an episiotomy if it looks as though you're going to end up with a severe tear or multiple tears. (Most health-care professionals these days believe it's best to let the tear occur naturally, if it's likely to be a minor one, and repair it after the fact. A minor tear is easier on the perineum than an episiotomy.)

perineal massage

Practising perineal massage in the weeks leading up to your baby's birth may help to increase the stretchiness of your perineum (the area between your anus and your vagina), reducing the likelihood that you will tear or require an episiotomy when you give birth. Perineal massage also gives you the opportunity to practise relaxing the muscles in your perineum when you experience the stretching, burning sensation you will feel when your baby's head starts to crown. (As you stretch your perineum during perineal massage, you'll get a sneak preview of what this sensation will be like.)

It's best to start perineal massage approximately six weeks before your due date. You can do it on your own or with some help from your partner.

ON YOUR OWN:

- Find a private place and get comfortable. You may discover that it works best if you get into a semi-seated position with plenty of pillows for back support. If you're finding it difficult to relax, take a warm bath or apply warm compresses to your perineum for five to ten minutes before you plan to begin your massage.
- Ensure that you've washed your hands thoroughly and that your fingernails are well trimmed (to minimize the risk of infection).
- Use plenty of lube (vitamin E oil, almond oil (unless you're allergic to nuts), olive oil, or a water-soluble jelly such as KY jelly). Apply it to your thumbs and your perineal tissues. Note: If you've got an abundance of natural lubricant, you can skip the lube. Avoid baby oil, mineral oil, petroleum jelly, and other oil- and mineral-based lubricants.
- Insert your thumbs 3 to 5 centimetres (1 to 2 inches) inside your vagina. Your thumbs should be resting on your perineum, pointing downward toward your anus. Press downward (toward your anus) and pull outwards (sideways) until you feel a

burning and stretching sensation. Try to hold this position for one to two minutes. Breathe slowly and deeply.

- Using your thumbs, massage the lower half of your vagina using a U-shaped motion. Breathe slowly and deeply.
- If you make a point to practise perineal massage for about four minutes, three to four times per week, you should notice that your perineal area soon becomes stretchier and experiences less burning during the stretching exercise.

WITH A PARTNER:

Ask your partner to follow the instructions above. Your partner may find it works best to use his or her index fingers rather than thumbs to apply the U-shaped downward pressure. Be sure to let your partner know how much pressure is enough and how much is too much.

Pain relief during labour

Something else you'll want to consider before the labour contractions kick in is what comfort measures and pain relief methods you intend to use during labour and birth. You may decide to stick with natural (non-medicinal) pain relief options, or you may decide to go straight for the hard stuff. Jennifer, a 31-year-old mother of two, opted for Plan B: "I knew I was having an epidural the moment the pregnancy test turned blue."

The Canadian *Maternity Experiences Survey*—the first-ever national survey of Canadian mothers' experiences with pregnancy, labour, birth, and post-partum—asked over 6,000 new moms what types of pain relief measures they relied upon when they were in labour. Seventy-four per cent used breathing exercises, 57 per cent used an epidural, and 69 per cent used a combination of medication and natural pain relief methods. Fifty-five per cent of women who used water (a bath or shower) found this method very helpful. You can find out more about the survey by visiting the Public Health Agency of Canada website: www.phac-aspc.gc.ca/rhs-ssg/survey-eng.php.

Here's what you need to know about the various methods of coping with pain during labour:

Comfort measures and other non-medicinal forms of pain relief

The following strategies have proven to be helpful to other women in labour. You may wish to experiment with these techniques ahead of time so that you'll have an idea about which techniques you may wish to draw upon when you're in labour. Be sure to let your partner and/or doula know which comfort measures you find most helpful. One more thing: be flexible. What works to relieve pain varies from woman to woman, labour to labour, and even labour stage to labour stage. The more techniques you have at your disposal, the better prepared you'll feel.

Note: One of the reasons that many women gravitate toward non-pharmacological methods of pain relief is that you can use more than one method at the same time—or rotate from method to method, to meet your changing needs as your labour progresses. The side effects of pharmacological methods of pain control make it difficult for you to incorporate other methods if you find that you need more assistance.

- **Acupressure.** The application of finger pressure or deep massage to traditional acupuncture points may help to reduce labour pain and promote progress.
- **Acupuncture.** Needles are inserted in your limbs or ears to help to block the corresponding pain signals.
- **Aromatherapy.** Aromatherapy involves using essential oils to reduce anxiety and promote relaxation. Aromatherapy is often combined with massage. It's best in early labour since women become sensitive to strong smells during transition.

endorphins

Endorphins are one form of pain relief you don't have to choose because you've already got them on-board, thanks to some smart planning on the part of Mother Nature. During late pregnancy, your placenta ramps up its production of endorphins—your "feel-good" hormones—so that you'll be better able to cope with the challenges of giving birth. And, during labour, your endorphin levels increase when you have contractions and while your cervix is effacing. Endorphins help to block pain signals before they reach your brain. They also help to regulate your mood during labour.

Even if you do need to rely on a medicinal form of pain relief during labour, you'll need less of it than you otherwise would, thanks to endorphins, the labouring woman's little helper.

Your endorphins may also help to ease the transition to life in the outside world for your newborn. Colostrum (the pre-milk food substance that is available to your newborn during the first few days of breastfeeding) is rich in endorphins, too.

- **Changing positions.** Positions that tend to work well include kneeling over a birthing ball or a pile of pillows, standing and leaning forward, sitting in a chair facing backward (using the back of the chair for support), squatting (with a birth bar or a partner; on a birthing stool), and sitting on the toilet. You want to find a position that puts gravity to work for you and that keeps your pelvis open (to give your baby maximum room to wriggle through). If you're experiencing back pain in labour, you may want to try supporting your abdomen while you are in a standing position. (Note: 1. Lock your fingers together and place your hands underneath your abdomen, right against your pubic bone. 2. Bend your knees slightly.) You may also want to ask your partner or doula to apply counter pressure to the area where you are experiencing back pain. While you are leaning forward against a dresser (with your head on a pillow), your partner or doula should press steadily and firmly in one spot on the lower back. A cold can of soda pop rolled over your lower back during contractions can be incredibly soothing. Penny Simkin, co-founder of DONA International, recommends keeping a six-pack in a bowl of ice so you'll always have a cold can handy.

- **Heat or cold.** Apply heat (in the form of a warm gel pack, a hot water bottle, hot, moist towels, or a heated rice pack) to sore or achy body parts. Applying cold (via a frozen gel pack, frozen moist cloths, cold cans of pop, or a bag of ice) can help to relieve lower back pain. Cool cloths applied to the face, chest, or the back of your neck can be very soothing if you're feeling hot from the hard work of labour.

- **Hydrotherapy.** Labouring in water relaxes you and helps to counteract the effects of gravity, something that can make labour less painful. Early in labour, taking a bath can help to relax you and give you a bit of a break from the early contractions, which tend to be more uncomfortable and annoying than out-and-out painful. When the contractions become more intense, labouring in warm (37°C to 38°C/99°F to 100°F) water can provide considerable relief from the pain—so much so that labouring in water has been proven to reduce the likelihood that an epidural will be requested. Being immersed in warm water (ahhhh) helps to bring down a labouring woman's blood pressure, makes the dilatation phase of labour less painful, reduces the need for pain medication or anaesthetic during both the dilatation phase and the pushing stage, and leaves mothers feeling more satisfied with their pushing efforts. If you're experiencing back labour (labour in which most of the mother's pain is felt in her back), directing a soothing jet of warm water on the part of your back that is affected can provide a great deal of relief.

- **Hypnosis.** Self-hypnosis techniques can be used to promote relaxation during labour, thereby reducing the amount of pain you experience. Some caregivers also have special training in the use of hypnosis during labour. Hypnotherapy is associated with a reduced need for pain medication, a reduced likelihood that oxytocin will be used to augment labour, increased maternal satisfaction with pain relief, and a shorter labour.

- **Massage and encouraging touch.** Light, firm stroking of your hands, feet, scalp, shoulders, back, or limbs helps to reduce pain, stress, and anxiety, and helps you to cope with labour. Not every woman likes to be touched during labour, however: some women find it extremely annoying, while others find certain types of touch very soothing. Let your partner and/or doula know whether or not it works for you. If you plan to try massage during labour, have massage oil, lotion, or powder on hand (to reduce friction).

- **Movement.** Walking, changing position, rocking (in a rocking chair) or swaying your body from side to side (while seated on a birthing ball, or while standing and leaning forward), and otherwise remaining active during labour is an effective method of pain relief. It also helps to shorten the first and second stages of labour (see Table 10.2) and reduces the likelihood of an instrumental or Caesarean delivery. Movement during labour also helps your uterus to contract more efficiently and your baby to rotate and descend more effectively. You don't have to use any complicated movements. Walking or slow dancing work just fine.

- **Relaxation and positive visualization.** Relaxation breathing and/or focusing on an object that you find calming can help to calm you during labour, and thereby reduce the amount of pain you experience. Some people react to pain by hyperventilating (breathing too quickly and deeply). Unfortunately, hyperventilating will heighten your sensations of pain and leave you feeling panicked because your muscles and your brain are receiving too little carbon dioxide. The solution is to breathe slowly and deeply. If you are anxious or exhausted, your perception of pain will be heightened. If you become severely distressed, your contractions may even stop. The solution is to have continuous support in place from your partner and/or a doula or other professional labour support person. This person can talk you through the difficult times, help you to remain calm and centred, and suggest position changes and other practical strategies for maximizing your comfort (such as progressive muscle relaxation, touch, massage, calming self-talk, or repeating calming and reassuring birth affirmations to you).

- **Rhythmic breathing.** Forget everything you've heard about complicated breathing exercises. That's not what this is all about. If you can breathe in and out in a slow, relaxed rhythm, you've got this breathing thing mastered. You may also want to practise variations on this theme, such as shallow, light breathing (which can come in handy in late labour, right before the pushing stage).
- **Transcutaneous electrical nerve stimulation (TENS).** A TENS machine stimulates the nerves in your lower back, which can help block the transmission of pain impulses to the brain. An evaluation of the effectiveness of TENS as method of pain relief during labour looked at eight trials involving 712 women. While no difference in pain scores was found between women who did and did not rely upon TENS during labour, there was a difference in the use of pain medication, with TENS users turning to pain medications less frequently.

Medicinal pain relief options

- **Sedatives.** Sedatives, tranquilizers, and sleeping pills can be used to reduce anxiety and encourage a labouring woman to relax. Unfortunately, these drugs cross the placenta and can affect the baby. Babies whose mothers use sedatives during labour may experience breathing and breastfeeding difficulties after the birth. They may also remain limp until the effects of the drug wear off.
- **Anti-nausea drugs.** Some labouring women take anti-nausea drugs like Gravol to combat nausea and vomiting triggered by either labour itself or by the use of narcotics such as Demerol or morphine. These drugs tend to cause sleepiness and dizziness in the mother.
- **Injectable narcotics and narcotic-like medications.** Narcotics such as Demerol, morphine, Nubain, and Stadol can provide up to two hours' worth of pain relief. Unfortunately, the doses given to labouring women tend to be relatively low and frequently fail to provide adequate pain relief. They tend to take the edge off your contractions, but you still feel pain. At the same time, they make it more difficult for you to cope with the contractions that you're experiencing because your brain is a little foggy. These drugs are narcotics, after all. To make matters worse, they interfere with endorphin production—your body's natural pain-relief and mood-regulation mechanism. And, what's more, narcotics can cause side effects ranging from drowsiness, nausea, and vomiting, to respiratory depression and low

blood pressure, to breathing difficulties in the newborn (if the drugs are used within two hours of the birth). There's also some evidence that Demerol may prolong labour, thereby increasing the likelihood that some other type of intervention will be required. Narcotics do have their purpose, however: they may be useful in providing "therapeutic rest" to women in early labour who have become exhausted and who need to rest up before dealing with the rest of the hard work of labour and giving birth.

"Medicating the pain away disrupts labour. If you can't feel the pain of contractions or the pressure of your baby's descent, you can't respond to it . . . Removing labour pain also prevents endorphin release, depriving you of the natural high of childbirth. Remove the pain at any point in the journey, and you remove the signals your body needs to keep labour progressing and to protect itself and your baby."

—JUDITH LOTHIAN AND CHARLOTTE DEVRIES,
THE OFFICIAL LAMAZE GUIDE: GIVING BIRTH WITH CONFIDENCE

- **Epidural.** An anaesthetic is injected into the space between the covering of the spinal cord and inside the bony vertebrae of your spine, numbing you from the waist down. An epidural provides full relief for 85 per cent of women, partial relief (for example, pain relief on one side of the body) in 12 per cent of women, and no relief in 3 per cent of women. The side effects of epidurals include a longer second stage of labour, very low blood pressure, a reduced ability to push (which may necessitate a forceps or vacuum extraction delivery), lack of mobility for a short time after the birth, difficulty passing urine, and fever. A 2011 Cochrane Review of the effects of epidurals noted, however, that "Epidural analgesia had no statistically significant impact on the risk of Caesarean section, maternal satisfaction with pain relief and long-term backache and did not appear to have an immediate effect on neonatal status as determined by Apgar scores."

    Not all epidurals were created equal:

    - Low-dose epidurals that allow you to be mobile during labour and to feel the urge to push reduce the full-dose epidural risks of stalled labour and assisted (forceps or vacuum) delivery. Note: These aren't available in all hospitals.

- A patient-controlled epidural puts you in charge of how much pain relief you are receiving. (Research has shown that the total dose ends up being lower and that patient satisfaction ends up being higher. Talk about a win–win.)
- Traditional epidurals lead to higher levels of instrument-assisted vaginal delivery. (These types of epidurals are associated with poor motor function in the mother.)

• **Spinal.** A spinal is similar to an epidural, except that anaesthetic is injected into the spinal fluid in the lower back, numbing you from the waist down. Spinals are usually used for elective Caesarean deliveries, in cases when the anaesthetic must be administered in a hurry (such as an emergency forceps delivery), if the placenta has been retained, or if you've experienced a severe tear that requires a difficult repair. They're not recommended for some women who have severe pre-eclampsia (only if the platelet count is very low) or who face a high risk of hemorrhaging (such as women with low blood platelet levels, placenta previa, or a major placental abruption). There's a chance that a spinal will cause low blood pressure, severe post-delivery headaches, temporary bladder dysfunction, nausea, and, in rare cases, convulsions or infection.

• **Inhalable analgesics (such as nitrous oxide).** Inhalable analgesics such as nitrous oxide numb the pain centre in the brain. The key advantage to this pain relief method is that it's administered by the woman as she needs it and can be used to help a woman to weather a difficult transition stage as she waits for the pushing stage to begin. The key disadvantages are that it can cause drowsiness and nausea, as well as claustrophobic feelings (you have to wear a mask tightly on your face), it does not provide pain relief in all cases (it is effective for about 50 per cent of women), it's only suitable for a short period of time (typically an hour or less), its effectiveness varies significantly from woman to woman, and, what's more, some studies have shown that women who use nitrous oxide during labour can aspirate (inhale the contents of their stomachs). Nitrous oxide isn't widely available in Canada.

• **Local anaesthetic.** Local anaesthetic can be injected into the tissues of the perineum so that an episiotomy can be performed or an episiotomy or tear can be repaired after the delivery. Some studies have demonstrated that injections of local anaesthetic may weaken the perineal tissue, which increases the likelihood of tearing in the event that an episiotomy isn't performed after all. Another form of local anaesthetic is a pudendal block—local anaesthetic that is injected into the middle of the vagina to numb the perineal nerves. A pudendal block can be helpful in a fast labour when a little pain medicine is needed close to delivery. It does not affect the baby.

- **General anaesthetic.** A general anaesthetic is sometimes used in emergency situations. It is no longer used routinely during delivery, as it was a generation ago, because of the high risk of breathing problems and extreme sleepiness in the newborn, and the small chance that the mother might aspirate (breathe in) the contents of her stomach while she's under the anaesthetic, causing potentially life-threatening complications.

While you should give some thought to the types of pain relief you hope to use during labour, it's important to go into labour with an open mind. If the speedy delivery you envisioned turns out to be a 30-hour endurance test, you might decide to rethink your stance on epidurals. Conversely, the epidural you had your heart set on might not be feasible or even necessary if you're already 8 centimetres dilated by the time you arrive at the hospital!

Marguerite found that the natural methods she had planned to use during the birth of her first child weren't particularly helpful: "I couldn't tolerate any of the planned massage or counting techniques," the 36-year-old mother of two recalls. "My poor husband had to remain silent, not touching me and not doing anything else either. I was very irritable and couldn't tolerate any distractions of any kind. All our practised breathing and massage and relaxation techniques were totally useless to me. I just needed to focus on myself."

Jane ended up changing her game plan when labour dragged on and on. "I expected a textbook labour, and mine wasn't," the 33-year-old mother of two explains. "I stayed at two centimetres after 24 hours of good strong labour. I don't know how common this is, but I didn't hear much about it from my midwife or from the classes. I became more and more frustrated and less and less able to cope with the pain as the hours went by and I still didn't progress. If I'd been moving forward bit by bit, I think I could have gone on longer without drugs. As it was, I had an epidural after 24 hours. I needed a rest from the pain. I was exhausted and I felt very, very out of control. The contractions had become scary and negative for me because they weren't getting me anywhere."

"I'm not going to say that giving birth was easy. It wasn't. But I was amazed by—and proud of—my ability to cope with the powerful contractions that were required to push my baby out into the world," recalls Marie, 36, mother of four. "Our childbirth instructor had used the phrase 'pain with a purpose' to talk about the type of pain we'd be experiencing during labour. She also stressed that each contraction took us one step closer to meeting our baby. I reminded myself of both of those things during each of my labours: that this was 'good pain'—productive pain—and that I would soon have my baby in my arms."

better maternity care

The *Maternity Experiences Survey* (conducted by the Public Health Agency of Canada in 2006 and published in 2009) revealed that just 53.8 per cent of Canadian women felt very positive about their maternity experiences, 65.4 per cent felt very satisfied with the compassion and care shown to them by their health-care providers, and that 61.8 per cent felt very satisfied by the information they received from their health-care providers throughout pregnancy, labour, and birth.

Mothers of Change (www.mothersofchange.com), the only national, non-profit consumer advocacy group in Canada to focus exclusively on maternity care, is working to make those numbers even higher: "The evidence is clear," states Asheya Hennessey, executive director and founder of Mothers of Change. "Our maternity care needs to change. Who will create that change? We will. We are mothers... We are birthing better maternity care. We are becoming mothers of change."

The Top Labour-Related Worries

Now that you're entering the home stretch of pregnancy, you're starting to think ahead to the birth. That gives you a whole bunch of new things to worry about! Time to take a stroll down Anxiety Avenue by looking at the most common labour-related worries.

I'm worried that I won't be able to tell when I'm really in labour and that I'll end up waiting too long before I get help. This is one of the most common fears of first-time mothers: that they won't clue in to the fact they're in labour until the baby's head is starting to crown.

Most women who've been through labour will tell you that, while it's hard to be sure at first whether or not it's actually begun, as time goes on you become more and more certain.

Here are a few guidelines to help you decide whether the moment of truth has arrived.

Don't be surprised if you end up experiencing a few false starts before labour actually begins. While there's nothing false about the way these labour contractions feel, you're said to be in pre-labour (sometimes referred to as false labour, although the term is falling out of favour) because these contractions don't cause the cervix to dilate. You're likely experiencing pre-labour rather than the main event if

- contractions are irregular and are neither increasing in frequency (the length of time between the start of one contraction and the next) nor severity (the amount of pain you experience);
- contractions stop if you change position, empty your bladder, or have two large glasses of water (becoming dehydrated can cause your uterus to become irritable, triggering contractions);
- the pain from the contractions can be felt in your lower abdomen rather than your lower back;
- the show is brownish rather than reddish, and so is more likely to be the result of a recent internal examination or sexual intercourse.

However, you should assume you're experiencing the real thing and take a moment to double-check that everything that you're going to need is handy or tucked into your labour bag (see Table 10.1) if you experience one or more of the following symptoms of true labour:

- contractions that seem to be falling into a regular pattern, that are getting longer, stronger, and more frequent, that intensify with activity, and that don't subside if you change position or drink two large glasses of water;
- contractions that start in your lower back and then spread to your abdomen and possibly your legs;
- abdominal cramping that feels as if you had a gastrointestinal upset;
- diarrhea or loose stool;
- show that's either pinkish or blood-streaked;
- the rupture of your membranes.

There's no such thing as a textbook labour, so you may find that it's not exactly crystal clear whether you're dealing with bona fide labour contractions or not. Sometimes it can be very hard to tell what's really going on.

Maria, a 35-year-old mother of two, had a hard time deciding whether or not she was actually in labour, even though her doctor had actually prescribed a cervical gel that was supposed to help ripen her cervix. "Everyone says that when you're really in labour, you'll know. Well, I'm here to tell you that's not always the case. The first time around, I had a prostaglandin gel applied to my cervix to soften it as a preparation for induction. I was told the gel sometimes gets labour rolling, but that it's not that effective in first-time mothers. I went home and started getting these killer menstrual cramps. I mean, they were just horrendous. I remember saying to my husband, 'God, it's so bad and I'm not even in labour yet. What's labour going to be like?' It was awful. I was on my

10.1 What to Take to the Hospital

Wondering what you should take to the hospital with you? Here are a few ideas:

Labour Bag	Suitcase
Your health insurance card and proof of any extended health benefits you may have (e.g., semi-private or private room coverage through your health plan at work)	Hairbrush
	Shampoo
	Soap
	Toothbrush
Your hospital pre-registration forms (unless you've already dropped them off at the hospital)	Toothpaste
	Deodorant
One or more copies of your birth plan	Highly absorbent sanitary pads (unless the hospital provides them)
Sponges (to help keep you cool)	
A tennis ball or rolling pin (ideally one that can be filled with hot or cold water) to massage your back	Books and magazines to read (including a good breastfeeding book)
A frozen freezer pack (small) wrapped in a hand towel	Birth announcements and a pen (fill out as many of these as you can ahead of time, and pre-stamp and pre-address the envelopes)
A picture or other object that you find comforting (you might wish to use it as your focal point during labour)	Earplugs (so you can get some sleep)
Unscented massage oil or lotion	A small gift for each of the baby's siblings (unless this is your first baby)
Cornstarch or other non-perfumed powder to reduce friction during massage	Two or more nightgowns (front-opening style if you're planning to breastfeed)
A hot water bottle	Bathrobe
Lip balm or petroleum jelly to relieve dry lips	Two or more nursing bras
A camera or video camera plus spare batteries or battery charger and maybe a disposable camera too	Five or more pairs of underwear (disposables or inexpensive ones that can be thrown away if they become badly stained)
Extra pillows in coloured pillow cases (so they won't get mixed up with the hospital pillows)	Two pairs of warm socks
	A pair of slippers
An iPod or MP3 player to listen to during labour	A going-home outfit for you (something that fit when you were five or six months pregnant)
Books, magazines, a deck of cards, a portable DVD player, a gaming device, etc.	A going-home outfit for the baby (ideally a sleeper or newborn nightie plus a hat)
Paper and pens	A receiving blanket
A cellphone and charger	A bunting bag and/or a heavy blanket if it's wintertime
A list of people to contact and their numbers or e-mail addresses	
Snacks and drinks	A diaper for your baby to wear home (just in case the hospital uses cloth diapers)
A bathing suit for your partner (so that your partner can accompany you into the shower or the Jacuzzi to help you to work through contractions)	Toiletries and a change of clothes for your partner

hands and knees trying to get some relief when I threw up all over the floor. And somewhere in the recesses of my brain, a little light went on. 'Oh,' I thought. 'Maybe I'm in labour after all.' Duh!'"

Maria was confused because her contractions seemed to defy the "rules" about how labour was supposed to progress (at least according to what she'd read): "My first labour was nothing like what I expected. I thought labour pains would be sharp and have a beginning and an end. My contractions were dull and grinding and never peaked. I swear, I had one five-and-a-half-minute contraction."

Like Maria, it took Bevin a while to clue in to the fact that she was really in labour: "I was in total denial for the first seven hours of my labour," the 27-year-old mother of one confesses. "It wasn't at all like how they said it would be in prenatal class. All the signs I was having seemed to point to false labour: my pains were centred in my belly, I had no back labour, very little pain, irregular contractions. But seven hours later when the really heavy pains set in, I knew it was really happening."

> "Our child was born in November. My husband was working on a Christmas present for his mom—a cross-stitch birth certificate for the baby. Just as we were about to leave for the hospital, he put it in his bag. I asked him why on earth he'd bring it with him, and he said it was to keep him busy during the slow times. I thought he was nuts, but there was my husband, sitting in the rocker cross-stitching away between contractions. Every time I had a contraction he'd neatly put it all down, come help me through the contraction, and then go back to working on it. He must have done that for a few hours."
>
> —STEPHANIE, 27, MOTHER OF ONE

I'm petrified that I won't make it to the hospital on time to have my baby. If you live in an urban area and you're giving birth for the first time, there's generally little cause for concern. Since a first labour typically lasts anywhere between 12 and 13 hours, you've got plenty of time to figure out that you're in labour, grab your labour bag, and head for the hospital. In fact, even women who are giving birth for the second or subsequent time tend to have time on their side: their labours typically last seven hours.

Things can, of course, be a little trickier if you live a little farther off the beaten path and the nearest hospital is a good hour or two away. While you're likely to have enough time to make it to the hospital, you may have to err on the side of caution and make the trip before you're 100 per cent sure that you're really in labour. Don't be surprised if you end up with a couple of false starts. Sometimes the only way to tell whether it's the real thing is to have your caregiver do an internal examination to see if your cervix has begun to dilate. While it can be frustrating and even a little embarrassing to be sent home from the hospital time and time again, it's better to be safe than sorry if you have a considerable distance to travel.

Something else we Canadians have to keep in mind is the possibility of bad weather. If you're due around the end of January—prime snowstorm season for certain parts of the country—you'll want to talk to your doctor or midwife about what arrangements would be made if the roads aren't passable. Would you need to call 911 to request assistance in getting to the hospital? Would the midwife make the trek to your home by snowshoe? Obviously, these are issues best discussed months before you actually go into labour.

Labour Guidelines: When to Call Your Caregiver

As soon as your labour is well established, you should touch base with your doctor or midwife to let her know that you're in labour—or you think you're in labour. If you're not sure or if you're worried about any symptoms you're experiencing, call right away. Your instinct that you need to call sooner should always trump any labour "rules" you read here or anywhere else.

If you're looking for some guidelines on when to place that first call (assuming you haven't placed an "are we in labour?" or "is this normal?" call in the meantime), you should plan to call when

- your contractions are regular, becoming increasingly strong, and occurring at increasingly shorter intervals (Note: Most caregivers will want to hear from you by the time your contractions are occurring at five-minute intervals—measured from the start of one contraction to the start of the next contraction—if not sooner.);
- your membranes have ruptured or you suspect they've ruptured (depending on your position and your baby's position, you might experience a large gush or a continuous trickle);
- you have lower back pain that doesn't go away;
- your past experience with labour tells you this is the real thing and you have this nagging gut feeling that it's time to call your caregiver.

Rather than letting a family member make the phone call for you, try to make the call yourself so that your caregiver can better assess how far your labour has progressed. She'll know that the contractions are getting pretty intense if you have a hard time talking during contractions.

Regardless of how well your labour is established, you'll need to notify your caregiver immediately if

- you experience a lot of bleeding (which can indicate premature separation of the placenta or placenta previa—see Chapter 9);
- you notice thickish green fluid coming from your vagina (which can indicate that your baby has passed meconium into the amniotic fluid and may be in distress; normal amniotic fluid is clear with white flecks);
- there's a loop of umbilical cord dangling from your vagina or you think you feel something inside your vagina (a possible indication of a cord prolapse). If you suspect you've experienced a cord prolapse (an emergency situation in which the cord is presenting in front of your baby's head, leading to a possible lack of oxygen), call 911 while you lie with your head and chest on the floor and your bottom in the air. This will help to prevent your baby's head from compressing the umbilical cord and interrupting the flow of oxygen while you wait for the ambulance to arrive.

WHEN TO GO TO THE HOSPITAL:

You should plan to head to the hospital when

- your contractions are four to five minutes apart, lasting one minute, and occurring consistently for one hour or more;
- your contractions are so painful that you have to rely on your relaxation breathing or other pain management techniques;
- you can no longer talk during a contraction;
- your membranes have ruptured (something that should be confirmed just in case antibiotics need to be started);
- you instinctively feel that it's time to go. If you live a significant distance from the hospital, you're giving birth in the middle of a snowstorm, or you have a history of rapid labours, you'll want to head out sooner rather than later.

I'm worried that my water will break when I'm out in public—like when I'm doing my grocery shopping. I can't imagine anything more embarrassing than that, short of giving birth right in the middle of the produce department! Here's a reassuring statistic, just in case this particular anxiety is keeping you awake at 3:00 a.m.: Only 10 per cent of women experience premature rupturing of the membranes (when they rupture before rather than during labour). So the chances of your water breaking in the middle of the grocery store are decidedly slim.

And even if your membranes do end up rupturing in a public place, you're more likely to experience a constant trickle of amniotic fluid rather than any sudden gushes. That's because your baby's head acts like a cork, blocking the exit to your uterus and slowing the escape of the amniotic fluid. So while you'll know something's happened (you tend to feel this weird popping sensation, followed by the telltale trickle of fluid down your leg), chances are no one else in the store is going to clue in. And because amniotic fluid doesn't have a particularly strong odour, you don't have to worry about smelling funny either.

If you're losing a lot of sleep over this one, there's an easy solution. Start wearing a maxi pad when you go out. It'll buy you some time to exit with grace if your membranes do decide to rupture at an inopportune time and you have to abandon your cart in the frozen-food aisle.

I'm worried that I won't know what to do when I'm in labour or when it's time to give birth. While it is helpful to be prepared for labour and birth, you shouldn't feel like you're cramming for an exam, trying to stuff as much information as possible into your brain so that you'll be ready for any and all possible scenarios. Instead, focus on developing a sense of trust in your body and yourself. Your body knows. Think about all the changes your body has experienced during pregnancy. You didn't have to tell your body what to do. Your body knew what it needed to do to care for and nurture your baby. And it will know exactly what it needs to do to help you give birth to your baby. You don't have to know exactly what labour will be like to feel prepared. Every labour is unique, after all. Know which comfort measures you intend to draw upon (so that you can work with your body, not against it, when you're dealing with particularly painful contractions). Envision yourself going with the flow of labour rather than fighting it. Talk through any worries or concerns you may have about giving birth with your health-care provider, your doula, or another trusted person who is knowledgeable about birth. Once you get these issues out into the open, others can help you to come up with ways of dealing with your worries and concerns. You will no longer feel controlled by fear.

It is much easier to cope with the challenges of labour when you feel confident that your body knows what it is doing, and when you understand that the pain that you are experiencing is contributing to the progress of labour and taking you closer to the birth of your baby. Here's a quick overview of what's happening to your body, the bodily sensations you may be experiencing, and how that "pain with a purpose" helps your labour to progress.

In the weeks leading up to labour your body releases additional prostaglandins to soften your cervix. You may notice strong uterine contractions. These contractions may even become rhythmic at times, but, unlike the labour contractions that result in the birth of a baby, these pre-labour contractions don't last.

Early labour contractions may feel like period-like cramps that originate in the abdomen and move downward toward the groin. If your baby's head is facing your back, you may simply experience these early contractions as back pain.

Your body ramps up the production of oxytocin, causing your contractions to become stronger and to occur closer together. As your contractions intensify, your cervix effaces (thins out) and dilates (opens up) while your baby inches downward in your pelvis. You are in active labour once your contractions are lasting for a minute, occurring at intervals of less than five minutes (measured from the start of one contraction to the start of the next), and they are becoming stronger from one contraction to the next.

Your body monitors the amount of oxytocin that is being secreted and the level of pain that you are experiencing and responds by releasing endorphins to help you cope. Endorphins dull pain perception, moderate the release of oxytocin, and help you to zone out a little.

When your baby has reached the right position and your body is ready for the next stage of labour, you will feel an urge to push. (Your body may decide to take a brief time out to rest after your cervix is fully dilated. If you don't feel the urge to push right away, be patient. When your body is ready, it will send you an unmistakable signal that it is ready for you to help push out that baby.)

You don't have to worry that you won't know what to do or how to push. The urge to push (or bear down) is a basic reflex, which means you don't have to practise it or learn it: it will be there when you need it. You'll probably find that you want to change positions once the urge to push arrives, that you're eager to find a position, like squatting, that encourages your pelvis to open up wide and that puts gravity to work for you and your baby.

Don't be surprised if you feel restless and anxious during the pushing stage. When you respond this way, Mother Nature gives you a shot of catecholamines (stress hormones) to help carry you though the final sprint portion of what may be starting to feel like a marathon event. These stress hormones will help you to focus on the task at hand—getting the baby out—while increasing your strength and endurance. It's the confidence and energy-booster you need, just when you need it. Your body is so smart.

Your baby gets the big squeeze as he travels through your vagina, a process that helps to extract amniotic fluid from his lungs. As he is born, a number of forces combine to encourage him to take that all-important first breath: the slightly cooler temperature in the room, the decrease in oxygen in his environment, and the stress hormones that have made him super-alert.

Your baby plays an important role in your immediate postpartum recovery—while you help to keep him warm. Having him on your abdomen, in close proximity to your breasts, encourages your uterus to contract and helps to promote breastfeeding. (You'll want to offer him the breast within the first hour after the birth, while he's wide awake.) At the same time, skin-to-skin contact with you helps to regulate his breathing, temperature, and heart rate.

I'm petrified that I won't be able to cope with the pain of labour. Given the scary stories pregnant women are subjected to by well-meaning (and not-so-well-meaning) friends and relatives, it's hardly surprising that many of us decide around the eight-month mark that we really don't want to give birth after all.

The best way to cope with your labour-related fears is to learn as much as you can about giving birth. Read up on the subject, take some childbirth classes, and talk to your doctor or midwife about comfort techniques and pain-relief options during labour. Come up with a plan for dealing with each possible scenario so you will know what to do even if there are changes.

In the meantime, don't underestimate your abilities. Labour is indeed a trial by fire, but you're up to the challenge. Generations of other women have walked this path before and lived to tell. (Heck, some of them even went back and had more babies!) So rather than feeling afraid that you can't do it, focus on the strength you can draw upon to meet this challenge. (I know this sounds all very crunchy-granola, but it's true: there's an inner reservoir of strength just waiting to be called upon when you're in the heat of labour. Trust me on this one, okay?)

I'm afraid that I'll lose control during labour. This is another tremendously common fear—that you'll do or say something unspeakably embarrassing during labour. You may worry that you'll swear or grunt or say something really bitchy to your partner, or that you'll end up pooping a bit while you're pushing out your baby.

Most of us spend our entire lives working at maintaining control, so it can be more than a little disconcerting to envision yourself in a situation where it's your body that's calling the shots rather than the rational, in-control part of your brain.

The first thing you need to realize is that the labour and delivery staff and your doctor or midwife have seen it all, and they certainly won't think any worse of you if you happen to lose control during labour. In fact, your caregiver may actually encourage you to moan or make grunting noises during contractions if that helps you to cope with the pain.

And as for your partner thinking any the less of you because of something you do or say during labour, you're overlooking one important detail: your partner will be busy witnessing a miracle.

I'm worried that my birth experience will be disappointing. So many women talk about how their birth wasn't what they wanted it to be. I'd hate for that to happen to me. When Ellen D. Hodnett of the Faculty of Nursing at the University of Toronto examined what was known about women's satisfaction with their birth experiences, she discovered that four factors are really key:

- expectations of the birth;
- the amount of support from caregivers;
- the quality of the caregiver-patient relationship; and
- the extent to which the woman is able to be involved in decisions about her care.

> "I felt powerfully connected to all my ancestresses down through all time. I could literally see the echoes of every woman who ever laboured to give forth a new life. I felt triumphant, filled with grace, utterly humbled by my own body and by the miracle that lay wet and sweet and messy on my belly. I was full to the skin with welcome for the new life that so suddenly became real to me."
>
> —HEATHER, 32, MOTHER OF ONE, QUOTED IN *THE UNOFFICIAL GUIDE TO HAVING A BABY* BY ANN DOUGLAS AND JOHN R. SUSSMAN, MD

If you have realistic and non-rigid expectations about the birth, you choose supportive caregivers (including a supportive birth partner and/or a doula who can provide you with continuous labour support), you have an excellent relationship with your caregiver, and you plan to be actively involved in making decisions about your care during labour and birth (something that requires researching key issues ahead of time, discussing key issues with your caregivers, and asking others to help you advocate for yourself during labour), your odds of having a positive birth experience increase dramatically.

I'm worried that there won't be anyone on hand to take care of my older child when I go into labour. Since it's impossible to predict exactly when you're going to give birth—unless, of course, you're having a scheduled induction or a Caesarean—the question of who will care for your older child during your labour can represent quite a challenge and a worry. You may have to come up with a whole roster of people who are available at various times of day or night. Hopefully, if you recruit enough friends and family members to the cause, you'll be able to reach at least one person on their cellphone when the moment of truth arrives.

Once you've made your arrangements, be sure to fill your child in on the details. She needs to know that she could wake up one morning to find Grandma or Uncle Bill sitting at the breakfast table instead of you. And be sure to explain that you'll be arranging for her to meet the new baby as soon as possible—that she'll be able to come and visit you while you're in the hospital, if you'll be sticking around for a day or two, or that you'll be bringing the baby home as soon as you can after the birth.

If you're intending to bring your child to the hospital with you for the birth, be sure to check to find out whether you'll be expected to bring along an extra adult to care for your child. Some hospital policies specify that there must be another adult on hand to care for children under a certain age.

Don't make the mistake of assuming that you won't need to arrange care for your older child if you're planning a home birth or if your child will be present at your hospital birth. Unless he's of the age where he can pretty much fend for himself (10 or older), you'll want to make sure there's someone else on hand to answer his questions about the birth and/or get him something to eat when mealtime rolls around. You certainly won't be up to the task yourself when you're in the heat of labour, and your partner is likely to have his or her hands full dealing with you.

I'm worried that I'll be subjected to some embarrassing procedure, like an enema or a perineal shave. First things first. Routine enemas and perineal shaves have pretty much gone the way of the dodo. I say "pretty much" because the *Maternity Experiences Survey* revealed that some Canadian hospitals are still performing these two procedures, even though there is no medical evidence that they lead to better outcomes for mothers or babies.

While doctors used to believe it was necessary to give a pregnant woman an enema in order to empty her bowels (it was thought that a large amount of stool might stop labour from progressing), we now know that Mother Nature takes care of this particular problem in her usual efficient manner. The diarrhea that most women experience during early labour ensures that there's very little left in the bowels by the time a woman is ready to give birth.

Perineal shaving has become similarly passé. While doctors used to believe that it was necessary to shave the perineal area in order to minimize the risk of infection, we now know that doing so actually increases the chances that an infection will occur. Besides, don't women who've just given birth have enough discomforts to contend with without having to cope with soreness and itching in this particular area?

As for other embarrassing or humiliating procedures, you lose your sense of modesty pretty quickly once you're in labour. Your focus shifts to finding the most comfortable position possible and focusing on your contractions. You couldn't care less about being naked (or if the entire birthing staff was naked, for that matter). Whatever. You've got other things on your mind.

I just tested positive for group B strep. I am really worried about how this will affect my plans for the birth. Group B strep is a strain of bacteria carried by 10 to 30 per cent of pregnant women. Most caregivers screen for the bacteria during late pregnancy because it can cause a serious, possibly even fatal, infection in the newborn if it's transmitted from mother to baby during labour. There is also at least a theoretical possibility that group B strep could be transmitted from you to your baby, even if your membranes are still intact. Approximately 2 per cent of babies born to mothers with group B strep will end up developing group B strep disease (a serious condition with a 5 to 9 per cent mortality rate). Diabetes during pregnancy is associated with higher rates of group B strep colonization. Fortunately, the vast majority of cases of group B strep can be prevented by administering antibiotics during labour.

If you happen to go into labour prematurely, you have previously given birth to a baby infected with group B strep, you develop a fever during labour, your membranes rupture more than 12 to 18 hours prior to delivery, you have an intra-amniotic infection, or you have not yet been screened for group B strep (or your group B strep culture result is unknown), your caregiver may decide to prescribe antibiotics during your labour whether or not you've been formally diagnosed with group B strep. An ounce of prevention is, after all, worth a pound of cure—especially where group B strep disease is concerned.

In terms of how this will affect your plans for the birth, you'll be receiving your antibiotics intravenously, which means you'll have to give birth at the hospital rather than at home or in a birthing centre, and you'll have to take your IV pole with you if you go for a walk in the birthing unit (and you'll need to park it outside the shower if you want to take advantage of the soothing properties of water while you're in labour). Unfortunately, you'll have to stick to the shower rather than the tub. Labouring in water is not recommended for women with group B strep.

Going Overdue

Your due date has come and gone and there's still no baby. Chances are you're feeling pretty cranky! After all, you thought you were signing a 40-week contract when you agreed to this whole pregnancy thing.

Here are some tips on maintaining what's left of your sanity until baby makes his grand entrance:

- Remind yourself that it's perfectly normal to be overdue. According to British anthropologist and childbirth expert Sheila Kitzinger, only 5 per cent of babies actually arrive on their due date, and of the 95 per cent who don't, just three out of ten arrive before the due date while seven out of ten come after it. And here's another statistic: nine out of ten babies manage to make an appearance within 10 days of their due date. (Just 7 per cent of pregnancies make it to week 42, or the 294th day of pregnancy.)
- Put technology to work for you. If you're sick of fielding all those annoying "haven't you had that baby yet?" phone calls, let your voice mail pick up the calls. Or better yet, do what one couple I know did and record a message that says, "We're just out. We're *not* having the baby!"
- Keep yourself busy. Go to a movie. Have lunch with a friend. Do whatever it takes to take your mind off the fact that your baby is L-A-T-E. And don't be afraid to make plans just because you might have to cancel on your friends. Having a baby is the best excuse ever for standing someone up.
- Pamper yourself. Take advantage of your final baby-free days to get your hair done, soak in the tub, or read incredibly trashy novels. You'll have days like this again, of course—but you'll have to wait another 18 years!
- Enjoy some special time alone with your partner. It may be weeks—even months—before you can both eat dinner at the same time again, so seize the moment!
- Don't expect your doctor or midwife to know how much longer you're going to be pregnant. As much as they'd like to pinpoint the time of your baby's arrival, they don't have a crystal ball.

Is my baby at risk?

You've no doubt heard all the scary stories about the dangers of being overdue—about the awful things that can happen if your baby ends up spending too much time in the womb. What you might not realize, however, is that there's a world of difference between being overdue (past your due date) and postdate (being more than two weeks overdue). If you're more than seven to ten days late your doctor or midwife will want to deliver your baby sooner rather than later. Here's why:

- The placenta may start to deteriorate. The placenta—your baby's life-support system while he's in the womb—is designed to work for about 40 weeks from the time of conception (until approximately the 42nd week of pregnancy, counted from the first day of your last menstrual period). Most placentas continue to function for longer than that, but in some cases the placenta will start to deteriorate and will no longer be able to provide the baby with the nutrients he needs to grow. This could result in a stillbirth.
- Amniotic fluid levels may drop. After about the 34th to 36th week of gestation, the amount of amniotic fluid that your baby is floating around in begins to decrease. If a pregnancy continues for too long, amniotic fluid levels can drop to the point that your baby is at risk of settling on the umbilical cord, causing an umbilical cord compression problem.
- Your baby could inhale meconium. The longer your baby stays in the womb, the greater the odds that he'll pass his first bowel movement—meconium—before birth. If this happens, the baby could end up breathing in some of this black, sticky, tar-like substance, which can result in breathing problems after birth.

While these things don't tend to become a problem until you are more than a week overdue, your doctor or midwife will want to monitor you closely once your due date comes and goes. If your caregiver concludes that your baby would be better off being born now than remaining in the womb much longer, the decision will be made to induce you.

To induce or not to induce?

According to the 2008 Canadian Perinatal Health Report, between one in four and one in five labours in Canada are induced. Despite what you may have heard about women being induced early so that their doctors don't miss out on important golf games, the decision to induce is rarely taken that lightly. According to the SOGC, elective induction (inducing labour when there is no specific medical reason for doing so) is associated with potential complications (prolonged labour, instrumental delivery, postpartum hemorrhage). In all cases of induction, the risks of induction must be balanced against the risks to mother and baby if the pregnancy is allowed to continue.

If your doctor does make the decision to induce, it will likely be for one of the following reasons:

- Your baby doesn't appear to be doing particularly well in the uterus and would likely be better off being induced early.
- You were diabetic before you became pregnant. (There is a high instance of stillbirth in women with pre-existing diabetes and this risk increases once your due date passes.)
- A test has indicated that the placenta is no longer functioning properly and that it would be better for the baby to be born as soon as possible.
- Your membranes have ruptured, but labour has not yet started. Note: Whether or not you'll be induced will depend on how much amniotic fluid has been lost and how close you are to your due date.
- You've developed pre-eclampsia or some other serious medical condition and an induction is necessary for the sake of the baby's health as well as your own.
- You have a history of rapid labour that puts you at high risk of experiencing an unplanned home birth.
- You live a considerable distance from the hospital and may not be able to make it there in time to deliver your baby once labour begins.

Before inducing you, the doctor will need to determine how ready your body is for an induction. (He or she will likely use the Bishop scoring system, which involves looking for evidence that your cervix has begun to efface and dilate, that your baby has begun to descend into your pelvis, that your cervix has begun to soften, and/or that your cervix is moving into the anterior or forward-pointing position. Basically, you're assigned a score of one, two, or three on each of these five criteria. If you score eight or higher, your body is considered to be ready for induction.) If your body isn't ready, you may need to be induced more than once—something no woman should have to endure! Your doctor also has to ensure that your baby is ready to be born. That means checking your prenatal records to confirm that your due date is accurate and, if there is reason to suspect that your due date may be wrong and your baby may actually be premature, possibly assessing the maturity of your baby's lungs by performing amniocentesis.

What to expect during an induction

Induced labours are not necessarily more painful than spontaneous labours. Studies have shown that women who are induced are no more likely to require epidurals than women who go into labour on their own.

If your doctor decides to induce you, he or she will likely use one of the following four methods:

- **Artificial rupture of membranes (amniotomy).** A piece of obstetrical equipment resembling a crochet hook is inserted through your cervix and used to tear a small hole in the amniotic sac. The procedure is virtually painless if you've already started to dilate, but can be quite painful if you're less than 1 centimetre dilated. What's more, if the induction fails, you'll have to be induced using another method. Once your membranes have been ruptured, there's no turning back.
- **Prostaglandin E suppositories or gel.** Prostaglandin E suppositories or gel are used to ripen the cervix. In 50 per cent of cases, the woman will go into labour on her own within the next 24 hours.
- **Pitocin.** Pitocin—the synthetic form of oxytocin (the naturally produced hormone that triggers uterine contractions)—is injected via an intravenous drip and the strength of your contractions is monitored to ensure that you're getting an appropriate dose. It can take a couple of attempts to induce labour with Pitocin.

stripping (or sweeping) membranes

Stripping membranes (sometimes referred to as sweeping membranes) involves gently separating the bag of water from the side of the uterus near the cervix. (Your doctor or midwife inserts her finger through your uterus to perform this procedure, which can be done in her office as part of a regular pelvic exam.) Because hormones are released by your body when the bag of water is separated from the uterus, stripping your membranes may help to send your body into labour—eventually. (It's not a guaranteed method of triggering labour and, even if it does work, it isn't effective right away. The hormones that are released when the bag of water is separated from the uterus take time to soften the cervix, trigger contractions, and encourage the cervix to start opening.) If you have your membranes stripped, you can expect to feel crampy and to experience mild contractions for about 24 hours after the procedure is performed—something that can cause you to miss out on sleep. You may also experience spotting (minor reddish, pink, or bright red bleeding) for up to three days after your membranes are stripped. (If you experience severe pain or bleeding, call your caregiver right away.)

What Labour Is Really Like

Now we come to the $10,000 question—one of the key reasons why you bought this book. You want to know what labour is really like. If I could come up with a nice pat answer, this would become the fastest-selling pregnancy book of all time. Doctors and midwives would be ordering it in by the truckload and giving copies to their patients. Maternity stores would be selling maternity T-shirts printed with my pithy definition of labour. It would show up on subway ads, the sides of buses, and the stickers on the apples in the grocery store. CBC Kids would feature public service announcements for children, offering tips on how to tell if Mom is really in labour. The spinoff possibilities would be endless.

I hate to disappoint you (to say nothing of my publisher), but that's not going to happen. The reason is simple. I'd have to catalogue about 1,000 descriptions of labour per day just to stay on top of things. You see, no two labours are exactly alike, and there are about 1,000 babies born in Canada each day, so, in the interests of scientific inquiry, I'd have to interview about 1,000 new moms a day. That would be exhausting, and this book would quickly turn into a multi-volume pregnancy book. (*Encyclopaedia Pregnanica,* I presume.) See the problem?

Since it's unlikely my publisher would agree to put out a 20-volume pregnancy book set, you're going to have to settle for the next best thing: an insider's look at what labour *may* be like for you. We'll start out by considering the three stages of labour. Then we'll look at what the handy-dandy chart that I've included won't actually tell you: the stuff only your most talkative girlfriends are willing to spill the beans about.

The three stages of labour

The first thing you need to know is that the labour process can be broken down into three distinct stages: the first stage (which lasts from the first contraction until your cervix is fully dilated), the second stage (the "pushing stage"), and the third stage (the delivery of the placenta). (See Table 10.2.) Some people include a fourth stage—postpartum recovery and involution (the return of the uterus to its pre-pregnant state).

What other mothers want you to know

Now let's get to the bottom line—the things other mothers want you to know about giving birth.

Your body doesn't pay attention to clocks while you're in labour. You'd be wise to follow your body's example. Keeping track of how long it's taking your cervix to dilate fully or how long you've been pushing can be an exercise in frustration—and it doesn't accomplish a thing.

Let your body do its work. Instead of obsessively over-thinking what your body is doing, relax and go with the flow.

Your birthing environment does matter—a lot. Giving birth in a place where you feel safe—where you will be supported by people who understand and who will respect your birth philosophies—makes a huge difference.

Partners need help to prepare for the birth, too. We expect them to be mind readers in the labour room—mind readers with little practical training. Make it easier for your partner to be your ideal labour support person: attend childbirth classes together and be specific about your hopes and dreams for the birth.

Birth is a journey you ultimately make on your own. Because you will be making the most challenging part of your journey on your own, you will want to be well prepared. Once you know what the journey will be like, and you have been reassured that countless other women have walked this path before you, you will be able to anticipate rather than fear the journey that lies ahead.

If you wait to experience each and every labour symptom before you call your doctor or midwife, you'll be giving birth on your kitchen floor. I can practically guarantee it! It could take you two, three, or even a dozen or more pregnancies to experience all these symptoms. Don't get greedy and expect to experience them all the first time around.

You have an almost endless supply of amniotic fluid. Don't expect it to disappear in one fell swoosh when your membranes rupture. It'll dribble . . . and dribble . . . and dribble. In fact, that endless dribbling of the amniotic fluid is one of the most annoying aspects of labour. It leaves you cold, wet, and, frankly, quite miserable.

Your contractions won't feel the way your best friend's did. There's no such thing as a textbook contraction. The type of pain you experience (a sharp, stabbing sensation versus a dull, aching or burning pain) depends on which type of nerve fibre triggers the impulse. Some women have "traditional" contractions with well-defined starts and finishes. Others find that one contraction kind of just blurs into the next.

It's possible to experience uterine contractions primarily as lower back pain. (This is particularly common if, like 10 per cent of babies, your baby is lying in the posterior position, meaning that the back of his head is up against

10.2 The Three Stages of Labour

What Happens During This Stage	How You May Be Feeling Physically	How You May Be Feeling Emotionally	Tips on Coping with This Stage
First Stage (From the Onset of Labour Until the Cervix Is Fully Dilated)			
Early or latent labour (when your cervix dilates from 0 to 3 centimetres)	Backache, menstrual-like cramping, indigestion, diarrhea, a feeling of warmth in the abdomen, bloody show (the passage of blood-tinged mucus from the vagina), and a trickling or gushing sensation if your membranes have ruptured.	Excitement, relief, anticipation, uncertainty, anxiety, fear.	Eat lightly and keep yourself well hydrated, continue with your normal activities as long as possible, ask your partner or labour support person to help you time contractions and to pack any last-minute items before you leave for the hospital or birthing centre (unless, of course, you're having a home birth).
Active labour (when your cervix dilates from 4 to 7 centimetres)	Increased discomfort from contractions (suddenly, it's more difficult to talk or walk through a contraction), pain and aching in your legs and back, fatigue, increased quantities of bloody show.	Anxiety, discouragement, highly focused on getting through this stage of labour.	Remain upright and active as long as possible, experiment with positions until you find one that works best for you when a contraction hits, rest between contractions, empty your bladder regularly (at least once an hour), allow your partner or labour support person to help you with labour breathing and/or relaxation techniques, continue to consume light fluids (as long as you've got your caregiver's go-ahead).
Transition (when your cervix dilates from 8 to 10 centimetres)	Increased quantities of show, pressure in your lower back, perineal and rectal pressure, hot and cold flashes, shaky legs, intense aching in your thighs, nausea or vomiting, belching, heavy perspiration.	Irritable, disoriented, restless, frustrated, like you can't take it any longer.	Change positions frequently to see if doing so will help your labour to progress and/or provide any measure of pain relief, apply a hot water bottle or cold pack to your back, have your partner or labour support person apply counter pressure to the part of your back that's hurting, or have him/her apply strong finger pressure below the centre of the ball of your foot (an acupressure point for pain relief). When you are in an upright position, your abdominal wall relaxes and your baby's head presses on your cervix (which triggers more frequent and more intense contractions).

Second Stage (The Pushing Stage)

Your cervix is fully dilated and your body is ready for the pushing stage (or will be soon: sometimes there is a short delay between full dilation and the onset of the urge to push)	Expect to experience a series of 60- to 90-second contractions at two- to five-minute intervals. Your baby's head needs to stretch the vaginal and pelvic floor muscles before the urge to push is triggered, so there can be a delay before you feel that urge (sometimes called the rest and descend phase). If you have had an epidural, pushing can be delayed for up to two hours (if you're giving birth for the first time) and up to one hour (if you're giving birth for the second or subsequent time). Once that urge kicks in, you'll likely experience increased rectal pressure, an increase in bloody show, an urge to grunt as you bear down, a burning or stretching sensation as your baby's head crowns in the vagina, and a slippery feeling as your baby is born. The bones in your baby's skull can overlap during birth, decreasing the size of your baby's head by 0.5 to 1 centimetres.	Excited and energetic, or tired, discouraged, and overwhelmed, depending on how your labour is going.	Have your partner or labour support person help you move into a squatting or semi-squatting position to make it easier for you to push your baby out. Push when you feel the urge, take short breaths rather than holding your breath and pushing through an entire contraction, and be prepared to stop pushing (pant or blow instead) if your caregiver tells you that your perineum needs time to stretch gradually in order to avoid an episiotomy or a tear. When you get the urge to push, do whatever comes naturally. Three to four short pushes (six to eight seconds each) per contraction is more effective and easier on your baby than going for a giant push and trying to hold your breath for 10 to 15 seconds. (When you hold your breath, there is decreased blood flow to the placenta.) If your baby is not responding well to pushing, the staff may suggest that you change positions and/or take a break from pushing before trying again. Your support team should be tuning in to the feedback from your baby and your body, not following a generic script that tries to dictate how birth should go. Note: Being upright (standing, squatting, sitting) leads to a shorter pushing stage and better outcomes for both mothers and babies. When you squat, your pelvis opens up (it becomes 28 per cent larger), which assists with your baby's engagement and descent.

continued

What Happens During This Stage	How You May Be Feeling Physically	How You May Be Feeling Emotionally	Tips on Coping with This Stage

10.2 The Three Stages of Labour (continued)

Third Stage (The Delivery of the Placenta)

What Happens During This Stage	How You May Be Feeling Physically	How You May Be Feeling Emotionally	Tips on Coping with This Stage
Your uterus expels the placenta	The uterus contracts on itself and starts shrinking down in size, a process known as involution. The placenta separates from the uterine wall. Mild contractions lasting for one minute or less will gently push the placenta out of your body. It feels small and slippery in comparison to your baby. Your caregiver will examine the placenta to make sure it's complete, since retained placental fragments can cause hemorrhaging. You'll experience heavy bleeding from the vagina and may pass some large blood clots when you go to the bathroom. (Be sure to tell your caregiver if they are any larger than a lemon.)	Distracted, happy, excited to finally be meeting your baby, exhausted from the delivery, cold, hungry.	Your caregiver may give you a shot of oxytocin to try to prevent any problems with postpartum hemorrhaging. Your baby's nose and mouth will be suctioned and the baby will be assessed using the Apgar test. This test evaluates the baby's appearance, pulse (heartbeat), grimace (response to stimulation), activity (movements), and respiration (breathing). The test is performed twice, at one minute and five minutes after birth. The baby is given up to two points for each attribute. A baby with a score of seven or over is doing well, a baby with a score of four to six may require resuscitation, and a baby with a score of three or less may be in serious trouble.

your spine. Most posterior babies make the 180-degree shift into the anterior position at some point during labour, but those that don't can either be delivered naturally or, if necessary, via forceps or vacuum extraction.) Back labour can be long and drawn out, and very discouraging. Counter pressure (having your labour support person apply pressure to your lower back), applying a heating pad or a hot water bottle to the affected area, and experimenting with various positions (side lying, tailor sitting, leaning forward while you are standing or sitting, or rocking your pelvis) may help to relieve the pain of back labour.

Sometimes labour can be painstakingly slow or grind to a halt altogether. This can happen if

- your contractions are weak and ineffective;
- there's some sort of fetal obstruction (for example, your baby is breech, posterior, lying in a transverse or sideways position, or lying in an oblique or diagonal position; your baby is presenting with its face or forehead first rather than the top of its head; your baby is large in relation to the size of your pelvis; you are delivering twins and they have become entwined; or your baby has a fetal anomaly such as hydrocephalus);
- there's some sort of maternal obstruction (for example, your pelvis is deformed or unusually small, you have pelvic tumours such as large fibroids or a large ovarian cyst, your uterus, cervix, or vagina is abnormal, or your uterus is contracting in a manner that causes a band of tight muscle tissue to prevent the uterus or cervix from contracting);
- you become overly anxious. Anxiety and fear can interfere with the progress of labour. That is why it is important to choose labour support people who help you to feel safe and supported and who will give you the time and space you need to give birth to your baby in a relaxed, unhurried way.

You may feel as though you're on another planet during the most intense part of your labour. Forget about looking lovingly into your partner's eyes while the two of you contemplate the impending birth of your child. You may be just plain zoned out. "Labour was a continual dull ache that consumed my entire being," confesses Bonnie, a 27-year-old mother of two. "I couldn't focus on anything except the next labour pain. I have no idea what was being said or who was in the room. It was almost a delusional state, like when you're very sick. You're in and out of consciousness, it seems."

Some women won't be completely honest about their birth experiences until after you've given birth. The reason is obvious. They don't want you to take the vow of celibacy! (Hey, if foot-long stretch marks and 30-hour labours were good enough for them, they're good enough for you, too.) "I think there's a bit of a conspiracy that you don't tell friends who haven't given birth how much it really does hurt because you don't want to scare them," admits Cheryl, 29, who is currently pregnant with her second child (and not saying a word about her first birth to any of her first-time pregnant buddies).

Pregnancy books are big on euphemisms. Take everything that you read with a grain of salt. "I had a girlfriend who experienced natural childbirth a few

breech birth

About 4 per cent of babies are in the breech position at term. (If a mother's first baby was breech, the odds of her second baby being breech are about 9 per cent.)

If a baby is in the vertex position—the head-down birth position that most babies assume before birth—the baby's head will be born first. If, however, a baby is in the breech position, the baby's feet or bottom are the presenting parts.

A breech birth—whether vaginal or Caesarean—carries a higher risk of complications, which is why many doctors will recommend a procedure known as an external cephalic version (ECV) (a procedure in which the doctor applies her hands to your abdomen and attempts to shift your baby from the breech position to the vertex position through a series of movements). The ECV will take place in the hospital so that the baby can be monitored—and in case you go into labour. The procedure can be quite uncomfortable, and even painful. (Talk to your doctor about pain relief options, should you choose to have an ECV.) In many cases, the baby reverts to the breech position following the ECV (something that can be extremely frustrating and disappointing for you).

While there are certain risk factors associated with giving birth vaginally when your baby is in the breech position—head entrapment, cord prolapse, and cord compression—according to the Society of Obstetricians and Gynaecologists of Canada, a vaginal breech delivery offers reasonable odds of success. About 60 per cent of women who attempt to deliver breech babies vaginally manage to give birth that way. And, if unanticipated complications arise during a vaginal breech birth, a Caesarean is performed immediately. Careful screening ahead of time can also help to identify some situations when a scheduled Caesarean would be the best option for Mom and Baby. Note: Not all obstetricians deliver breech babies vaginally. Your doctor may end up referring you to a high-risk pregnancy specialist who specializes in this type of delivery.

months before me," explains Joyce. "Fortunately she tipped me off to this problem. She told me, 'You know that part in the books that tells you that the mother
may experience some burning when the baby's head is crowning? Well, believe
me—it's not just a mild burning sensation; it's more like a f—ing blowtorch!'"

**The pushing stage is different than the active stage of labour, but it's not
exactly a vacation.** Think about it. You're trying to push a 8-pound (3.5-
kilogram) baby out through an opening that's generally snug enough to hold a
tampon in place. You think that's going to be easy? Not according to Cheryl:
"I didn't expect it to be so hard to push the baby out. It's a real physical effort
and it was exhausting." Marinda, a 30-year-old mother of two, agrees: "I was
overwhelmed by the pain of the pushing stage. I thought it was hell. For a short
time, I didn't even care if I got a baby out of it. I just wanted the pain to end."

Every labour is unique. Ditto for the amount of pain a woman experiences
during labour. Labour pain is mild in 15 per cent of cases, moderate in 35 per
cent, severe in 30 per cent and extreme in 20 per cent. Pain is likely to be more
intense the first time a woman gives birth and for women who have a history
of painful periods or a fear of pain. Women who have taken childbirth classes,
experience complications during pregnancy, wish to breastfeed, and are older
and of higher socio-economic status tend to experience less severe pain.

You'll amaze yourself with your strength and resilience. Your body is doing
the hard work involved in opening up and pushing your baby out into the
world. The more you are able to focus on the purpose behind the pain, the
more manageable the pain becomes and the more confident you feel about
your ability to cope with the remaining contractions. You'll also dazzle your
partner. Joyce was very apprehensive about giving birth, but, in the end, she
was pleasantly surprised by her own abilities: "I was so sure I'd be afraid, but
what amazed me was how 'natural' the whole thing turned out to be: how
we as females and the givers of life have such a reserve of strength we didn't
know existed until it's called upon."

The great Caesarean debate

Until now we've been focusing on vaginal birth. Since a significant number of
babies are born through Caesarean section—more than one in four Canadian
babies are delivered via Caesarean—it's important to know what a Caesarean
involves, even if you're almost positive that you'll be delivering vaginally.

According to the 2008 *Canadian Perinatal Health Report*, the Canadian Caesarean rate has been on the rise for the last three decades. The rate has been rising for a variety of reasons. Mothers are giving birth later in life (which has led to an increase in the birth rate of multiples), a larger percentage of births are to first-time moms, and more moms are obese during pregnancy—all of these factors increase the likelihood of a Caesarean. What's more, changes in medical practise, such as greater use of electronic fetal monitoring during labour (which can lead to an increased Caesarean birth rate), and an increased use of Caesareans for breech births have contributed to the increased rate as well.

At first glance, you might think that a Caesarean is the perfect way to have a baby. After all, you get to avoid all those gut-wrenching contractions, to say nothing of that annoying third-trimester "Am I really in labour or not?" guessing game. But having a Caesarean section isn't exactly a picnic. I mean, this is major abdominal surgery we're talking about here, complete with a less-than-enjoyable recovery. We're talking killer gas pains, stitches in your abdomen, and—if you require a general anaesthesia—feeling somewhat dopey and drowsy when you finally get the chance to meet your baby. And then there are all the possible complications: infection, problems related to the anaesthesia, blood clots caused by reduced mobility after surgery, bladder and bowel injuries, maternal hemorrhage, and fetal respiratory problems. So a Caesarean shouldn't be treated as a no-fuss option to a vaginal delivery. Unfortunately, society seems to be treating them as such, which may explain why a recent survey of Canadian women reported that 8.4 per cent of them requested a Caesarean section at some point during their last pregnancy. Reasons for requesting a Caesarean when there are no maternal or fetal indications for having one include fear of losing control, fear of labour pain, a previous negative birth experience, a desire to control the timing of the birth, fear of something happening to the baby, or a mistaken belief that Caesarean birth is better for the mother's body. (The Canadian Term Breech Trial, which studied planned Caesarean section versus planned vaginal birth, did not find any differences with regard to long-term sexual function, urinary or fecal incontinence, pelvic pain, or postpartum depression.) If you have specific fears related to the birth, it is important to talk through your feelings with someone you trust.

In their *Position Statement on Elective Cesarean Section* (issued in June 2004), the Canadian Association of Midwives spoke out against elective Caesareans (procedures performed when there is no medical reason to warrant the surgery):"This trend both reflects and serves to construct a mechanical and fragmented vision of the body and birth and also of the pregnant woman and her unborn baby. It is a product of our society's 'culture of fear' around childbirth and demonstrates the extent to which the 'epidemic of risk' is reflected in maternity care . . . Presenting interventions such as c-sections as 'options' puts maternity care providers and women in a consumerist relationship and treats childbirth as a problem to be solved rather than a process to be respected."

That's not to say Caesareans are a terrible thing. They've helped save the lives of countless mothers and babies and prevented many birth-related injuries, after all. It's elective Caesareans that are the concern.

What you can do to decrease your odds of requiring a Caesarean section

Start your family sooner rather than later. The older you are when you have your baby, the greater your risk of requiring a Caesarean.

Embark on pregnancy at a healthy weight. And avoid gaining an excess amount of weight during pregnancy. Obese mothers face an increased risk of requiring a Caesarean section.

Don't head to the hospital too soon. Arriving at the hospital too soon (for example, if your cervix is 3 centimetres dilated or less) may result in a diagnosis of dystocia. You can end up having labour induced before your body is ready, something that can ultimately result in a Caesarean section.

Don't agree to labour interventions when they aren't medically necessary. Just because we have the technology doesn't necessarily mean we should use it every time. Continuous electronic fetal monitoring (EFM) is not recommended for low-risk labours, but, in some hospitals, it is used in every labour nonetheless. The net result? More interventions, including Caesareans. Here's why: EFM limits your ability to be up and about during labour, something that reduces the efficiency of your labour contractions and increases your perceptions of the amount of pain you are experiencing. You may become discouraged and exhausted if your labour fails to progress, leading to a diagnosis of dystocia. That, in turn, could lead to attempts to induce labour before your cervix is ready. If those attempts were unsuccessful, you could end up with a Caesarean when all you needed was to be mobile in early labour and to be given time and space to go with the flow of labour.

What happens during a Caesarean

Even if you're planning for a vaginal delivery, it's important to understand what's involved in giving birth via Caesarean. There's always the chance that a pregnancy or birthing complication could arise, necessitating a change in plans. You might also want to talk to your health-care provider about what you would want in the event of a Caesarean birth. For example, would you want to have your baby placed on your chest as soon as possible after the birth—or handed to your partner? Hospitals are trying to be more sensitive to the needs of mothers giving birth via Caesarean section. The more you talk to your health-care provider about your options upfront (whether you think you're having a Caesarean or not) the greater your odds of having these options available to you, should you need them.

---

the natural Caesarean

Researchers from the Imperial College London and the University of Queensland in Australia have been researching what they are calling "the natural Caesarean"—a Caesarean technique that attempts to emulate as closely as possible the woman-centred aspects of "natural" vaginal birth when a woman has a Caesarean. "Increasing evidence shows that women undergoing Caesareans have a less satisfactory childbirth experience than those delivering vaginally and are more prone to postnatal depression, bonding difficulties and unsuccessful breastfeeding," the researchers note. Reporting on their findings in the April 7, 2008, issue of the *British Journal of Obstetrics*, the researchers noted that their technique—which involves lowering the surgical drape and raising the head of the table after the uterine incision has been made so that the mother can watch the birth, and encouraging immediate skin-to-skin contact following the birth—is suitable for healthy mothers having healthy babies at term, but that it is not suitable for emergency procedures or Caesareans involving preterm or breech presentations.

Before the delivery

- Your doctor will give you medication to dry the secretions in your mouth and upper airway. He or she will also give you an antacid to reduce the acidity of your stomach contents—important if you end up inhaling some of the contents of your stomach during the delivery.
- Your doctor may give you a single dose of antibiotics to guard against the possibility of infection.
- Your lower abdomen will be washed and possibly shaved as well.
- A catheter will be inserted into your bladder to reduce the risk of injury during the delivery. (A full bladder can be injured more easily.)
- An intravenous needle will be inserted into your hand or arm so that you can be given medications and fluids during the delivery.
- You'll be given an anaesthetic—either an epidural, a spinal, or a general. (General anaesthetic is used when an emergency Caesarean is required

and it is important to administer anaesthesia quickly, when an epidural or spinal block cannot be placed, or when a woman cannot be given a regional anaesthetic because doing so would pose a risk to her health (she is on blood thinners or has an infection in her back, for example).)

- Your abdomen will be swabbed with antiseptic solution and covered with a sterile drape.
- A screen will be put in place to keep the surgical field sterile. It also helps to block your view of the delivery. Note: If you would like to watch your baby being born, ask if it would be possible to have a mirror angled so that you witness this powerful moment.

During the delivery

- An incision will be made through both the wall of your abdomen and the wall of your uterus as soon as the anaesthetic has taken effect. You may still be able to feel some pressure, but you won't feel any pain.
- The amniotic sac will be opened and amniotic fluid will pour out.
- Your baby will be lifted from your body. You may feel a slight tugging sensation if you've had an epidural (an obstetrician I know says the pressure and sensation you feel during a Caesarean delivery is similar to what you experience when you touch your face or tongue after the dentist has frozen your mouth), but you're unlikely to feel any such sensation if you've had a spinal. You may also experience some nausea and vomiting because tugging on the peritoneum—the layer that coats your internal organs—can trigger this reaction in some women.

After the delivery

- The umbilical cord will be clamped and the placenta will be removed from your uterus.
- Your baby's nose and mouth will be suctioned and the baby will be assessed using the Apgar test.

---

the big squeeze

Worried that a baby born through Caesarean section is at a disadvantage because he doesn't get the same "squeezing" as babies born vaginally? Most obstetricians agree this is a myth. A fair bit of squeezing occurs as the baby is delivered through the incision in your uterus, something that—like a vaginal delivery—helps to clear amniotic fluid from the baby's lungs and stimulate the baby's circulation.

- Your uterus and abdomen will be stitched up and you'll be given the opportunity to hold your baby if both you and the baby are feeling up to it.
- You'll be taken to the recovery room so that your vital signs can be monitored and you can be checked for excessive bleeding and other possible post-delivery complications.
- You may be given antibiotics and/or pain medications at this time.
- You'll be moved to the postpartum floor to continue your recovery.
- About six to eight hours after the delivery, your catheter will be removed and you'll be encouraged to get out of bed.
- You'll be given intravenous fluids for one to two days, until you're able to start eating again. (Basically, you'll be kept on intravenous fluids the entire time you're receiving intravenous drugs and you'll continue to receive these fluids until you're feeling well enough to drink enough fluids to keep your body adequately hydrated.)
- You'll be able to leave the hospital within three to five days after the delivery, unless unexpected complications arise.
- You may have difficulty breastfeeding comfortably, but position changes for feeding and lots of cushions for support can help reduce the discomfort.

Vaginal birth after Caesarean (VBAC)

Doctors used to live by the motto, "Once a Caesarean, always a Caesarean." That's not the case today. More and more often, doctors are encouraging their patients to consider vaginal births after Caesarean (VBACs). And why not? According to the Society of Obstetricians and Gynaecologists of Canada, the success rate of a trial of labour after Caesarean ranges from 50 per cent to 85 per cent. If you required a Caesarean in a previous pregnancy because of issues such as fetal malpresentation (the baby's position) or gestational hypertension (pregnancy-related high blood pressure) that may not necessarily recur in a subsequent pregnancy, your odds of a successful VBAC are particularly good. If you have previously experienced a successful vaginal delivery, they are even higher.

There are clearly many advantages to attempting a VBAC—vaginal deliveries are generally less risky than Caesareans, take less time to recover from, and allow you to play a more active role in your baby's birth—but there are also some risks involved. There's always the chance, however slight, that the uterine scar tissue from your previous incision may split—a potentially life-threatening complication for both you and your baby. (Your odds of experiencing this sort of complication when you've had a single Caesarean delivery are approximately 1 in 600.)

Your doctor is unlikely to encourage you to attempt a VBAC if

- you had a vertical rather than a horizontal uterine incision, since there's a higher risk of uterine rupture (Note: The incision on your uterus may not necessarily be in the same direction as the incision on your skin);
- your baby is in either the breech or transverse position;
- you are showing signs of placenta previa or another condition that would make a Caesarean section a safer choice;
- your baby is showing signs of fetal distress;
- you will be giving birth within 24 months of your previous Caesarean. According to the Society of Obstetricians and Gynaecologists of Canada, women who give birth within 24 months of a previous Caesarean section should be informed that the risk of a uterine rupture is greater than in mothers who wait a little longer before attempting a VBAC.

You might be interested to know that carrying multiples should not prevent you from attempting a VBAC. According to the SOGC, success rates of 69 per cent to 84 per cent have been reported for VBACs in multiple pregnancy—and without any increased reports of harm to mother or baby. Similarly, the SOGC does not consider diabetes mellitus (pre-existing diabetes as opposed to gestational diabetes, the kind of diabetes that develops during pregnancy), fetal macrosomia (carrying a large baby), or being postdate (at 42 weeks of pregnancy or beyond) to be sufficient cause to rule out a VBAC.

The SOGC recommends that VBACs take place in a hospital. They also recommend continuous electronic fetal monitoring during labour. "The most reliable first sign of uterine rupture is a non-reassuring fetal heart tracing. This may be sudden in onset and may not be related to contractions," the SOGC notes in its 2005 VBAC clinical guidelines.

Birth trauma

You don't hear much about women being traumatized by their birth experiences—or experiencing flashbacks to earlier traumas while they are giving birth. That doesn't mean that the phenomenon isn't real. Major studies conducted in Australia and the UK indicate that between 1 per cent and 6 per cent of women will develop symptoms of post-traumatic stress disorder following childbirth. Unfortunately, a diagnosis of PTSD is frequently delayed or missed in women who have experienced birth trauma. And even when it is diagnosed, women struggling with birth trauma don't receive a lot of support. "The problem is trivialized and women are blamed," says Penny Christensen, Executive Director of Birth Trauma Canada (www.birthtraumacanada.org). "The attitude is that you survived and your baby survived: be grateful."

This dismissive attitude ignores the debilitating fallout of a traumatic birth: flashbacks (vivid memories of the event), feelings of fear and panic, nightmares, and difficulty sleeping. Women may avoid situations that remind them of their birth experience. They may detach emotionally to avoid re-experiencing emotions related to trauma. They may become hypervigilant in order to try to protect themselves or their loved ones from any potential future trauma. Unresolved trauma can have far-reaching consequences for a new mother and her family. It can affect her physical and emotional well-being and her relationships with other people. And, if the feelings of hopelessness and helplessness that typically accompany PTSD are not addressed, the new mother remains vulnerable and is more susceptible to future trauma.

Being denied the opportunity to make informed decisions about birth traumatizes women. That's one of the key findings to emerge from a research review conducted by the School of Nursing and Midwifery at the University of Western Sydney in Australia, and reported on in the May 2010 issue of the *Journal of Advanced Nursing*. "Healthcare professionals must recognize women's need to be involved in decision-making and to be fully informed about all aspects of their labour and birth to increase their sense of control," the authors wrote.

And as for what helps mothers to heal from trauma, the study highlighted two key strategies: Mothers should be encouraged to talk about their birth experiences and to access trauma therapy. And mothers who have experienced birth trauma should receive extra breastfeeding support.

How you may feel about meeting your baby

After months of anticipation, your baby is finally here. You may feel over the moon with excitement or so tired you can hardly even process the fact that this tiny human being belongs to you. While you may worry that you'll be setting your child up for a lifetime of psychological problems if you don't manage to bond in the first few minutes after the birth, that's simply not the case.

Lori, a 29-year-old mother of four, remembers what it was like after her first baby arrived: "I wasn't prepared to be as tired as I was. By the time my daughter was born, pain aside, I'd been awake for 32 hours and was completely exhausted. Being in pain and going through labour just intensified that feeling. So by the time my baby was born, all I could think about was sleep."

Stephanie, a 27-year-old mother of one, had a different experience, although it started out the same. "I was so exhausted that I could hardly keep my eyes open," she said. "I remember thinking, 'What's wrong with me? This is my child and I, at this moment, don't even care if I hold her. I just want to sleep.' I took her on my chest and then the midwife came over and helped me to start breastfeeding her. That was the magical moment—to see her instantly take my breast and start sucking. I nursed her for almost half an hour and it was the bonding moment for me."

Alexandra remembers feeling as though she'd just been handed someone else's baby. "I couldn't believe that the little baby on my tummy was mine," the 33-year-old mother of two recalls. "I actually asked the nurses if I could touch her. Although I felt overwhelming love toward my baby, it took a couple of days for me to actually bond with her."

Janet, 32, felt much the same way when her daughter was born. "I was immediately fascinated by her, but I didn't feel like she belonged to us until several days—maybe even a week—after her birth. Initially she seemed like a novelty item of some sort, and it did not sink in that she was with us permanently."

Some women, like Jennifer, do experience that magical, mystical, love-at-first-sight bonding that you hear so much about. "I was amazed at how quickly I bonded with my babies," the 31-year-old mother of two recalls. "There was an instant connection and I felt immediately like their mommy."

Christina, 25, also felt overcome with emotion when she met each of her three children for the very first time. "I felt an instant bond with my children when they were born. It didn't matter that they were wrinkled and funny looking. They were the most beautiful sight in the world to me. When I held my son in my arms for the first time, I felt something I'd never felt before: unconditional love and an amazingly strong protective instinct."

In the words of Jennifer, 32, mother of one, "There isn't necessarily a bright light or a wave of emotion or a band playing when you hold your new child for the very first time. Don't force the situation. Just allow yourself to be happy, tired, relieved, scared—whatever."

Parting Words

I can't believe we've already come to the end of this book. I still feel as though I have so much left to say. But given that the book is already 50,000 words over length (again), my publisher would like me to turn off my computer. I hope you'll send me your comments about the book and drop by the official website for updates and news on other related titles (www.having-a-baby.com). In the meantime, I wish you and your baby all the best in your journey to birth and beyond.

Glossary

Active labour The period of labour during which the cervix dilates from 4 to 10 centimetres.

Adrenal gland A small gland situated above each kidney that secretes sex hormones and other hormones, including cortisone and adrenaline.

Afterbirth Another name for the placenta—your baby's physiological support system in utero.

Alpha-fetoprotein (AFP) testing A prenatal blood test performed between 15 and 18 weeks of pregnancy to screen for both neural tube defects (high levels of AFP) and Down syndrome (low levels of AFP). If it's combined with measurements of both human chorionic gonadotropin (hCG) and unconjugated estriol, the test is referred to as maternal serum screening. These tests are screening tests rather than diagnostic tests. In other words, they can't definitely state whether or not your baby is affected by a particular problem; they can only state whether it is likely that your baby is affected.

Amniocentesis A procedure that involves inserting a needle through the abdominal wall and removing a small quantity of amniotic fluid from the sac surrounding the developing baby. The amniotic fluid is then used to test for fetal abnormalities, to determine the baby's sex, or to assess lung maturity and overall fetal well-being. Alpha-fetoprotein levels can also be measured using a sample of amniotic fluid.

Amniotic fluid The protective liquid, consisting mostly of water, which surrounds the baby inside the amniotic sac.

Amniotic sac (or amnion) The thin-walled sac within the uterus that houses the baby and the amniotic fluid.

Androgens The name given to a general class of male sex hormones, one of which is testosterone.

Andrology The study of the male reproductive system.

Anencephaly A birth defect involving a malformed brain and skull. Anencephaly leads to stillbirth or death soon after birth.

Anomaly A malformation or abnormality in any part of the body. Some anomalies are relatively minor; others can be serious, even fatal.

Anovulation The total absence of ovulation. It's still possible to menstruate during an anovulatory cycle.

Anovulatory bleeding The type of menstruation most often associated with anovulatory cycles. It tends to be either scanty and of short duration or abnormally heavy. The pattern of bleeding tends to be irregular.

Apgar score The numerical result of the Apgar test. Up to two points are given to each of the following attributes: appearance, pulse (heartbeat), grimace (response to stimulation), activity (movements), and respiration (breathing). A baby with a score of seven or over is doing well; a baby with a score of four to six may require resuscitation; and a baby with a score of three or less may be in serious trouble.

Apgar test An assessment of a newborn's early response to the stress of birth and life outside the womb. The test is performed one minute and five minutes after birth. A poor test result on the one-minute test can be due to the stress of the delivery process. The result on the five-minute test is more meaningful in terms of the infant's long-term outcome. An infant with a poor Apgar score is re-tested every five minutes until a score of at least six is obtained.

Areola The flat, pigmented area encircling the nipple of the breast.

Artificial insemination (AI) Any method of insemination other than sexual intercourse.

Assisted reproduction The use of any new reproductive technology (NRT) for the purpose of overcoming infertility to produce a child (e.g., in vitro fertilization, assisted insemination, donor insemination).

Basal body temperature (BBT) The female partner's temperature taken upon rising first thing in the morning. In 95 per cent of cases, BBT readings can be used to determine if ovulation has occurred.

Bed sharing Sharing a bed with a baby. (Sometimes called co-sleeping.) Room sharing is recommended by Health Canada (as opposed to bed sharing).

Binovular twins *See* fraternal twins.

Biopsy Surgical removal of a sample of tissue for analysis.

Blastocyst The name given to the cluster of cells that will eventually form the fetus.

Blood pressure There are two readings: the systolic pressure (the upper figure) and the diastolic pressure (the lower figure). You're generally considered to have high blood pressure if the reading exceeds 140/90. (Generally, elevations in diastolic pressure are considered to be most dangerous.)

Bloody show The mucus discharge—often tinged with blood—that may indicate the cervix is effacing and/or dilating.

Braxton Hicks contractions Irregular contractions of the uterus that occur during pregnancy and that are felt most strongly during the late third trimester. Braxton Hicks contractions neither efface nor dilate the cervix.

Breast abscess A condition in which pus accumulates in one area of the breast.

Breast engorgement When the breasts become swollen and full of milk.

Breech presentation When the fetus is positioned buttocks or feet down rather than head down.

Caesarean section A surgical procedure used to deliver a baby via an incision made in the mother's abdomen and uterus.

Campylobacter A common bacterial cause of intestinal infections.

Cephalopelvic disproportion When the presenting part of the baby's head is too large for the mother's pelvis and birth canal.

Cerclage A procedure in which a stitch is inserted into and around the cervix early in the pregnancy, usually between weeks 12 to 14, and then removed toward the end of pregnancy when the risk of miscarriage has passed.

Cervical dilation A measure of how wide the cervix has opened up prior to or during labour. Cervical dilation is measured in centimetres (from 0 to 10). When you're 10 centimetres dilated, you're fully dilated and ready to push.

Cervical effacement The thinning out of the cervix before and during labour. When the cervix is fully effaced, it is paper-thin.

Cervical incompetence A congenital defect or injury to the cervix that causes it to open prematurely during pregnancy, resulting in miscarriage or a premature birth without labour.

Cervical mucus Mucus produced by the cervix. Cervical mucus aids in the movement of sperm from the cervix to the uterus and Fallopian tubes. The mucus increases in volume and acquires an egg white–like consistency during the days leading up to ovulation.

Cervix The entrance to the uterus.

Chadwick's sign A dark blue or purple discolouration of the vagina and cervix during pregnancy. In the days before pregnancy tests, it provided your doctor with an important clue that you could be pregnant. Sometimes called Jacquemin's sign, after the French doctor who first discovered these changes.

Chlamydia A common sexually transmitted infection that can render a woman infertile if left untreated. Antibiotics can be used to treat the infection.

Chloasma Extensive brown patches of irregular shape and size on the face or other parts of the body that can occur during pregnancy. Sometimes referred to as the "mask of pregnancy."

Chorioamnionitis An inflammation of the membranes surrounding the fetus.

Chorion The outer sac enclosing the fetus within the uterus.

Chorionic villus sampling (CVS) A prenatal diagnostic test in which a few placental cells are extracted via a fine hollow needle or catheter inserted into the womb through the abdomen or the cervix. Like amniocentesis, CVS can be used to detect a variety of genetic disorders and to determine the sex of the fetus. CVS can be done as early as the eighth or ninth week of pregnancy, and the results are usually known within a week.

Chromosomal abnormalities Problems that result from errors in the duplication of the chromosomes—the thread-like structures in the nucleus of a cell that transmit genetic information.

Circumcision Surgical removal of the foreskin of the penis.

Cleft lip A condition in which there is a separation of the upper lip that can extend into the nose.

Cleft palate A condition in which the roof of the mouth is incompletely formed.

Clubfoot A condition in which the baby is born with the sole of one or both feet facing either down and inward or up and outward.

Colostrum The first substance secreted from the breasts following childbirth. Colostrum is high in protein and antibodies. A clear type of colostrum is also secreted in small amounts during pregnancy.

Conception When the sperm penetrates the egg.

Congenital anomaly An abnormality that is present at birth. A congenital anomaly is acquired during pregnancy but is not necessarily genetic in origin.

Congenital defect A defect that is present at birth. A congenital defect is acquired during pregnancy but is not necessarily hereditary.

Conjoined twins Identical twins who have not separated completely. More commonly known as Siamese twins.

Contraction A painful, strong, rhythmic squeezing of the uterus.

Contraction stress test A test that assesses the baby's well-being by monitoring its response to uterine contractions. If you're not already in labour when the test is performed, you will be given enough synthetic oxytocin to cause three contractions in a 10-minute period. A "positive" result on the test means that your baby's heart rate dropped near the end of or after a contraction.

Cord prolapse A rare obstetrical emergency that occurs when the umbilical cord drops out of the uterus into the vagina before the baby, leading to cord compression and oxygen deprivation.

Corpus luteum The cyst that forms in the ovary at the site of the released egg and that's responsible for the production of the hormone progesterone during the second half of the normal menstrual cycle.

Cytomegalovirus (CMV) A group of viruses from the herpes virus family that can affect and harm the unborn baby.

Diastasis recti Separation of abdominal muscles.

Diethylstilbestrol (DES) A synthetic form of estrogen that was given to women between the 1940s and 1970s to inhibit miscarriage. DES was later discovered to have serious effects on women and children, including cancer, infertility, and miscarriage. Both male and female offspring can be affected.

Dilation and curettage (D&C) A surgical procedure in which the cervix is dilated and the lining of the uterus is scraped using an instrument called a curette.

Dislocated hip A condition that occurs when the ball at the head of the thigh bone doesn't fit snugly enough into its socket in the hip bone.

Dizygotic twins *See* fraternal twins.

Donor insemination The process of inserting donor sperm into a woman's vagina or uterus by means other than sexual intercourse.

Doppler A hand-held device that uses ultrasound technology to enable the caregiver to monitor the fetal heart rate.

Doula Someone who assists a woman and her family during labour and the postpartum period.

Due date The date on which a baby's birth is expected, calculated by adding 279 days to the first day of the woman's last menstrual period (LMP) or 265 days to the date of ovulation, if known. Medically known as the estimated date of confinement (EDC). A simpler way to estimate your due date is to subtract three months and add seven days to the date of the first day of your last menstrual period (a calculation known as Naegele's rule).

Dysmenorrhoea Painful menstruation.

Early neonatal death A live-born infant who dies before the seventh day following birth is classified as having experienced an "early neonatal death."

Eclampsia A serious but rare condition that can affect pregnant or labouring women. It is a severe form of pre-eclampsia. Symptoms of eclampsia include hypertension, edema, and protein in the urine. An emergency delivery may be necessary if the eclampsia is severe enough.

Ectopic pregnancy A pregnancy that occurs outside the uterus, most often in the Fallopian tube.

EDC/EDD Estimated date of confinement or estimated date of delivery. Medical jargon for your due date.

Edema The accumulation of fluid in the body's tissues, resulting in swelling.

Egg donation The donation of one woman's egg(s) to another woman.

Ejaculate Sperm plus fluid from the seminal vesicles and prostate gland that is ejaculated through the penis.

Electronic fetal monitor (EFM) An electronic instrument used to record the heartbeat of the fetus as well as the mother's uterine contractions. Fetal monitors can be either external (placed on the abdomen) or internal (attached to the baby's scalp via the vagina).

Embryo The term used to describe the early stages of fetal growth, from conception through the third month of pregnancy.

Embryo transfer A procedure that involves introducing an embryo into a woman's uterus. Part of IVF treatment.

Endometrial biopsy The extraction of a small sample of endometrial tissue (tissue from the uterine lining) for examination.

Endometriosis Presence of endometrial tissue (the uterine lining) in abnormal locations such as the ovaries and the Fallopian tubes. May cause painful menstruation and infertility.

Endometrium The mucous membrane lining the uterus.

Engagement When the baby's presenting part (usually the head) settles into the pelvic cavity.

Engorgement Congested or filled with fluid. This term refers to the fullness or swelling of the breasts, which can occur between the second and seventh postpartum day when a woman's breasts first start to produce milk.

Epididymis The organ that stores and nourishes sperm as they develop and make their way from the testes to the vas deferens. Sperm acquire motility (the ability to move) within the epididymis.

Epidural A local anaesthetic that is injected into the epidural space at the level of the spinal cord that you wish to numb. The most popular form of pharmacological pain relief during labour and often used for Caesarean sections as well.

Episiotomy A small incision made into the skin and the perineal muscle at the time of delivery to enlarge the vaginal opening and make it easier for the baby's head or body to emerge or to insert birthing instruments such as forceps.

Erythromycin ointment Ointment that is applied to a newborn baby's eyes within a couple of hours of the birth.

Estimated date of confinement (EDC) The medical term for due date.

Estrogen A group of hormones that are produced in the ovaries and that work with progesterone to regulate the reproductive cycle. Estrogen is produced in all phases of the cycle, whether or not you ovulate.

External version A procedure in which the doctor turns the baby or babies in the uterus by applying manual pressure to the outside of the mother's abdomen.

Face presentation A labour presentation that occurs when the baby's head is down but its neck is extended as if it were looking down through the birth canal.

Fallopian tubes The long, narrow tubes that carry eggs from the ovaries to the uterus.

False labour When you experience regular and/or painful contractions that neither dilate nor thin the cervix.

Fertilization *See* conception.

Fetal hypoxia When the fetus is deprived of oxygen.

Fetal monitor *See* electronic fetal monitor.

Fetus The medical term used to describe the developing baby from the end of the third month of pregnancy until birth.

FH or FHR Fetal heart or fetal heart rate.

Fibroid tumour A benign tumour of fibrous tissue that may occur in the uterine wall. It may be totally without symptoms or it may cause abnormal menstrual patterns, abdominal pressure and swelling (if the tumours are very large), infertility problems, and recurrent miscarriage.

Fimbriae The finger-like outer ends of the Fallopian tubes that seek to capture the egg when it's released from the ovary.

Floating The baby's head is not yet engaged.

Follicle The structure in the ovary that has nurtured the ripening egg and from which the egg is released.

Follicle-stimulating hormone (FSH) A hormone produced in the anterior pituitary gland that stimulates the ovary to ripen a follicle for ovulation.

Fontanelle The soft spots on a baby's head where the skull bones do not completely cover the brain. The absence of bone tissue in these two areas make it possible for your baby's head to be moulded to allow for passage through tight quarters while your baby is being born. The posterior fontanelle typically closes over by the time a baby is six weeks of age. The anterior fontanelle typically closes over by the time a baby is eighteen months of age.

Forceps A tong-like instrument that may be placed around the baby's head to help guide it out of the birth canal during a vaginal delivery.

Fraternal twins Twins who are the result of the union of two eggs and two sperm.

FSH (Follicle-stimulating hormone) A hormone produced in the anterior pituitary gland that stimulates the ovary to ripen a follicle for ovulation.

Fundal height The distance from the upper, rounded part of a pregnant woman's uterus to her pubic bone. On average, the measurement in centimetres is equal to the number of weeks of pregnancy, but it may vary by as many as 3 to 4 centimetres (1.2 to 1.6 inches) or more, depending on the mother's height, weight, and body shape; the position of the baby; and, of course, the size of the baby and the amount of amniotic fluid. Note: Measuring fundal height is a rather inexact science. Different caregivers can get different measurements on the same day. The measurement is most reliable when it is consistently taken by the same caregiver. Also called symphysis fundal height.

Gamete The mature male or female reproductive cell (sperm are the male gametes; eggs are the female gametes).

Gastroesophageal reflux The movement of stomach contents up the esophagus.

Genetic screening Screening tests designed to indicate which couples may be at increased risk of passing along an inherited trait or disease to their baby.

German measles *See* rubella.

Gestational diabetes Diabetes that is triggered by pregnancy. It typically occurs after the 24th week of pregnancy.

Giardia lamblia A parasite in the stool that causes bowel infections.

Gland A hormone-producing organ.

Glucose tolerance test A blood test used to detect gestational diabetes. Blood is drawn at specified intervals after you drink a sugary beverage. Unfortunately, the test isn't considered to be terribly useful: you can get different results by taking the test on different days.

Gonadotropin A hormone capable of stimulating the testicles or the ovaries to produce sperm or an egg, respectively.

Gonadotropin-releasing hormone (GnRH) A hormone released from the hypothalamus that controls the synthesis and release of the pituitary hormones FSH and LH.

Gonorrhea A bacterial infection spread through sexual contact that can lead to infection of the reproductive tract, infertility, serious illness in the mother, and injury to the developing baby.

Group B strep A bacteria found in the vagina and rectum of approximately 15 per cent of pregnant women. Women who test positive for group B strep may require antibiotics during labour to protect their babies from picking up this potentially life-threatening infection.

hCG *See* human chorionic gonadotropin.

HELLP syndrome A severe form of pre-eclampsia that can be associated with liver dysfunction and clotting abnormalities. The syndrome can be life-threatening to both mother and baby and won't disappear until after the delivery.

Hemorrhoids Swollen blood vessels around the anus or in the rectal canal that may bleed and cause pain, especially after childbirth.

HIV test A blood test to detect the presence of antibodies to the AIDS virus.

Human chorionic gonadotropin (hCG) The hormone manufactured by the placenta in early pregnancy that causes your pregnancy test to be positive.

Hydrocephalus An excessive increase in the fluid that cushions the brain—something that can result in brain damage.

Hyperemesis gravidarum Very severe nausea, dehydration, and vomiting during pregnancy.

Hypospadias A condition in which a baby is born with the urethral opening on the underside of the glans of the penis. The penis may curve downward.

Hypothalamus The portion of the base of the brain that controls the release of hormones from the pituitary.

Hypothyroidism A condition caused by an inadequate thyroid gland. If undetected or untreated, it can lead to intellectual disabilities.

Identical twins When twins are the result of the fertilization and subsequent splitting of a single egg and single sperm. Note: The preferred term is now monozygotic twins.

Imperforate anus When the anus is sealed, either because there is a tiny membrane of skin over the opening to the anus or because the anal canal failed to develop properly.

Impetigo An infection of the skin that is characterized by yellow pustules or wide, honey-coloured scabs.

Implantation The embedding of an embryo into the endometrium (the lining of the uterus).

In vitro fertilization (IVF) A procedure wherein a number of eggs are removed from the ovary and fertilized by sperm outside of the body. The resulting embryos are given the opportunity to divide in a protected environment for three to five days before being transferred to the uterus. Note: The embryo may also be transferred to another woman.

Incomplete abortion A miscarriage in which part, but not all, of the contents of the uterus are expelled.

Infertility The inability to conceive a child.

Internal version The act of adjusting a baby's position in the uterus by placing one hand in the mother's vagina and the other on her abdomen.

Intrauterine contraceptive device (IUCD or IUD) A plastic or metal birth control device inserted into the uterus to prevent fertilization or implantation.

Intrauterine death The death of a fetus within the uterus.

Intrauterine growth restriction (IUGR) When the baby's growth is less than what would normally be expected for a baby of that gestational age. It can be symmetric (e.g., both the head and the body are small) or asymmetric (e.g., just the body is small).

Intrauterine insemination (IUI) The placement of washed sperm (from partner or donor) into the uterus via a fine tube.

Kangaroo care Skin-to-skin contact between parent and baby.

Kegels Exercises that work the muscles of the pelvic floor.

Labour The process of childbirth, including the dilation of the cervix and the delivery of the baby and the placenta.

Late neonatal death A live-born infant who dies on or after the seventh day following birth, but before the 28th day.

LHRH Luteinizing hormone. *See* gonadotropin-releasing hormone.

Lightening A change in the shape of the pregnant woman's uterus a few weeks before labour. It generally occurs when the presenting part of the baby engages in the mother's pelvis.

Linea nigra A dark line running from navel to the pubic area that may develop during pregnancy.

LMP The first day of your last menstrual period.

LOA Left occipito-anterior. A term that refers to the position of the crown of the baby's head (i.e., occiput) in relation to your body. In this case, your baby is "left" and "anterior" (toward your front). See also LOP, ROA, ROP.

LOP Left occipito-posterior. A term that refers to the position of the crown of the baby's head (i.e., occiput) in relation to your body. In this case, your baby is "left" and "posterior" (toward your back). See also LOA, ROA, ROP.

Low birth weight Babies who weigh less than 5 pounds, 8 ounces (2.5 kilograms) at birth. A baby who weighs less than 3 pounds, 5 ounces (1.5 kilograms) at birth is considered to be a very low birth weight baby.

Luteal phase The phase of the menstrual cycle that lasts from ovulation through the start of menstruation.

Luteal phase defect A shortened luteal phase or one in which there is inadequate progesterone production.

Luteinizing hormone (LH) A hormone produced by the pituitary gland. It plays an important role in ovulation and implantation.

Mask of pregnancy *See* chloasma.

Maternal serum screening A screening test used to determine the probability that a particular woman is carrying a fetus with certain types of abnormalities. It involves taking a blood sample.

Meconium The greenish substance that builds up in the bowels of a growing fetus and that is normally discharged shortly after birth. A baby who passes meconium before birth may be in distress, so it's important to let your caregiver know immediately if your membranes rupture and the amniotic fluid that leaks out has a greenish tinge.

Meningitis An inflammation of the membranes covering the brain and the spinal cord.

Miscarriage Spontaneous loss of the fetus or embryo from the womb, usually during the first trimester of pregnancy, but at any point prior to the 20th week of pregnancy, or when the baby weighs less than 500 grams (17.5 ounces). The medical term for a miscarriage is "spontaneous abortion"—a term that many women find offensive.

Missed abortion A situation that arises when the embryo or fetus dies in utero but the body fails to expel the contents of the uterus. It is typically diagnosed by ultrasound.

Mittelschmerz Pain that coincides with release of an egg from the ovary.

Molar pregnancy A pregnancy that results in the growth of abnormal placental cells rather than a fetus. Also known as a hydatidiform mole or gestational trophoblastic disease.

Monovular twins *See* identical twins.

Monozygotic twins *See* identical twins.

Mucus plug The plug of thick and sticky mucus that blocks the cervical canal during pregnancy, protecting the baby from infection.

Multigravida You're pregnant for the second or subsequent time.

Multipara You've given birth one or more times before your current pregnancy.

Mumps An illness that is characterized by flu-like symptoms and an upset stomach followed by tender swollen glands beneath the earlobes two or three days later.

Neonatal death The death of a live-born infant between birth and four weeks of age.

Neonatal intensive care unit (NICU) An intensive care unit that specializes in the care of premature, low-weight babies and seriously ill infants.

Neural tube defects Abnormalities in the development of the spinal cord and brain in a fetus, including anencephaly, hydrocephalus, and spina bifida.

NICU *See* neonatal intensive care unit.

Non-stress test A non-invasive test in which fetal movements are monitored and recorded using an electronic fetal monitor, along with changes in fetal heart rate.

Oligohydramnios A shortage of amniotic fluid.

Oocyte The reproductive world's term for the egg that's produced by the ovary.

Ovaries The female sexual glands responsible for producing estrogen and progesterone, and for housing the developing egg prior to its release at ovulation. There are two ovaries: one on either side of the pelvis.

Ovulation The point in the menstrual cycle in which a mature egg is released from the ovaries into the Fallopian tubes.

Ovum The egg cell produced in the ovaries each month. Another word for oocyte.

Oxytocin The naturally occurring hormone that causes uterine contractions. A synthetic form of this hormone (Pitocin) is often used to induce or augment labour.

Pap test The popular name for the Papanicolaou test, which involves examining cervical cells under a microscope to look for any abnormalities.

Paraphimosis An emergency situation that can occur if the foreskin gets stuck when it's first retracted.

Pelvic floor muscles The group of muscles at the base of the pelvis that help support the bladder, uterus, urethra, vagina, and rectum.

Pelvic inflammatory disease (PID) An infection that can affect the uterus, Fallopian tubes, ovaries, and other parts of the reproductive system. It can be caused by sexually transmitted infection or other organisms and can lead to infertility.

Percutaneous umbilical cord sampling (PUBS) A diagnostic test that involves drawing blood from the fetus's umbilical cord prior to birth to test for abnormalities and genetic conditions. This procedure is performed only in a couple of Canadian hospitals.

Perineum The name given to the muscle and tissue located between the vagina and the rectum.

Phenylketonuria (PKU) A recessive genetic disorder in which a liver enzyme is defective, making it impossible for an individual to digest an amino acid known as phenylalanine. PKU is detected through a blood test done at birth and may be controlled by a special diet. If untreated, PKU results in intellectual disabilities.

Pituitary A gland located at the base of the human brain that is responsible for secreting a number of important hormones related to normal growth and development of fertility.

Placenta The organ that develops in the uterus during pregnancy, providing nutrients for the fetus and eliminating its waste products.

Placenta previa A condition in which the placenta partially or completely blocks the cervical opening. It necessitates delivery by Caesarean section and can be associated with pregnancy loss and massive hemorrhaging. (In rare cases, a hysterectomy may be required to control the bleeding.)

Placental abruption The premature separation of the placenta from the uterus.

Placental infarction The death of part of the placenta. It is caused by a loss of blood supply to part of the placenta, which, if extensive enough, can cause stillbirth.

Pneumonia An infection of the lungs.

Polycystic ovarian syndrome (PCO) A condition that involves the development of multiple cysts in the ovaries. Its cause is uncertain, but it appears to be linked to insulin resistance.

Polyhydramnios An abnormal condition of pregnancy characterized by an excess of amniotic fluid.

Postdate A baby born after 42 completed weeks' gestation. Note: other terms for this are "post-term" or "post-mature."

Postpartum blues The hormone-driven wave of emotion that tends to come crashing down on you three to five days after the birth, leading to temporary mild depression. This type of depression often lasts only a few days and typically occurs within one to two weeks of the delivery. If the feelings of depression last longer than this or are particularly severe, you may be suffering from postpartum depression.

Postpartum depression (PPD) Clinical depression that can occur at any point during the year following the delivery. Postpartum depression is characterized by sadness, impatience, restlessness, and—in particularly severe cases—an inability to care for the baby. Postpartum anxiety is another type of perinatal mood disorder.

Postpartum hemorrhage The loss of more than 450 millilitres (15 ounces) of blood during a vaginal delivery or 1,000 millilitres (34 ounces) during a Caesarean section.

Pre-eclampsia/toxemia A serious condition marked by sudden edema, high blood pressure, and protein in the urine.

Pregnancy-induced hypertension (PIH) A pregnancy-related condition in which a woman's blood pressure is temporarily elevated. Her blood pressure returns to normal shortly after she gives birth.

Pre-implantation diagnosis The diagnosis of genetic disorders or the determination of the sex in an embryo formed through IVF before it's transferred to the uterus. The Society of Obstetricians and Gynaecologists of Canada is strongly opposed to using pre-implantation diagnosis for sex-selection purposes.

Premature baby A baby born before 37 completed weeks of pregnancy.

Premature rupture of the membranes (PROM) When the membranes rupture before the onset of labour.

Prenatal diagnosis (PND) Testing before birth to determine whether a fetus has a particular type of malformation or disorder and/or to determine the sex of the fetus.

Presenting part The part of the baby's body that is likely to come through the cervix first.

Primary lactation failure A rare condition that is typically diagnosed if you fail to experience any breast changes during pregnancy.

Primigravida You are pregnant for the first time.

Primipara You are giving birth for the first time.

Progesterone A hormone secreted by the ovary after ovulation has occurred. It helps to prepare the uterus for pregnancy and maintains the endometrium in early pregnancy until the placenta takes over progesterone production.

Prolactin The hormone responsible for milk production and for suppressing ovulation in a nursing mother. Prolactin is released following the delivery of the placenta and the membranes.

Prostate The gland responsible for producing much of the seminal fluid.

Quickening The term used to describe the moment when a pregnant woman first detects fetal movement (typically between the 20th and 24th weeks if you are having your first baby, and between the 16th and 20th week of pregnancy if you are having your second or subsequent baby).

Renal disease Kidney disease.

Rh antibodies Antibodies capable of crossing the placenta and destroying the baby's red blood cells. Rh antibodies can be produced if your blood type is Rh-negative and the baby's blood type is Rh-positive, and some of your baby's blood leaks into your circulation during pregnancy, birth, or in the event of a miscarriage. This sensitization doesn't cause a problem in the first pregnancy, but it can cause a problem during the next pregnancy. That's why you'll require an RhoGAM injection immediately following delivery, a miscarriage, an abortion, or amniocentesis. Note: Some caregivers give RhoGAM injections at 28 weeks to prevent early sensitization.

Rheumatic fever A serious disease that can result in heart damage and/or joint swelling.

ROA Right occipito-anterior. A term that refers to the position of the crown of the baby's head (i.e., occiput) in relation to your body. In this case, your baby is "right" and "anterior" (toward your front). See also LOA, LOP, ROP.

ROP Right occipito-posterior. A term that refers to the position of the crown of the baby's head (i.e., occiput) in relation to your body. In this case, your baby is "right" and "posterior" (toward your back). See also LOA, LOP, ROA.

Round ligament pain Pain caused by the stretching of ligaments on the sides of the uterus during pregnancy. It increases in severity with each pregnancy.

Rubella (German measles) A mild, highly contagious viral disease that can cause serious birth defects in the developing baby, particularly during the first trimester. Most people are immunized against this disease as children, but it's possible to lose your immunity to the disease, which is why your caregiver will check your immunity if you're planning a pregnancy.

Ruptured membranes The loss of fluid from the amniotic sac. If it happens prematurely it is called the premature rupture of membranes or PROM. If it happens preterm, it is known as the preterm premature rupture of membranes or PPROM.

Sciatica Pain in the leg, lower back, and buttock caused by irritation of the sciatic nerve.

Scrotum The pouch of skin and thin muscle tissue that holds the testes.

Seminal fluid Fluid produced by the prostate and seminal vesicle that contains sperm.

Sepsis A serious infection caused by bacteria that has entered a wound or body tissue. Commonly known as "blood poisoning."

Shingles A disease that is characterized by a rash with small blisters that begin to crust over, resulting in itching and intense and prolonged pain.

Show *See* bloody show.

Siamese twins *See* conjoined twins.

Sickle-cell anemia An inherited blood disease.

Single gene abnormalities Genetic problems that are inherited from one or both parents.

Skin tags Small, soft, flesh-coloured or pigmented growths of skin.

Soft spot *See* fontanelle.

Spermatozoa (sperm) The fully developed male reproductive cells.

Spider nevi Thin, dilated blood vessels that are spider-like in shape and that radiate outward from a central red spot.

Spina bifida A condition in which the spinal column fails to close properly during the early weeks of embryonic development. It can result in malformations of the spinal cord or brain.

Spinal anaesthesia A regional anaesthetic that is injected into the spinal fluid. Generally used for Caesarean sections.

Spontaneous abortion *See* miscarriage.

Stale air Air that has been previously breathed in.

Startle reflex *See* Moro reflex.

Station An estimate of the baby's progress in descending into the pelvis. Generally, negative numbers mean that the presenting part is unengaged and positive numbers mean it is engaged.

Stem cells The bone marrow components that are responsible for producing red cells, white cells, and platelets.

Stillbirth A fetal death that occurs after the 20th week of gestation.

Stress test A test that records the fetal heart rate in response to induced mild contractions of the uterus.

Stretch marks Reddish streaks on the skin of the breasts, abdomen, legs, and buttocks that are caused by the stretching of the skin during pregnancy. Stretch marks fade over time but don't disappear entirely.

Sudden infant death syndrome (SIDS) The sudden and unexpected death of an apparently healthy infant under 1 year of age that remains unexplained after all known and possible causes have been ruled out through autopsy, death scene investigation, and review of the medical history.

Teratogens Agents such as drugs, chemicals, and infectious diseases that can cause birth defects in the developing baby.

Terbutaline A medication used to stop contractions in preterm labour.

Testes The male sexual glands. Contained in the scrotum, they produce the male hormone (testosterone) and the male reproductive cells (sperm).

Testosterone A male sex hormone produced in the testicles.

Tetanus A disease that can lead to muscle spasms and death.

Thalassemia An inherited blood disease.

Threatened abortion Bleeding during the first trimester of pregnancy that is not accompanied by either cramping or contractions.

Toxoplasmosis A parasitic infection that can cause stillbirth or miscarriage in pregnant women and congenital defects in babies.

Transition The third or final phase of the first stage of labour when the cervix goes from 7 to 10 centimetres dilation. When transition ends, the pushing stage begins.

Transverse lie When the fetus is lying horizontally across the uterus rather than in a vertical position.

Tubal ligation A permanent sterilization procedure that involves blocking off a woman's Fallopian tubes to prevent conception.

Tubal pregnancy A pregnancy that occurs in the Fallopian tube.

Ultrasound A technique that uses high-frequency sound waves to create a moving image, or sonogram, on a television screen.

Umbilical cord The cord that connects the placenta to the developing baby, removing waste products and carbon dioxide from the baby and bringing oxygenated blood and nutrients from the mother through the placenta to the baby.

Umbilical hernia A small swelling close to the belly button that becomes more prominent when a baby is crying.

Undescended testicles Testicles that have not yet descended from the abdomen into the scrotum by the time a baby boy is born.

Uterus The hollow muscular organ that protects and nourishes the fetus prior to birth.

Vacuum extraction A process in which a suction cup is attached to a vacuum pump placed on a baby's head to aid in delivery.

Vaginal birth after Caesarean (VBAC) A vaginal delivery that occurs when a woman has previously delivered a baby or babies by Caesarean section.

Varicella zoster immune globulin A type of immune globulin that is given to prevent or minimize the severity of chicken pox.

Varicocele A collection of varicose veins in the scrotum. Varicoceles can elevate scrotal temperature, contributing to fertility problems.

Varicose veins Abnormally swollen veins, usually on the legs.

Vas deferens The tube connecting the epididymis with the seminal vesicles.

Vascular disease Heart disease.

VBAC *See* vaginal birth after Caesarean.

VDRL test Test of syphilis (also referred to as RPR).

Vena cava The major vein in the body that returns unoxygenated blood to the heart for transport to the lungs.

Ventricular septum The dividing wall between the right and left pumping chambers of the heart.

Vernix caseosa A greasy white substance that coats and protects the baby's skin before birth.

Vertex Head-down presentation.

Zygote A cell formed by the union of egg and sperm.

Planning for Your Birth

Multi-page birth plans have been replaced by one- to two-page birth plans or wish lists that highlight the points that matter most to you. That way, instead of getting bogged down by minutiae, your caregiver and the other people who will be supporting you and helping you to advocate for yourself at your birth can zero in on what matters most to you. This document is intended as a brainstorming tool: to give you ideas about what to include in your much shorter summary. When you've decided what you want to include, you can simply list those points in a letter and give a copy to your doctor or midwife, attach it to the pre-registration form that you fill out at the hospital (assuming, of course, that you're planning a hospital birth), tuck it into your labour bag (if you're giving birth in the hospital), or stick it in your night-table drawer (if you're planning to give birth at home) so that you'll have an extra copy handy during labour.

Note: Even if you're planning to give birth at home, you should spend some time thinking about the items in the hospital section of this document. It's always possible that you may end up delivering in the hospital after all.

BIRTH WISHES

Personal information

Name: _____

Partner's name: _____

Home phone number: _____

Due date: _____

_____ We have attended or are planning to attend prenatal classes.
Details: _____

_____ We have taken or are planning to take a hospital tour.
Details: _____

About your labour support team

Name and phone number of doctor/midwife:

_____

_____

Name and phone number of doula or other labour support person(s):

_____

_____

Name and phone number of baby's doctor:

_____

_____

Names and ages of any children who will be attending the birth:

_____

_____

Labouring environment

While I am in labour, I would like . . . [check as many as apply]

_____ to have the lights dimmed.

_____ to have noise and distractions in the area where I am labouring kept to a minimum.

_____ to labour in the bathtub, Jacuzzi, or shower (circle the appropriate choices).

_____ to have access to the following birthing equipment during labour:

    _____ birthing bed

    _____ birthing stool

    _____ birthing chair

    _____ squatting bar

    _____ birthing pool/tub

    _____ a mirror so that I can view my baby's birth.

_____ to be able to listen to music.

_____ to be able to wear my own clothes or no clothing at all.

_____ to have my partner and/or other support person(s) with me at all times, unless an emergency situation arises.

_____ to leave my contact lenses in place throughout my labour, unless it becomes necessary for me to undergo anaesthesia.

_____ to take photographs and/or videos taken of my labour and my baby's birth.

Choices about the labour

If my labour . . .

_____ has not yet started when my water breaks, I'd like to wait at least 24 hours before an induction is attempted.

_____ has not yet started and I'm two weeks overdue, I'd like to be induced.

_____ has not yet started and I'm two weeks overdue, I'd prefer not to be induced.

_____ has not progressed very far when I arrive at the hospital, I'd like to be given the option of returning home until my labour is further along.

Labouring positions

While I am in labour, I would like . . .

_____ to walk around as much as possible, and to be free to experiment with a number of different labouring positions.

_____ to labour on my side.

_____ to labour in a squatting position (either using a squatting bar or sitting on the toilet).

_____ to be offered the option of having a massage.

_____ to eat and drink as I need during my labour until it becomes medically necessary to stop.

Pain relief

I'm planning to use the following pain-relief measures during my labour (and have practised them, where necessary):

_____ Relaxation

_____ Breathing techniques/distraction

_____ Frequent changing of positions

_____ Labouring in water (shower and/or bathtub):

     _____ alone; or _____ with my partner

_____ Heat or cold therapy

_____ Massage

_____ Acupressure

_____ Acupuncture

_____ Hypnosis

_____ Vocalization

_____ Pain medications (provide details) _____

_____ Anaesthetic gases (provide details) _____

_____ An epidural

_____ Other (please specify) _____

Induction/augmentation of labour

If it becomes necessary to induce or augment my labour, I would prefer that the following technique(s) be used, if possible:

_____ Natural methods of getting labour started (walking and sexual intercourse)

_____ Nipple stimulation

_____ Prostaglandin gel

_____ Synthetic oxytocin (Pitocin)

_____ Stripping membranes

_____ Amniotomy (rupturing the membranes)

_____ Other (please specify) _____

Delivery

I am intending to deliver my baby in the following position:

_____ Sitting

_____ On my side

_____ Squatting

_____ On all fours

_____ On my back

After the birth

Once the baby has been delivered, I would like . . .

_____ my baby's hands to remain unwashed until I've had a chance to initiate breastfeeding.

_____ to have my baby placed skin-to-skin on my chest as soon as possible, or, if I am not available to do this, to have our baby placed skin-to-skin on my partner.

_____ to delay umbilical cord clamping (to allow the placenta to transfer more oxygenated blood, nutrients, and stem cells to my baby).

_____ to have my partner cut the umbilical cord.

_____ to breastfeed my baby as soon as possible.

_____ to avoid any unnecessary separation from my baby.

_____ to have 24-hour rooming-in (sharing a room) with my baby.

_____ to be present myself or have my partner present for any tests my baby may require (e.g., PKU/TSH heel prick blood test).

_____ to receive instruction on routine baby-care procedures such as diapering, bathing, and so on, after I have enjoyed some time getting to know my baby.

Caesarean section

If I have a Caesarean, I would like to have . . .

_____ my partner present at the delivery.

_____ my labour support person present at the delivery.

_____ a screen placed in front of my face to block my view of the delivery.

_____ as much information as possible about what's happening on the other side of the screen.

_____ as little information as possible about what's happening on the other side of the screen.

_____ the delivery photographed or videotaped.

_____ an opportunity to hold my baby right after the delivery (or to have my partner hold my baby, if that is not possible).

_____ my partner cut the cord.

_____ the opportunity to breastfeed as soon as possible and to enjoy skin-to-skin time with my baby.

_____ Other (please specify)

Circumcision

If my baby is a boy, I am intending to . . .

_____ have him circumcised.

_____ not have him circumcised.

Length of stay (if you're having a hospital birth)

I'm intending to leave the hospital within . . .

_____ 6 hours of the delivery

_____ 12 hours of the delivery

_____ 24 hours of the delivery

_____ 48 hours of the delivery

_____ 2 to 5 days of the delivery

Birthing philosophies

You may wish to include a statement or two about your childbirth philosophies. These prompts may help you to get started:

I hope that my birth . . .

_____

_____

I believe that birth . . .

_____

_____

My birth will be a joyous experience for me if . . .

_____

_____

I will be satisfied with my birth if . . .

_____

_____

It is important to me that . . .

_____

_____

You can support me in birthing my baby by . . .

_____

_____

I hope to welcome my baby to this world by . . .

_____

_____

We have written this birth plan according to our wishes for our baby's birth. We understand that medical emergencies may require us to modify our plans, but, as much as possible, we would like everyone who is present at our baby's birth to respect the choices we have outlined here.

Emergency Childbirth Procedures

Emergency childbirth supplies to have on hand

- A flashlight
- A pen
- Pillows
- Clean sheets
- Clean towels or newspapers
- A face cloth
- A couple of dishpans or large bowls
- Soap and water
- A suction bulb
- Sterile rubber gloves
- A large container

How to deliver your baby if you're alone and without assistance

Getting help

- Try to remain calm.
- Call the emergency response number in your community and ask the person who takes the call to send out an emergency response team and to notify your doctor or midwife that you're about to deliver your baby.
- Ask a friend or neighbour to stay with you until the emergency response team arrives. (If you're able to find someone, they should follow the tips below on helping a mother who's about to give birth.)

Preparing for the birth

- Wash your hands and your vulvar area with mild detergent or soap and water.
- Spread a shower curtain, a plastic tablecloth, clean towels, newspapers, or sheets on a bed, a sofa, or the floor, and then lie down until someone arrives to assist you.

Coping during labour

- If you feel the urge to push, try panting instead. It will help you to hold off on pushing until someone arrives to help deliver your baby.
- If your baby starts coming before help arrives, gently ease your baby out of your body by pushing each time you feel the urge and catching the baby with your hands.

After the birth

- Lay the baby across your abdomen or put the baby to your breast if the umbilical cord is long enough to reach.
- Don't try to pull the placenta out. If the placenta is delivered before help arrives, wrap it in towels or a newspaper and keep it elevated above the level of the baby.
- Do not try to cut the cord on your own. Wait until help arrives.

How to assist a woman who's about to give birth

What to do first

- Remain calm. Focus your energy on comforting and reassuring the mother.
- Call the emergency response number in your community and ask the person who takes the call to send out an emergency response team and to notify the mother's doctor or midwife that she's about to deliver her baby.

Preparing for the delivery

- Wash your hands and the mother's vulvar area with mild detergent or soap and water.
- Spread a shower curtain, a plastic tablecloth, clean towels, newspapers, or sheets on a bed or table.
- Help the mother sit at the edge of the bed or table with her buttocks hanging off and her knees apart. Support her head with one or two pillows.
- If she's in active labour and in too much pain to climb onto the bed or table, place a stack of newspapers or folded towels under her buttocks so that she'll be far enough off the floor for you to be able to deliver the baby's shoulders easily.
- If you're in a vehicle, help the mother lie down on the seat. Then help her to position herself so that she has one foot on the floor and the other on the seat.

Assisting the mother during labour

- If the mother needs to vomit, help her turn her head to the side so that her mouth and airway will remain clear.
- Use a dishpan or basin to catch the amniotic fluid and blood.
- Encourage the mother to start panting if she feels the urge to push. This may aid in delaying the birth until help arrives.

Delivering the baby

- Once the baby's heard starts to crown (i.e., to emerge through the tissues at the opening of the vagina), encourage the mother to pant or blow. This will help to slow the baby's exit from the birth canal. Then, to keep the baby's head from emerging too quickly, you should apply gentle counter-pressure to the baby's head.
- If you see a loop of umbilical cord around the baby's neck, gently pull on it and lift it over the baby's head.
- If the baby's amniotic sac is intact when the baby's head emerges, puncture the sac with a clean fingernail or a ballpoint pen, being sure to hold the pen away from the baby's face, and carefully move the sac away from the baby's mouth.
- Take the baby's head in your hands and press it slightly downward, asking the mother to push at the same time. Then help to ease the baby's shoulders out one at a time. Once the baby's shoulders have been delivered, the rest of the baby should slip out easily.
- Clear the baby's mouth and nose immediately after the birth, using a bulb syringe and gauze pad (if you have them) or by gently stroking the sides of the baby's nose in a downward direction and the neck and underside of the chin in an upward direction to help expel mucus and amniotic fluid. You can also try holding the baby's head lower than its body to use gravity to drain away the fluid. Once the baby starts crying vigorously, you can return the baby to an upright position.

After the birth

- Wrap the baby in a clean blanket or towel and lay it across the mother's abdomen or place it at her breast if the cord is long enough.
- Don't try to pull the placenta out. If the placenta is delivered before help arrives, wrap it in towels or a newspaper and keep it elevated above the level of the baby.
- Do not try to cut the cord before help arrives.

Keep the mother comfortable and the baby warm and dry until help arrives.

Prenatal Record

The prenatal record that follows can be used to record the information that is gathered during your prenatal checkups. Prenatal appointments are generally scheduled

- every four to six weeks during early pregnancy,
- every two to three weeks after 30 weeks, and
- every one to two weeks after 36 weeks

unless you're expecting multiples or your health-care provider is monitoring your pregnancy extra closely for another reason.

During your initial prenatal checkup, your caregiver will

- confirm your pregnancy;
- estimate your due date;
- perform a blood test to check for anemia, hepatitis B, hepatitis C, HIV (if you request it), syphilis, antibodies to rubella (German measles), and—depending on your ethnic background and family history—certain genetic diseases;
- take a vaginal culture to check for infection;
- do a Pap smear to check for cervical cancer or precancerous cells;
- do a breast exam;
- check your urine for signs of infection, blood sugar problems, and excess protein;
- weigh you to establish a baseline so that your weight gain during pregnancy can be monitored;
- take your blood pressure;
- talk to you about how you and your partner feel about the pregnancy and ask whether you have any questions or concerns.

See Chapter 4 for additional information on what to expect during your initial prenatal checkup.

PRENATAL RECORD

Name:

Due Date:

Date	Week of Pregnancy	Weight	About You	About Your Baby	Special Test Results	Notes and Comments
			Blood pressure: Urine (protein): Urine (glucose):	Fetal heart rate: Height of fundus (top of uterus): Presentation and position:		
			Blood pressure: Urine (protein): Urine (glucose):	Fetal heart rate: Height of fundus: Presentation and position:		
			Blood pressure: Urine (protein): Urine (glucose):	Fetal heart rate: Height of fundus: Presentation and position:		
			Blood pressure: Urine (protein): Urine (glucose):	Fetal heart rate: Height of fundus: Presentation and position:		
			Blood pressure: Urine (protein): Urine (glucose):	Fetal heart rate: Height of fundus: Presentation and position:		
			Blood pressure: Urine (protein): Urine (glucose):	Fetal heart rate: Height of fundus: Presentation and position:		

continued

Date	Week of Pregnancy	Weight	About You	About Your Baby	Special Test Results	Notes and Comments
			Blood pressure:	Fetal heart rate:		
			Urine (protein):	Height of fundus:		
			Urine (glucose):	Presentation and position:		
			Blood pressure:	Fetal heart rate:		
			Urine (protein):	Height of fundus:		
			Urine (glucose):	Presentation and position:		
			Blood pressure:	Fetal heart rate:		
			Urine (protein):	Height of fundus:		
			Urine (glucose):	Presentation and position:		
			Blood pressure:	Fetal heart rate:		
			Urine (protein):	Height of fundus:		
			Urine (glucose):	Presentation and position:		
			Blood pressure:	Fetal heart rate:		
			Urine (protein):	Height of fundus:		
			Urine (glucose):	Presentation and position:		
			Blood pressure:	Fetal heart rate:		
			Urine (protein):	Height of fundus:		
			Urine (glucose):	Presentation and position:		
			Blood pressure:	Fetal heart rate:		
			Urine (protein):	Height of fundus:		
			Urine (glucose):	Presentation and position:		

	Blood pressure:	Fetal heart rate:	
	Urine (protein):	Height of fundus:	
	Urine (glucose):	Presentation and position:	
	Blood pressure:	Fetal heart rate:	
	Urine (protein):	Height of fundus:	
	Urine (glucose):	Presentation and position:	
	Blood pressure:	Fetal heart rate:	
	Urine (protein):	Height of fundus:	
	Urine (glucose):	Presentation and position:	
	Blood pressure:	Fetal heart rate:	
	Urine (protein):	Height of fundus:	
	Urine (glucose):	Presentation and position:	
	Blood pressure:	Fetal heart rate:	
	Urine (protein):	Height of fundus:	
	Urine (glucose):	Presentation and position:	
	Blood pressure:	Fetal heart rate:	
	Urine (protein):	Height of fundus:	
	Urine (glucose):	Presentation and position:	

Note: You can either write down specific values for the various tests listed above (e.g., amount of protein in urine) or you can use a checkmark to indicate that your test results were within the normal range.

Acknowledgements

While my name may be the one that's splashed on the front cover of this book, The Mother of All Pregnancy Books was anything but a solo effort. Writing a book of this size and scope requires assistance from a huge number of people— people I'd like to take a moment to thank right now.

First edition

First of all, I'd like to thank the parents who agreed to share intimate details about their lives with me while I was researching this book: Stephanie Anderson, Mike Arless, Kim Arnott, Rita Arsenault, Claudia E. Astorquiza, Gustavo F. Astorquiza, Josie Audet, David Austin, Sadia Baig, Aubyn Baker, Ken Barker, Nicole Barker, Christina Barnes, Kristi-Anna Beaudry, Michael Beaudry, Kim Becker, Lorinda Beler, Lori Bianco, Janelle Bird, Janet Bolton, Susan Borkowsky, Carolin Botterill, David Botterill, Lanny Boutin, Alison Briggs, Julie Burton, Rosa Caporicci, Stacey Couturier, Alex Crump, Jennifer Crump, Julie Cunningham-Marrows, Elvi Dalgaard, Marguerite Daubney, Marinda deBeer, Claudio Dinucci, Julie Dufresne, Rod Dufresne, Don Estabrook, Stephanie Estabrook, Maria Ferguson, Susan Fisher, Jane Fletcher, Cyndie Forget, Deirdre Friedrich, Jiri Fuglicek, Anne Gallant, Daniel Gallant, Sean Gallaway, Shannon Gallaway, Carrie Gallo, Susan Gibson, Cheryl Gilleshammer, Andrea Gould, Jeff Gould, Joyce Gravelle, Susan Gray, Line Hamelin, Bonnie Hancock-Moore, Terri Harten, Lynn Hawrys, Jennifer Henderson, Kevin Henderson, Charlie Hendren, Mark Higgins, Richard Higgins, Brian Holmes, Lisa Holmes, Tracey Hrvoyevich, Kathy Ireland, Mark Ireland, Jodi Jaffray, Robert Jaffray, Debbie Jeffery, Jennifer Johnston, Teagan Jones, Chris Kapalowski, Maria Latham-Foley, Brian Lavender, LeeAnne Lavender, David Lindensmith, Kimberly Long, Janis Louie, Liz Luyben, Lana Luzny, Warren Luzny, Jeff MacDonald, Jennifer MacDonald, Myrna MacDonald, Stephanie MacDonald, Lara MacGregor, Pandora D. MacMillan, Alexandra Marocchino, Heather McElroy, Melanie McLeod, Colleen Melsted, Jennifer Millenor, Kirk Millenor, Christopher Moore, Carissa Nicholson, Chris Nicholson, Erika Nielsen, Beverley North, Tammy Oakley, Chrystelle Pasquet, Yves Pasquet, Ken Pawlitzki, Maria Phillips, Tina Pilon, Heather Polan, Julie Pyke, Angelina Quinlan, Scott Ridley, Jennifer Kathleen Roos, Regan Ross, Lynn Rozon, Donna Sanders, Russ Sanders, Chris Schneider, Denice Schneider, Brenda Scott, Collin Smith, Jennifer

Smith, Charlie Sousa, Elizabeth Sousa, Jenna Stedman, Ben Stephenson, Bevin Stephenson, Elizabeth Taylor, Jasmine Taylor, Lori Voth, Jane Walden, Amanda Walker, Darci Walker, Garth Walker, Jennifer Walker, Dorothy Williamson, Henry Williamson, Chrystal Workman, Laura Young, and Susan Yusishen.

I'd also like to thank the technical reviewers who agreed to review relevant portions of the manuscript of this book to ensure that my facts were bang-on: Susan Hubay, public health nutritionist, Peterborough County-City Health Unit; Kathryn MacLean, Sidelines Canada Prenatal Support Network; and Jenna Stedman, professional fitness and lifestyle consultant and certified personal fitness trainer.

I owe a huge debt of gratitude to Margaret Lightheart, MD, FRCSC (OB/GYN), part-time assistant clinical professor in obstetrics and gynecology at McMaster University in Hamilton, Ontario, for reviewing the manuscript for accuracy and offering countless helpful suggestions. Her detailed comments on the book arrived by fax and e-mail at all hours of day and night—basically anytime she found herself with a lull between deliveries!

I would be remiss if I didn't acknowledge the contribution of Tracy Keleher of Canadian Parents Online, who helped me to recruit multitudes of parents to interview for the book.

I am also forever indebted to my husband, Neil, for the countless hours he spent holding down the fort and entertaining a tribe of wild children so that I could (almost) meet my book deadline.

Finally, I'd like to thank all the people who played an important role behind the scenes while I was researching and writing this book: my research assistants Janice Kent and Brenda May, and the numerous unsung heroes on the editorial, production, and marketing teams at CDG Books. Last but not least—I wish to thank Robert Harris and Joan Whitman, who believed in this book from the moment the idea was first conceived and who served as its midwife right through delivery day.

Second and third editions

Updating a book of this magnitude requires the assistance of many and the patience of even more. I owe a huge debt of gratitude to my current agent, Hilary McMahon of Westwood Creative Artists; my former agent, the late Ed Knappman of New England Publishing Associates; and my trademark agent, Valerie Edward of Ballagh and Edward LLP. And thank you to my new team at HarperCollins Canada for making me and The Mother of All series so welcome in our new home.

I'd also like to thank the members of the technical review panel, who agreed to review some or all of the manuscript for this edition in an effort to improve the book's accuracy and relevancy: Jon Barrett, MD, the head of maternal-fetal medicine at Sunnybrook Health Sciences Centre and a World Health Organization advisor on maternal health; Virginia Collins, a childbirth educator and doula who specializes in high-risk pregnancy support; Janice Johnston, RN, and Jennifer Vickers-Manzin, RN, public health nurses with a passion for maternal-child health; Marla Good and Jennifer Lawrence, mothers, writers, and technical reviewers extraordinaire; Karen Nordahl, MD, a family physician who practices obstetrics at BC Women's Hospital in Vancouver, and who has a special interest in exercise during pregnancy; and Wendy Cohen Reingold, RD, a private practice dietitian in Thornhill. Thank you so much for your invaluable comments and insights. Thanks also to Laura Apps, physiotherapist; and Marie Lane-Smith, postpartum depression research assistant for answering specific questions related to the third edition.

I can't even begin to express how thankful I am to my family and friends for their friendship, love, and support during The Mother of All revision processes. For once, I find myself at a loss for words.

Finally, I would like to thank every parent who cared enough about *The Mother of All Pregnancy Books* to write to me to pass along your comments about how the book might be improved; or to tell what the book has come to mean to you and your family. Knowing that you (or someone like you) was waiting to pick up the second edition is what kept me inspired during the four years it took to revise this book. Thank you for your past support and for your silent encouragement during the revision process—for being "the reader in my head."

Index